Gynecologic Oncology Handbook

Gynecologic Oncology Handbook
An Evidence-Based Clinical Guide

Michelle F. Benoit, MD
Seattle, Washington

**M. Yvette
Williams-Brown, MD, MMS**
*Baylor College of Medicine
Houston, Texas*

Creighton L. Edwards, MD
*Baylor College of Medicine
Houston, Texas*

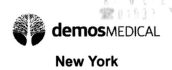

demosMEDICAL

New York

Visit our website at www.demosmedpub.com

ISBN: 9781620700051
e-book ISBN: 9781617051678

Acquisitions Editor: Richard Winters
Compositor: S4Carlisle

Library of Congress Cataloging-in-Publication Data

Benoit, Michelle F., author.
  Gynecologic oncology handbook : an evidence-based clinical guide / Michelle F. Benoit, Marian Yvette Williams-Brown, Creighton L. Edwards.
      p. ; cm.
Includes bibliographical references and index.
ISBN-13: 978-1-62070-005-1
ISBN-10: 1-62070-005-0
ISBN-13: 978-1-61705-167-8 (e-book)
I. Williams-Brown, Marian Yvette, author. II. Edwards, Creighton L., author. III. Title.
[DNLM: 1. Genital Neoplasms, Female—therapy—Handbooks. 2. Genital Neoplasms, Female—diagnosis—Handbooks. 3. Intraoperative Complications—Handbooks. 4. Postoperative Complications—Handbooks. 5. Pregnancy Complications, Neoplastic—Handbooks. WP 39]
RC280.G5
616.99'465--dc23   2013004085

Printed in the United States of America by Gasch Printing.
13 14 15 16 17 / 5 4 3 2 1

In Memoriam
Dr. Edward V. Hannigan

An amazing mentor, a consummate clinician, and a gentle soul.
non omnis moriar

Contents

Preface

This handbook is structured to provide comprehensive care for the gynecologic cancer patient. It is directed toward clinicians at all levels of training and the chapters are tiered in this fashion. Basic diagnosis, workup, staging, and treatment are outlined first. Specific surgical and adjuvant therapies are then recommended reflecting current standards of care. Finally, the evidence-based medicine is summarized in support of recommended treatments. Thus, the medical student can have a dedicated overview, the resident can refer to directed patient care protocols, and the fellow and practicing physician can support their clinical decisions with easily accessible literature.

It has been our honor to put together this handbook for our friends and colleagues. We acknowledge the dedication it has taken from the physicians, support staff, and especially our patients, to design and participate in the trials that have advanced our knowledge of these difficult gynecologic cancers. We hope the information provided herein can continue to guide high-quality care and reflect our commitment to the subspecialty.

Gynecologic Oncology Referral Parameters

I. Endometrial Cancer

A. Biopsy confirmed endometrial cancer of any grade

II. Pelvic Mass

A. Presence of, or concern for, advanced disease:

1. Omental caking
2. Pleural effusion
3. Ascites

B. A clinically suspicious pelvic mass:

1. Larger than 8 cm
2. Complex
3. Fixed
4. Nodular
5. Bilateral
6. Excrescences
7. Solid components

C. Premenarchal girls with a pelvic mass

D. Postmenopausal women with a suspicious mass or elevated tumor markers. Suspicious findings include: a solid mass, a simple mass greater than 8–10 cm, or a complex mass. ACOG recommends referral for a CA-125 above 35.

E. Perimenopausal women with an ovarian mass, particularly when associated with an elevated CA-125. ACOG recommends referral for a CA-125 above 200 in pre- or peri-menopausal women.

F. Young patients who have a pelvic mass and elevated tumor markers (CA-125, AFP, hCG, LDH)

G. A suspicious pelvic mass found in a woman with a significant family or personal history of ovarian, breast, or other cancers (one or more first-degree relatives).

III. Cervical Cancer

A. A biopsy (conization or directed) confirming invasive carcinoma

B. Women with suspicious cervical lesions should be referred but can be biopsied before referral.

IV. Vaginal Cancer

A. All women with invasive vaginal cancer

B. Depending on practitioner's comfort level:

    1. Women with unexplained abnormal cytology after colposcopy and biopsy

    2. Women with VAIN 3 lesions (suspicious of invasion) who require treatment

V. Vulvar Cancer

A. Biopsy confirmed invasive vulvar cancer

B. Women with a suspicious vulvar lesion should be biopsied before referral. These suspicious lesions include:

    1. Nonhealing ulcers

    2. Areas of chronic pain or pruritus

    3. Areas of pigment change

    4. Grossly enlarged lesion

C. Depending on practitioner's comfort level:

    1. Women with multifocal, complex, and/or recurrent VIN 3

    2. Women with Paget's disease of the vulva

VI. Gestational Trophoblastic Disease

A. Referral should occur after evacuation of the molar pregnancy if there is evidence of persistent trophoblastic disease/gestational trophoblastic disease (GTD):

    1. GTD (low or high risk)

    2. Choriocarcinoma

    3. Placental site trophoblastic tumor

If there is evidence of metastatic disease at initial diagnosis, referral should occur immediately.

Preinvasive Disease

I. Cervical Intraepithelial Neoplasia (CIN)

CIN is asymptomatic; Pap smear screening is the main means of detection with a median age of 23 years old at diagnosis (1). CIN is classified according to the amount of epithelium involved: CIN 1 demonstrates atypia in the lower third of epithelium; CIN 2 demonstrates atypia up to the middle third of epithelium; and CIN 3 demonstrates atypia throughout the entire epithelium. The microscopic appearance of CIN is nuclear atypia, disorganization/depolarization, parakeratosis, and abnormal mitotic figures. Most lesions occur in the transformation zone.

A. Risk of progression for dysplastic lesions:

Lesion	% Regression	% Persistent	% Progress to CIN 3
CIN 1	57%	32%	11%
CIN 2	43%	35%	22%
CIN 3	32%	35%	NA

B. Risk factors for dysplasia are human papillomavirus (HPV) infection, immunosuppression, smoking, a history of STDs, and multiple sexual partners. A diet low in vitamins A, C, and beta-carotene/retinol has also been linked to higher rates of cervical dysplasia and cancer. Immunosuppression can significantly contribute to increased rates of dysplasia and cancer: for those infected with HIV, the relative risk is 9.2 times higher; for transplant patients, the relative risk is 13.6 times higher.

C. Diagnosis is via Colposcopic directed biopsy obtained after the application of 3% acetic acid to the cervix for 5 minutes. An endocervical curettage (ECC) should be done if the patient is not pregnant. Histologic confirmation with biopsy should occur before ablative therapy is performed (i.e. cryotherapy).

D. Pathologists cannot distinguish between CIN 3 and carcinoma in situ (CIS); thus, it is recommended that CIS terminology not be used. Terminology has become two-tiered: CIN 1 is categorized as a low-grade lesion and CIN 2 to 3 are combined into the category of high-grade lesions.

E. Glandular precancerous changes include adenocarcinoma in situ (AIS). This is histologically represented as: crowding of cells, atypia, pseudostratification, and increased mitotic activity. To distinguish atypia versus adenocarcinoma in situ (AIS), the degree of mitotic activity and pseudostratification should be taken into account. To diagnose an invasive lesion, atypical glands extend beyond the depth normally involved by endocervical glands, which is approximately 5 to 6 mm from the surface.

F. Treatment of CIN 1 can vary. In the ASCUS/LSIL Triage Study for Cervical Cancer (ALTS) study, 41% of CIN 1 diagnoses were downgraded to normal, and 13% were upgraded to CIN 2/3. In one study, 90% of women with CIN 1 spontaneously regressed in 24 months (2). If CIN 1 is diagnosed after a Pap test that showed HSIL or ASC-H, more aggressive management should be considered. If CIN 1 is diagnosed after an ASC-US or LSIL Pap, HPV testing every 12 months or repeating a Pap smear every 6 months can be considered.

   If the CIN 1 persists for 2 years, a loop electrosurgical excision procedure (LEEP) can be considered. Before using any ablative (cryo or laser) therapy, a negative ECC should be obtained.

G. Treatment for CIN 2/3 is usually excisional with conization. This can be done with a LEEP, cold knife conization, or CO_2 laser. Cryotherapy is usually preserved for geographical areas with fewer resources. For the conization procedure, it is necessary to remove 5 to 7 mm of cervical stroma and perform an ECC. There is evidence of skip lesions and multifocality, especially in glandular lesions, so one should, therefore, not solely remove the acetowhite lesion.

H. Indications for conization include the following: treatment of CIN 2/3, treatment of a positive ECC, evaluation of microscopic invasive cancer, treatment of Stage IA1 cervical cancer, evaluation of significant cytologic/histologic discrepancy, and evaluation of an unsatisfactory colposcopic exam. Cold knife conization may be a more favorable procedure for glandular lesions.

I. Follow-up after conization should include HPV testing at 6 to 12 months or cytology at 6-month intervals. After 2 negative Pap tests, routine screening can be reinitiated for the next 20 years. For positive margins after conization, either colposcopy with ECC at 4 to 6 months or re-excision can be considered. There is data to support the spontaneous resolution of positive margins in 56% of women.

J. Histologic guidelines can be found at:
www.asccp.org Histology Algorithm
www.nccn.org NCCN Guidelines for Detection, Prevention, and Risk Reduction; Cervical Cancer Screening

II. Vulvar Intraepithelial Neoplasia

A. **Characteristics**: Vulvar dysplasia/vulvar intraepithelial neoplasia (VIN) can present with pruritus, a mass lesion, or hyperpigmentation. It can also be asymptomatic. The median age at diagnosis is 46 years old. VIN is classified according to the amount of epithelium involved: VIN 1 demonstrates atypia in the lower third of epithelium; VIN 2 demonstrates atypia up to the middle third of epithelium; and VIN 3 demonstrates atypia throughout the entire epithelium. 3% to 4.8% of VIN 3 patients who receive treatment can still progress to cancer. 88% of untreated patients have been found to develop invasive disease (3). 12% to 23% of women with VIN 3 are found to have invasive disease at the time of VIN 3 excision (4); however, most of these diagnoses have less than 1-mm depth of invasion. One-third of invasive cancers have coexisting VIN 3. Solitary lesions have the highest risk of progression. Spontaneous regression has occurred with a range of 10% to 56%. But, because this is a precancerous lesion, treatment is the standard of care. Recurrence is higher when associated with positive margins, ranging from 17% to 46%.

B. Risk factors for VIN are a history of other genital tract dysplasia (25% have another lower reproductive tract dysplasia), smoking, immunosuppression, and a history of other STDs.

C. The Vulvar Oncology Subcommittee of the International Society for the Study of Vulvar Diseases (ISSVD) classifies VIN into two categories:

1. VIN usual type: This encompasses former VIN 2-3 subtypes, warty type, basaloid type, and mixed types. The microscopic appearance of the basaloid type is thickened epithelium with

a flat, smooth surface, numerous mitotic figures, and enlarged hyperchromatic nuclei. The warty type is condylomatous in appearance, and microscopically cells contain numerous mitotic figures with abnormal maturation. The usual type is the most common, typically occurring in younger, premenopausal women. Risk factors include HPV, smoking, and immunosuppression. Lesions are often multifocal.

2. VIN differentiated type: This encompasses the former category of simplex type. These lesions comprise less than 5% of VIN. They typically occur in postmenopausal women and are associated with lichen sclerosis, but not HPV. Lesions are usually unifocal and p53 positive. This lesion is probably a precursor to HPV-negative vulvar cancer.

D. Most often VIN lesions are found between 3 and 9 o'clock on the vulva, in non-hair-bearing areas. The lesions are often multifocal and can be macular, papular, warty, white, red, gray, or brown. Diagnosis is with colposcopy and biopsy using 3% acetic acid applied to the perineum for 5 minutes.

E. Treatment is varied. Wide local excision with 5-mm margins (skinning vulvectomy) is appropriate, as is CO_2 laser ablation, or Cavitron ultrasonic surgical aspiration (CUSA). Topical treatment for VIN with 5-FU (5% 5-FU cream once daily per week; may increase to two or three times weekly as tolerated by the patient as this medication can cause a significant chemical burn) or imiquimod 5% cream (three times a week, i.e. Monday, Wednesday, Friday, but may decrease frequency to once per week if significant vulvar swelling reaction occurs) has also been shown to be effective in nonimmunocompromised patients.

F. Recurrent disease is common, approaching 50% if margins are positive, versus 15% if negative margins are obtained.

G. Benign lesions can mimic vulvar dysplasia. It is imperative to biopsy these lesions to confirm the histologic diagnosis prior to any treatment.

1. Warty lesions are of 3 main types: condyloma acuminatum, sessile plaques, and keratotic verruca vulgaris. Of patients with vulvar warts, 22% to 32% have concomitant CIN; therefore, screening colposcopy of the entire lower genital tract is recommended. Treatment can be with topical solutions,

such as imiquimod or TCA; laser ablation; CUSA; or surgical resection.

2. Micropapillomatosis labialis is asymptomatic and can appear as small areas of mucosal papillomas. No HPV DNA has been isolated in these lesions. Treatment is not necessary.

3. Lichen sclerosis can present with pruritus. The vulvar skin is paper thin and biopsy shows blunted rete pegs. Treatment is with clobetasol steroid cream to the perineum twice daily for 6 weeks. To promote thickening of the vulvar skin, applying a 2% compounded testosterone cream twice weekly may also be useful. There is an increased risk for malignant transformation to a well-differentiated squamous cell cancer with this lesion.

4. Hyperplastic dystrophy can also present with pruritus. Biopsy shows thickened and widened rete pegs and hyperkeratosis. Treatment is with 1% hydrocortisone cream to the perineum twice daily.

III. Vaginal Intraepithelial Neoplasia (VAIN)

A. Most patients are asymptomatic. Occasionally, patients complain of vaginal discharge or postcoital or postmenopausal bleeding. Most lesions are found because of an abnormal Pap smear.

B. Risk factors are HPV infection, other genital tract dysplasia, and immunosuppression.

C. VAIN is classified into three tiers: VAIN 1 demonstrates atypia in the lower third of the epithelium, VAIN 2 demonstrates atypia into the middle third of the epithelium, and VAIN 3 involves atypia of the entire epithelium. Microscopic abnormalities include nuclear atypia, cellular depolarization, parakeratosis, and abnormal mitotic figures.

D. The most common location of vaginal dysplasia is the posterior vaginal fornix. VAIN is often multifocal. Diagnosis is made with colposcopic directed biopsy after application of 3% acetic acid for 5 minutes.

E. There is data to suggest an association of VAIN in posthysterectomy women in whom surgery was done for cervical dysplasia: 5% developed VAIN within 10 years.

F. Treatment can be with laser ablation, surgical excision, or topical suppository creams: 5% 5-fluorouracil cream can be used. There are many regimens, but our recommended dosing for 5-FU is once weekly for 10 weeks. This may be decreased to once every 2–3 weeks if the patient becomes symptomatic due to development of a vaginal chemical burn. Monthly maintenance dosing can be considered. Recurrence rates range from 0% to 38%. Compounded 2.5% imiquimod cream can also be applied via an intravaginal applicator every other night for 16 weeks. It may be necessary to decrease the dosing frequency to once per week if significant vaginal swelling reaction occurs.

G. No large long-term follow-up studies have been done to evaluate the risk of VAIN and progression to vaginal cancer. One study from Finland evaluated 23 patients and showed a 78% rate of regression, 13% persistence, and 8% progression to cancer. Another study evaluated vaginectomy specimens and showed a 28% incidence of cancer (6). An 18% incidence of recurrence was demonstrated after vaginectomy.

IV. Dysplasia and HIV

A. One-third of people with HIV are infected heterosexually. Cervical dysplasia in women with HIV has a more negative outcome. Screening for cervical cancer in HIV-positive women is recommended every 6 months for 2 visits. If 2 consecutive normal Pap smears are obtained, annual Pap smears can follow. In HIV-positive women, CIN was found in 14% of women with a normal Pap versus 3% if HIV negative.

B. Current guidelines suggest measuring a baseline (pretreatment) viral load. A drug is considered efficacious if it lowers the viral load by at least 90% within 8 weeks. The viral load should continue to drop to less than 50 copies within 6 months. The viral load should be measured within 2 to 8 weeks after treatment is started or changed, and every 3 to 4 months thereafter. Anyone with a viral load over 100,000 should be offered treatment, as should anyone with an AIDS-defining illness, or a CD4 count less than 200.

C. Highly active antiretroviral therapy (HAART) includes at least 3 active antiretroviral medications. Typically 2 drugs are a nucleoside or nucleotide reverse transcriptase inhibitor (NRTI) plus a third medication. This third medication can be a nonnucleoside reverse transcriptase inhibitor (NNRTI), a protease inhibitor (PI), or another NRTI such as abacavir (Ziagen).

D. If CIN 1 is diagnosed, some clinicians treat immediately. Others may delay treatment if the Pap was a non-HSIL Pap prior to biopsy confirmation of CIN 1. It is important to check the viral load and CD4 counts. If there is a high viral load and a low CD4 count, delay in treatment can be detrimental. For a diagnosis of CIN 2/3, conization should be performed.

E. Analysis of 2 large studies (HIV Epidemiology Research Study [HERS] Group, and Women's Interagency HIV Study [WIHS]) showed that there was a 45% immediate failure rate/disease persistence at 6 months for HIV-positive women treated for CIN 2/3 by LEEP. For those who had a normal Pap smear at 6 months, there was a 56% recurrence rate. The median recurrence-free period was 30 months. About 60% of persistent or recurrent disease was low grade. 73% of patients in this study were not on HAART.

F. Conization margins are very important in HIV-positive patients. Those patients with positive margins had 100% recurrence versus a 30% to 50% recurrence with negative margins. This is compared to an 8% to 15% recurrence rate in HIV-negative women with negative margins. There is an association with a decreased recurrence rate with the use of HAART and higher CD4 counts in 2 studies (one for each factor). If the CD4 is greater than 500, 30% were found to regress.

G. 7% of HIV-positive women with condyloma in the perineal or pararectal area can develop VIN 2/3 within a 3-year period. HIV-positive women are 7 times more likely to develop VIN than HIV-negative women.

REFERENCES

1. Castle PE. A descriptive analysis of prevalent vs incident cervical intraepithelial neoplasia grade 3 following minor cytologic abnormalities. *Am J Clin Pathol.* 2012;138(2):241–246.
2. Schlect NF. Human papillomavirus infection and time to progression and regression of cervical intraepithelial neoplasia. *J Natl Cancer Inst.* 2003;95(17):1336–1343.
3. Jones RW. Vulvar intraepithelial neoplasia III: a clinical study of the outcome in 113 cases with relation to the later development of invasive vulvar carcinoma. *Obstet Gynecol.* 1994;84(4):741–745.

4. Modesitt SC. Vulvar intraepithelial neoplasia III: occult cancer and the impact of margin status on recurrence. *Obstet Gynecol.* 1998;92(6): 962–966.

5. Sideri M. Squamous vulvar intraepithelial neoplasia: 204 modified terminology ISSVD Vulvar Oncology Subcommittee. *J Reprod Med.* 2005;50(11):807–810.

6. Ireland D. The management of the patient with abnormal vaginal cytology following vaginal hysterectomy. *BJOG.* 1988;95(10):973–975.

7. Massad L, Stewart MD, Fazzari J. Outcomes after treatment of cervical intraepithelial neoplasia among women with HIV. *J Low Genit Tract Dis.* 2007;11(2):90–97.

Cervical Cancer

I. **Characteristics:** There are approximately 400,000 new cases of cervical cancer worldwide annually. In 2013 there were 12,340 anticipated new cases identified with approximately 4030 deaths in the United States.

A. The most common symptom of cervical cancer is abnormal vaginal bleeding—specifically, postcoital and intermenstrual bleeding, menorrhagia, and postmenopausal bleeding. Other symptoms include pelvic fullness/pain, unilateral leg swelling, bladder irritability, and tenesmus. Cervical cancer is also commonly asymptomatic, found only following an abnormal Pap smear, colposcopic exam, or cervical biopsy.

B. Common signs of advanced cervical cancer are a fungating cervical mass, unilateral leg edema, and obstructive renal failure.

C. Cervical cancer results from persistent infection with high-risk HPV types (most commonly 16 and 18). Risk factors associated with cervical cancer are: prior history of sexually transmitted diseases (STDs), early age of first coitus, multiple sexual partners, multiparity, nonbarrier methods of birth control, and smoking.

D. Cervical cancer primarily spreads by direct extension from the cervix to the parametria, vagina, uterine corpus, and the pelvis. Other routes of spread include lymphatic and hematogenous dissemination, as well as direct peritoneal seeding.

E. Lymph node (LN) metastasis usually occurs in a sequential fashion, traveling first to the parametrial lymph nodes, then to pelvic (obturator, internal, and external iliac), common iliac, para-aortic, then scalene LN.

II. **Pretreatment Workup:** The pretreatment workup of cervical cancer begins with a history and physical exam. Laboratory studies to assess hematologic, renal, and liver functions should be performed. Imaging studies should also be performed to include pelvic imaging and a CXR.

A. FIGO-approved imaging studies include barium enema, intravenous pyleogram, and chest x-ray. Other modalities such as CT (to assess LNs and evaluate for hydronephrosis), MRI (to assess integrity of tissue planes and extent of cervical disease), or PET/CT (to evaluate for distant metastasis) are non-FIGO-approved staging tests due to the poor availability of these imaging modalities in medically underserved countries.

B. Cervical conization should be used to evaluate microscopic disease. Conization can differentiate between microinvasive vs. invasive early-stage disease.

C. For lesions that are macroscopic, an office examination or an examination under anesthesia with cystoscopy and proctoscopy is indicated.

D. If patients cannot tolerate an office exam, or if there is ambiguity about the staging in an office setting, an examination under anesthesia (EUA) should be performed. There are data to suggest that EUA can significantly change clinical staging: 23% were upstaged, most to IIA or IIB disease. Patients were downstaged less often (9%) to IB2 and IIB. Proctoscopy was not found to be helpful, but cystoscopy identified 8% of patients with Stage 4A disease, and a chest x-ray was abnormal in 4% of patients (1).

E. Multiple studies have supported the use of PET scans. An analysis of 15 published FDG-PET studies on cervical cancer showed that the pooled sensitivity and specificity of FDG-PET for detecting pelvic LN metastasis were 79% (95% CI, 65%–90%) and 99% (96%–99%), compared with 72% (53%–87%) and 96% (92%–98%), for MRI, and 47% (21%–73%) for CT (specificity not available). The pooled sensitivity and specificity of FDG-PET for detecting PALNs were 84% (95%, CI 68%–94%) and 95% (89%–98%) (2). A study from Israel (3) revealed a sensitivity of 60%, a specificity of 94%, an PPV of 90%, and an NPV of 74%. PET-CT may not pick up lesions smaller than 1.5 cm. There is data to suggest that treatment modification can occur in 25% of patients based on PET-CT results.

III. Histology: There are several different histologic types of cervical cancer, the most common being squamous (85%). Other types include adenocarcinoma (15%–20%), verrucous carcinoma, adenosquamous carcinoma, clear cell carcinoma, neuroendocrine carcinomas, and undifferentiated types.

A. Adenocarcinoma: 15% have no visible lesion because the lesion arises from the endocervical canal, forming a "barrel-shaped" lesion.

B. Verrucous carcinoma: This is a well-differentiated squamous cell carcinoma. It is known to recur locally, but does not metastasize. Historically, these tumors should not be treated with radiotherapy because radiation can cause anaplastic transformation; however, recent evidence does not support this. It is associated with HPV6b.

C. Adenosquamous carcinoma: This is a mixed glandular and squamous carcinoma. It behaves similar to adenocarcinoma.

D. Glassy cell carcinoma: This is a poorly differentiated type of adenosquamous carcinoma.

E. Clear cell carcinoma: This is a poorly differentiated carcinoma. It is nodular and reddish in gross appearance. It has a hobnail cell shape microscopically. It can be associated with intrauterine DES exposure.

F. Neuroendocrine carcinoma: This includes the small cell and carcinoid carcinomas. Small cell is the most common neuroendocrine tumor in the cervix. It contains adenoid basal cells with scarce myoepithelial differentiation.

G. Papillary squamous cell: This is a variant of squamous cell carcinoma. It appears as transitional or cuboidal cells on microscopy.

IV. Staging:

A. FIGO Staging

Stage I: Confined to the cervix

- Stage IA1: Stromal invasion is $\leq$ 3 mm in depth. Diameter of lesion is $\leq$ 7 mm
- Stage IA2: Stromal invasion $>$ 3 mm and $\leq$ 5 mm in depth. Diameter of lesion is $\leq$ 7 mm
- Stage IB1: Lesion $\leq$ 4 cm
- Stage IB2: Lesion $>$ 4 cm

Stage II: Extends beyond the cervix but not to pelvic sidewall or lower third of vagina

- Stage IIA: No parametrial involvement
  - Stage IIA1: $\leq$ 4 cm
  - Stage IIA2: > 4 cm
- Stage IIB: Parametrial involvement

Stage III: Extension to the pelvic side wall with no cancer-free space between the tumor and pelvic wall. Tumor involves the lower third of the vagina. All cases of renal failure due to tumor or hydronephrosis are staged III.

- Stage IIIA: No extension to the pelvic sidewall but the lower third of the vagina is involved
- Stage IIIB: Extension to the pelvic wall, hydronephrosis, or nonfunctioning kidney due to tumor compression/obstruction of ureters

Stage IV: Tumor has extended beyond the true pelvis or involved adjacent organs

- Stage IVA: Spread to adjacent organs and involving the mucosa of the bladder or rectum
- Stage IVB: Spread to distant organs

B. AJCC Staging

Tumor:

TX: Primary tumor cannot be assessed

T0: No evidence of primary tumor

Tis: Carcinoma in situ

T1: Carcinoma confined to the uterus

- T1A: Diagnosed only by microscopy. Maximum stromal depth of invasion 5 mm and maximum diameter spread 7 mm
  - T1A1: Maximum stromal invasion $\leq$ 3 mm and maximum horizontal spread $\leq$ 7 mm
  - T1A2: Maximum stromal invasion > 3 mm and $\leq$ 5 mm with horizontal spread $\leq$ 7 mm
- T1B: Clinically visible lesion confined to the cervix or microscopic lesion > T1A

- T1B1: Clinically visible lesion ≤ 4 cm in diameter
- T1B2: Clinically visible lesion > 4 cm in diameter

T2: Tumor invades beyond the uterus but not to the pelvic wall or lower vagina

- T2A: Without parametrial invasion
  - T2A1: Clinically visible lesion ≤ 4 cm diameter
  - T2A2: Clinically visible lesion > 4 cm diameter
- T2B: With parametrial invasion

T3: Tumor invades to pelvic wall and/or lower third of the vagina.

Tumor causes hydronephrosis or nonfunctioning kidney

- T3A: Tumor involves lower third of the vagina but no extension to the pelvic wall
- T3B: Tumor invades to pelvic wall and/or causes hydronephrosis or nonfunctioning kidney

T4: (T4A) Tumor invades bladder or rectal mucosa or invades beyond the true pelvis

Nodes:

NX: Cannot be assessed

N0: No evidence of LN metastasis

N1: Pelvic or inguinal LNs positive

Metastasis:

MX: Cannot be assessed

M0: None

M1: (T4B) Distant metastasis

TNM Grouping:

Stage I: T1 N0 M0

Stage IA: T1A N0 M0

- Stage IA1: T1A1 N0 M0
- Stage IA2: T1A2 N0 M0

Stage IB: T1B N0 M0

- Stage IB1: T1B1 N0 M0
- Stage IB2: T1B2 N0 M0

Stage II: T2 N0 M0

- Stage IIA: T2A N0 M0
- Stage IIA1: T2A1 N0 M0
- Stage IIA2: T2A2 N0 M0
- Stage IIB: T2B N0 M0

Stage III: T3 N0 M0

- Stage IIIA: T3A N0 M0
- Stage IIIB: T3B Any N M0, or T1-3 N1 M0

Stage IV:

- Stage IVA: T4 Any N M0
- Stage IVB: Any T any N M1

V. Overall survival by stage:

IA: 100%

IB1: 90%

IB2: 80%

IIA: 70%

IIB: 65%

IIIA: 37%

IIIB: 53%

IVA: 29%

IVB: 5% to 15%

VI. Treatment: The treatment of cervical cancer may involve the use of surgery, chemotherapy, radiotherapy, or a combination of therapies. 70% of newly diagnosed patients with invasive carcinoma of the cervix have disease limited to the uterine cervix and are, therefore, potential operative candidates. 54% to 84% of these patients will need adjuvant therapies for intermediate or high-risk factors, however, so thorough investigation of the full extent of disease should be performed. NCI statements support treatment with the fewest number of interventions; thus, if high-risk factors are found on conization, which predict a high probability for the need of adjuvant therapies, it may be prudent to not perform surgery.

A. Treatment options by stage:

    1. Stage IA1:

    A simple hysterectomy or cold knife cone (if fertility-sparing treatment is desired) are adequate therapies. Intracavitary radiotherapy can be used alone. If there is < 3 mm stromal invasion but LVSI is identified, a radical hysterectomy should be considered.

    2. Stages IA2, IB1, and IIA1:

    A type II or III radical hysterectomy and pelvic LN dissection can be offered. Similar outcomes have been seen with both types of radical hysterectomy (4). Surgical candidates are those with lesions that are not bulky or barrel shaped. Definitive treatment can also be primary radiotherapy with concurrent chemotherapy. Similar cure rates are seen with either radical surgery or radiotherapy (5).

    3. Stages IB2, and IIA2 to IVA:

    A combination of radiotherapy with chemotherapy is the standard of care. Patients with large cervical lesions staged IB2 have a high rate of needing adjuvant therapies. Surgery can be considered as adjuvant therapy in certain situations; e.g., if there is residual tumor after definitive chemotherapy–radiation.

    4. Stage IVB:

    Chemotherapy should be used for disseminated disease and radiotherapy can be considered for pelvic tumor control or palliation of symptoms including bleeding.

B. Most randomized trials included 5% to 8% of patients with adenocarcinoma, so they are applicable to cite in treating adenocarcinoma of the cervix.

C. Margin status is important in conization. In one study evaluating adenocarcinoma in situ (6), 33% of patients with negative margins had residual disease at the time of hysterectomy and 14% had invasive cancer; 53% of those with positive margins had residual disease and 26% were found to have invasive cancers. In another study which reviewed patients with invasive squamous cell cancer on conization (7), 24% of patients had residual disease if they had negative margins and 60% were found to have residual disease if they had positive margins.

D. The incidence of positive LNs with squamous cell and adenocarcinomas is 5% for Stage 1A2, 15% for Stage 1B1, 30% for Stage 1B2, 45% for Stage 2B, and 60% for Stage 3B.

E. The incidence of adnexal metastasis with adenocarcinoma is 1.7% compared to 0.5% for squamous cell lesions. According to GOG 49 (8), this is a nonsignificant difference, and all patients with ovarian metastasis had evidence of other extra-cervical disease.

F. The rate of an aborted radical hysterectomy for grossly positive LNs is approximately 7% to 8% (9). Per GOG 49, the rate of abandoned radical hysterectomy was 8.3%.

G. If a positive LN is found at the time of radical hysterectomy, there are 2 management options: completion of, or abortion of, radical hysterectomy.

   1. Some proceed and complete the radical hysterectomy. The rationale is that removal of bulky lymph nodes leaves less residual tumor for radiation to sterilize.

   2. Another study showed that the local recurrence and distant recurrence rates were not significantly different for LN positive aborted vs. completed radical hysterectomy patients. The PFS was 74.9 months vs. 46.8 months ($P = .106$) and the OS was 91.8 months vs. 69.4 months ($P = .886$) (11). Potter (12) found similar outcomes and the trend favored definitive radiotherapy. Leaving the uterus in situ can help with treatment planning and can move the small bowel out of the treatment field. Debulking of LN greater than 2 cm prior to abortion of hysterectomy may be beneficial.

   3. The number of positive LN affects OS. The 5-year survival (YS) decreases for each additional positive LN: 1 node (79%), 2 to 3 nodes (63%), 4+ nodes (40%) (13).

H. Surgical staging in locally advanced cervical cancer may be beneficial. In one study, surgical staging of women with locally advanced cervical cancer was suggested to improve overall clinical outcome, as those with positive LNs had a modification in standard radiation fields in up to 43% of patients (14).

I. LN debulking can potentially improve the 5 YS in patients with locally advanced cervical cancer (10). One study showed that if grossly metastatic lymph nodes were resected, the survival of women in that group approached the level of those women who had microscopic lymph node involvement only

(50%, 5 YS), which was significantly higher than the women with unresectable lymph nodes (0%) (10). There was a 10.5% incidence of severe radiation-related morbidity and a 1% incidence of treatment-related deaths due to combined therapies.

J. A cut through hysterectomy refers to a cancer either found incidentally on final pathology or resected without radical surgery. Treatment of a "cut through" can include adjuvant radiotherapy or a radical parametrectomy. There is data to suggest that the 5 YS is better with adjuvant radiation vs. radical parametrectomy with a 68.7% vs. a 49% 5 YS. This is stage and margin dependent. The 5 YS for women staged 1A2 and IIA was 96% (15), but was much lower for women Stage IIB or higher who had a 5 YS of 28%.

K. Hydronephrosis found on imaging predicts a worse OS and PFS. Relief of ureteral obstruction has been associated with improved survival. Management with stenting via cystoscopy from below, or antegrade from above, is beneficial (16).

VII. Surgical Treatment:

    A. Hysterectomy types: Piver classification: I–V is based on the degree of resection of vagina, parametria, cardinal ligaments, and uterosacral ligaments (17).

        1. Class I radical hysterectomy is the same as a simple hysterectomy. It is indicated for Stage IA1 cervical cancers without lymphovascular space involvement.

        2. Class II radical hysterectomy is a modified radical hysterectomy. It involves resection of the medial half of the cardinal and uterosacral ligaments. The uterine artery is taken at its junction with the ureter. The upper one-fourth (or 1 to 2 cm) of the vagina is also removed. This results in a wider local treatment margin than a simple hysterectomy.

        3. Class III radical hysterectomy is also called a Wertheim/Meigs-Okabayashi hysterectomy. Originally, Wertheim did not include lymphadenectomy, whereas Meigs and Okabayashi did. In this procedure, the cardinal and uterosacral ligaments are completely transected and one-third to one-half of the vagina is removed. The uterine artery is taken at its origin. The autonomic nerves for bladder and rectal function are also resected, which can result in a high incidence of prolonged or permanent bladder dysfunction.

4. Class IV radical hysterectomy is reserved for larger bulky lesions. This procedure involves completely transecting the cardinal and uterosacral ligaments at their origin. One half of the vagina is removed; therefore, sexual dysfunction occurs from the shortened vagina. The superior vesical artery is sacrificed and all periureteral tissue is removed.

5. Class V radical hysterectomy is reserved for tumors that invade to the lower urinary tract. It involves the removal of involved portions of the bladder as well as the distal ureters.

B. There is data to suggest (4) for early-stage (IB to IIA) cervix cancer that there is no difference in recurrence rate or survival rate between class II or III radical hysterectomy. Surgeries took longer for the type III hysterectomies.

C. A scalene LN dissection is done if there is a question about distant metastasis. There is data to suggest (18) that 10.7% of patients with positive para-aortic LNs have positive scalene nodes. PET scanning may be a reasonable alternative to a scalene LN dissection.

1. The boundaries of the neck are the anterior and posterior triangles.

a. The anterior triangle is bordered by the sternocleidomastoid, the mandible, and the midline of the neck.

b. The posterior triangle is bordered by the sternocleidomastoid, the clavicle, and the trapezius. This is the larger triangle of the neck in which the scalene triangle lies.

c. The boundaries of the scalene triangle are the inferior belly of the omohyoid muscle, the sternocleidomastoid, and the subclavian vein. The scalenus anterior muscle lines the floor of the triangle. The phrenic nerve runs through the scalene triangle, as does the thoracic duct. If the duct is transected, it must be ligated at both ends to prevent a fistula.

D. Other surgical techniques and indications:

1. Radical vaginal hysterectomy (Schauta-Amreich procedure) is performed in two stages. The first stage involves a retroperitoneal pelvic LN dissection, most commonly via laparoscopy. The second step is to perform a vaginal radical hysterectomy.

2. Laparoscopic radical hysterectomy. This can also be approached with robotic assistance.

3. Radical trachelectomy is indicated for patients who desire fertility with tumors that are Stage IB1 or lower and that are < 2 cm in maximum diameter. Care should be taken with aggressive histological types. A radical trachelectomy involves the radical dissection and removal of the uterine cervix. This can be performed by either an abdominal approach or via the Schauta-Amreich vaginal approach. The cervix is amputated from the uterine corpus about 1 cm below the isthmus. An ECC is performed and sent for frozen pathology. If the ECC is positive, the hysterectomy is completed. If it is negative, a McDonald's or Shirodkar cerclage is usually placed at the time of surgery due to the risk of preterm labor from creating a shortened cervix. A Saling procedure, which advances the vaginal mucosa to cover the external os, can be performed at 14 weeks to reduce the risk of ascending infection. A separate LN dissection can be accomplished via laparoscopic, extraperitoneal abdominal, or intraperitoneal abdominal approach. Only the parametrial nodes can be removed during the vaginal portion of the surgery.

E. Specific indications for surgical therapy and not radiotherapy include a current pelvic abscess, the presence of a pelvic kidney, or a history of prior radiotherapy for other indications.

F. Ovarian transposition can be considered in some patients who wish to preserve their fertility or preserve their ovarian function. Studies have shown 41% to 71% of patients maintained their ovarian function after radiotherapy with ovarian transposition (19).

VIII. Radiotherapy:

A. Total dosing is prescribed to defined anatomical points. Please refer to the Chapter 7B "Radiation Therapy" for an involved discussion. The point A total dose should be at least 80 to 90 Gy. The point B dose is at least 50 to 60 Gy. External beam pelvic radiotherapy is usually dosed at 45 to 50.4 Gy. Brachytherapy provides a dose with LDR of 40 Gy, or with HDR of 30 Gy. The HDR rates are $0.6 \times$ the LDR rate.

B. The duration of treatment with radiation affects outcomes in cervical cancer. As treatment time lengthens, the overall survival decreases. The goal is completion of treatment within 56 days. There is a 1% per day decrease in survival if treatment goes beyond 56 days.

Stage	Treatment Time, Weeks	10-Year Pelvic Failure, Percent	10-Year DSS, Percent
Stage IB	≤ 7	5	86
	7.1–9	22	78
	> 9	36	55
Stage IIA	≤ 7	14	73
	7.1–9	27	41
	> 9	36	43
Stage IIB	≤ 7	20	72
	7.1–9	28	60
	> 9	34	65

C. Chemotherapy is usually given concurrently with radiation. It can be given as cisplatin monotherapy dosed weekly at 40 or 50 mg/m^2 with a maximum of 70 mg/m^2, or as combination chemotherapy with cisplatin dosed at 40 or 50 mg/m^2 on day 1 and 5-FU dosed at 1000 mg/m^2/day as a continuous infusion for 4 days every 3 weeks.

D. There is a 25% chance of needing adjuvant radiotherapy following radical hysterectomy for intermediate risk factors in patients with Stage IB1 disease. For Stages IB2 and IIA disease, this possibly increases to about 80%. There is data to suggest (5) that 54% of patients with a tumor less than 4 cm will need adjuvant radiotherapy. For those with lesions greater than 4 cm in size, approximately 84% will need adjuvant radiotherapy. Adjuvant radiation recommendations were based on pathological data to include: positive lymph nodes, positive parametria, close margins, and less than 3 mm uninvolved stroma.

E. The rate of radiotherapy complications increases in dual therapy patients. In GOG 92 there was a 7% incidence of grade 3 to 4 hematologic, GI, or GU complications in patients who had pelvic radiotherapy after radical hysterectomy vs. 2% who received NFT after radical hysterectomy (20). In the Landoni study, there was a 28% complication rate after radical hysterectomy with adjuvant radiation compared to 12% for definitive radiotherapy alone.

IX. Adjuvant Posthysterectomy Treatment: Adjuvant therapies are initiated by 6 weeks postoperatively. Risk factors are based on observational data from GOG 49 (21).

A. Intermediate risk factors GOG 92 (20): Radiation therapy is recommended for intermediate risk factor patients.

CLS*	Stromal Invasion	Tumor Size
Positive	Deep one-third	Any
Positive	Middle one-third	≥ 2 cm
Negative	Deep or middle one-third	≥ 4 cm
Positive	Superficial one-third	≥ 5 cm

*Capillary lymphatic space involvement.

B. High-risk factors GOG 109 (22): Patient must have two or more of the following risk factors: LN metastasis, positive margins, or positive parametria. Combination chemotherapy (every-3-weeks cisplatin and 5-FU, or weekly cisplatin alone) and radiation are indicated for patients following primary surgical treatment with high-risk factors.

C. A hemoglobin (Hg) goal of at least 9.4 g/dL has been shown to increase the 5 YS by 9% for patients undergoing radiotherapy (23) but the use of red cell stimulants has been associated with a 2 times higher risk of DVT. Use of transfusion can also increase the Hg but this can be associated with immunosuppression, in addition to the TACO or TRALI reactions. In head, neck, and breast cancers, the aggressive use of transfusion and growth factors has been associated with a poorer survival. GOG 191 (24) randomized patients to aggressive transfusion or red cell stimulation for patients undergoing concurrent chemotherapy and radiation to maintain hemoglobin at or above 12 g/dL compared to the standard level of 10 g/dL. This study was closed early due to higher DVT/VTE complications.

X. Advanced Disease: Treatment options for Stage IVB cervical cancer are limited. Chemotherapy alone or chemotherapy with palliative pelvic radiotherapy are the two main options. Chemotherapy can include cisplatin in combination with a taxane, topotecan, gemcitabine, or vinorelbin.

XI. Recurrent Disease: A full metastatic workup should be performed. If local recurrence alone is demonstrated, different surgical options exist. If there is extensive recurrent pelvic disease or distant metastasis, patients are best treated with chemotherapy and/or palliative radiotherapy.

A. Most recurrences are diagnosed within the first 2 years: 50% in the first year; 75% in the second year; 95% of recurrences are diagnosed in the first 5 years.

B. "Triad of Trouble": Signs of recurrence which indicate that a mass has reached the pelvic sidewall are:

  1. Sciatica (compression/invasion into the sciatic nerve)

  2. Lower extremity edema (compression of pelvic lymphatics)

  3. CVA tenderness (causing hydronephrosis from compression of the ureter)

C. The recurrent cervical cancer patient can be managed differently based on site of location, prior therapies given, and patient co-morbidities.

  1. Surgery:

   a. Radical hysterectomy: Can be considered if the recurrent tumor is < 2 cm and limited to the cervix. The rate of complications is high, however, with fistula occurring at 50%, and patients having a 5 YS of 62%.

   b. Pelvic exenteration: Total, anterior, or posterior. The 5 YS with positive pelvic LNs is 15% to 20% and this must be weighed with the morbidity of the procedure. There are certain patient selection factors that are important when considering exenteration: local extension, positive LNs, peritoneal disease, or malignant ascites are adverse factors related to decreased survival. One study found the following 3 risk factors predicted survival at 18 months: time to recurrence; size; preoperative pelvic sidewall fixation.

  2. Chemotherapy: Cisplatin and paclitaxel showed an improved response rate compared to cisplatin alone. Topotecan and cisplatin showed improvement in PFS and OS over cisplatin alone (25).

  3. Radiation:

   a. For radio-therapeutic curative-intent retreatment, patients can be broken down into 3 categories: central disease, limited peripheral disease, and massive peripheral disease. The central and limited peripheral disease patients are good candidates for curative intent, having a 30% to 70% chance for survival.

b. Patients who are candidates for salvage re-irradiation include those who are medically inoperable, those who refuse surgery, or in whom surgery is not feasible.

c. External beam doses of 39 to 72 Gy, brachytherapy doses of 60 to 89 Gy, or combination radiotherapy doses up to 90 Gy can be used. This yields 57% control for external beam, 67% for brachytherapy, and 44% for combination therapy (26). For recurrence in the para-aortic region, external beam radiotherapy can be delivered, but success rates for adenopathy greater than 2 cm are low. Therefore, resection with combination chemotherapy and radiation can be considered.

d. Interstitial radiotherapy implants placed via laparotomy guidance (27) have been reported to yield a 71% rate of local control with 36% of patients having no evidence of disease at follow-up.

e. In the palliative setting, RTOG protocols have given 3.7 Gy twice daily for 2 consecutive days at 3- to 6-week intervals repeated up to 3 times.

f. For palliative intent retreatment, the response rates are low and have a short duration. Combined modality retreatment with chemotherapy in addition to radiation can be considered. Platinum compounds, taxanes, and ifosfamide have a response rate of 20% with a median duration of 4 to 6 months.

XII. Survival:

   A. 5 YS by stage and histology:

     Stage I: Squamous 65% to 90%; adenocarcinoma 70% to 75%

     Stage II: Squamous 45% to 80%; adenocarcinoma 30% to 40%

     Stage III: Squamous 60%; adenocarcinoma 20% to 30%

     Stage IV: Squamous $< 15\%$; adenocarcinoma $< 15\%$

XIII. Prognostic Factors for Survival:

   A. Stage I:

     LVSI (predicts LN metastasis)

     Size of tumor

     Depth of invasion (greater than half the thickness of cervix)

     Tumor volume (> 500 mm^3)

     Presence of LN metastasis (decreases survival by 50% per stage)

B. Stages II–IV:

Stage

LN metastasis

Tumor volume

Age

Performance status

XIV. Follow-Up:

A. Every 3 months for the first 2 years

Every 6 months for years 3 to 5

Annually thereafter

B. During follow-up the visit may include:

A directed physical examination

Pap smear with each exam: A Pap smear is not performed within the first 3 months following radiotherapy due to radiotherapy-associated changes.

Consideration can be given to CT scan of the abdomen and pelvis every 6 to 12 months.

PET scanning can also be considered.

XV. Notable Trials in Cervical Cancer

A. GOG 49 (28) was a prospective surgical pathological study of Stage I squamous carcinoma of the cervix. 1120 patients with Stage IA2 or IB tumors were evaluated, 940 patients were eligible, 732 squamous cell tumors were investigated, and 645 patients underwent PPLND. Four risk factors were found on multivariate analysis as independently associated with a higher risk of pelvic LN metastasis: > one-third cervical stromal invasion, LVSI, tumor size > 4 cm, and age ≤ 50 years. On univariate analysis, parametrial involvement and grade were also found to be significant.

B. GOG 71 (29) showed that there is no improvement in survival with the addition of hysterectomy after radiotherapy. This study evaluated 256 patients with exophytic or barrel-shaped tumors, measuring ≥ 4 cm, who were randomized to EBRT and brachytherapy, or attenuated EBRT followed by extrafascial hysterectomy. 25% of the patients had tumors > 7 cm. There was a 27% vs. 14% decrease in the local recurrence rate, but there was no difference in the OS. The 5-year PFS was 53% for the radiotherapy arm vs. 62% for the radiotherapy with adjuvant hysterectomy arm ($P = .09$). Disease progression occurred in 46% of patients in the radiotherapy arm vs. 37% for the radiotherapy with adjuvant hysterectomy arm ($P = .07$). Radiotherapy dosing was 80 Gy to point A in the radiotherapy arm, whereas the adjuvant hysterectomy arm received 75 Gy to point A. The primary criticism of this study was that the adjuvant hysterectomy arm was underdosed. The study was powered for OS, with PFS as a secondary endpoint. For the subgroup with cervical lesions of 4 cm, 5 cm, or 6 cm, there was a borderline significance for PFS and OS in the adjuvant hysterectomy arm. Paradoxically, cervical tumors of 7 cm or greater had a worse survival when treated with adjuvant hysterectomy.

C. GOG 92 (20) with 12 years of follow-up (30) looked at 277 patients with at least 2 of the following intermediate risk factors: > one-third stromal invasion, positive lymphovascular space invasion, or large clinical tumor diameter. These were all Stage 1B patients who underwent radical hysterectomy with LN dissection and who had negative LNs and negative margins. 70% had tumors > 3 cm. 137 patients were randomized to adjuvant radiotherapy (50.4 Gy) and 140 patients received no further therapy. Patients with any combination of 2 or more risk factors who were treated with radiotherapy were found to have a decreased risk of recurrence. The recurrence rate was 15% with radiation vs. 28% for those who were observed over 2 years, yielding a 47% decrease in recurrence risk. At 12 years follow-up, essentially the same decrease in recurrence was seen except for those patients with adenocarcinoma who had a significantly different recurrence of 9% vs. 44%. There was no significant difference in OS.

Lymphovascular Space Involvement	Depth of Stromal Invasion	Tumor Size, cm
Yes	Deep one-third	Any
Yes	Middle one-third	2 or more
No	Deep or middle one-third	4 or more
Yes	Superficial one-third	5 or more

Adapted from Sedlis et al. 1999;73:177.

D. GOG 123 (31) evaluated 369 bulky Stage IB (at least 4 cm) patients who were randomized to radiotherapy followed by hysterectomy vs. radiotherapy and concurrent chemotherapy followed by hysterectomy. Radiation dosing was 45 Gy EBRT followed by brachytherapy to a total dose of 75 Gy to point A for both groups. An extrafascial hysterectomy was performed 3 to 6 weeks after radiation. Chemotherapy was dosed with cisplatin at 40 mg/m^2 weekly for a maximum of 6 doses. With a median follow-up of 36 months, the 3 YS was 79% vs. 83% with concurrent chemotherapy. The OS was 74% vs. 83% with concurrent chemotherapy. The relative risk of death was 0.54. The recurrence rate was 37% vs. 21% for the concurrent chemotherapy arm with a relative risk of recurrence of 0.51, favoring chemo-radiation. Fewer patients in the concurrent chemotherapy arm had residual disease in the uterus.

E. GOG 85 (32) evaluated 388 patients with Stages IIB–IVA disease. Patients were randomized to either radiotherapy with hydroxyurea at 80 mg/kg twice weekly during radiation, or radiotherapy with cisplatin at 50 mg/m^2 and 5-FU at 1000 mg/m^2 × 96 hr infusion every 28 days. All had negative para-aortic LN dissections. The relative risk of progression or death was 0.79 (95% CI 0.62 to 0.99) in the cisplatin/5-FU (CF) group. There was also a decreased incidence of lung metastasis from 9% to 6% when platinum therapy was given. Survival was significantly better for the patients randomized to CF ($P = .018$).

F. GOG 120 (33) evaluated 526 patients with Stages IIB to IVA with negative para-aortic LNs who were randomized to 3 arms. Radiotherapy was administered concurrently with either hydroxyurea alone, hydroxyurea–5-FU–cisplatin, or cisplatin alone. The dose of hydroxyurea was 2 g/m^2 twice weekly when in combination and 3 g/m^2 twice weekly when given alone. The dose of cisplatin when used alone was 40 mg/m^2 weekly, and the dose of cisplatin with 5-FU was 50 mg/m^2 days 1 and 29. 5-FU was dosed as a 96-hr infusion of 1000 mg/m^2. The relative risk of PFS or death was 0.55 to 0.57 for the cisplatin-containing groups. There was also a lower rate of lung metastasis with a rate of 3% to 4% vs. 10% favoring the cisplatin-containing arms. The OS rate was significantly higher in the cisplatin groups than in the hydroxyurea alone group with relative risks of death of 0.61 and 0.58, respectively.

G. GOG 109 (22) evaluated 243 patients staged as IA2 or IB. All were status-post radical hysterectomy and had high-risk factors to include: positive nodes (85%), positive margins (15%), or positive parametria (15%). Patients were randomized to pelvic EBRT dosed at 49.3 Gy or pelvic EBRT with concurrent chemotherapy consisting of cisplatin at 70 mg/m^2 and 5-FU of 1000 mg/m^2/day for 4 days every 3 weeks for 4 cycles, 2 cycles of which were given after completion of radiation. The projected 4-year PFS was 80% vs. 63% favoring concurrent chemotherapy, yielding a hazard ratio of 2.01 for PFS and 1.96 for OS. The projected OS rate at 4 years was 71% with radiation alone and 81% with chemo-radiation. The toxicity was higher (22% vs. 4%) in the concurrent chemotherapy arm. A reappraisal of the data (34) suggested that concurrent chemotherapy was beneficial specifically for cervical lesions $\geq$ 2 cm and for patients with 2 or more positive LNs. The absolute improvement in 5 YS for adjuvant chemo-radiation in patients with tumors $\leq$ 2 cm was only 5% (77% vs. 82%), while for those with tumors $>$ 2 cm it was 19% (58% vs. 77%). Similarly, the absolute 5 YS benefit was less evident among patients with 1 nodal metastasis (79% vs. 83%) than when at least 2 nodes were positive (55% vs.75%). Furthermore, this study also found that there was a significant difference with respect to histologies. Adenocarcinoma subtypes had a better PFS when treated with combination chemotherapy and radiation therapy.

H. GOG 136 (35) evaluated 86 patients with confirmed para-aortic LN metastases clinically staged I to IVA. Radiation doses were whole pelvic 39.6 to 48.6 Gy, point A intracavitary doses 30 to 40 Gy, point B doses 60 Gy combined with a parametrial boost. Extended field radiation was dosed at 45 Gy given with concomitant chemotherapy consisting of 5-FU 1000 mg/m^2/day for 96 hours and cisplatin 50 mg/m^2 weeks 1 and 5. The 3-year OS was 39% and the 3-year (Y) PFI was 34%. Extended field radiation therapy with concomitant chemotherapy is feasible with a 3 Y PFI of 33%. 90% of the patients completed the study.

I. GOG 165 (36) evaluated clinically staged IIB, IIIB, and IVA cervical cancer patients who were treated with 45 Gy whole pelvic radiotherapy with a parametrial boost of 5.4 Gy to 9 Gy using HDR or LDR. Standard therapy was weekly cisplatin 40 mg/m^2, and experimental therapy was prolonged venous infusion of

5-FU (PVI-FU) at 225 mg/m^2/d for 5 d/wk for 6 cycles concurrent with radiotherapy. The study was closed prematurely when an analysis indicated that PVI-FU/RT had a higher treatment failure rate (35% higher) (relative risk [RR] unadjusted, 1.29) and a higher mortality rate (RR unadjusted, 1.37). There was an increase in the failure rate at distant sites in the PVI-FU arm. The 4 Y PFS for the cisplatin group was 57% compared to 50% with the PVI-FU group (NS). The 4 Y pelvic failure rate was 16% and 14% in the cisplatin and PVI-FU arms. The distant failure rate (including abdominal, para-aortic region, bone, liver, and lung) was higher in the PVI-FU group (29% vs. 18%). The PVI-FU group had a higher failure rate for lung metastases (9% vs. 5%) and abdominal failures (11% vs. 3%). Para-aortic failure occurred in only 7% and 5% of patients in the PVI-FU and cisplatin arms, respectively, despite the fact that only 18% of patients were surgically staged in the para-aortic region.

J. RTOG 79-20 (37) evaluated 337 patients with Stages IB, IIA, and IIB disease without clinically or radiologically involved para-aortic LN who were randomized to external beam whole pelvic radiation dosed at 45 Gy or whole pelvic radiation with 45 Gy plus extended field dosed at 45 Gy. 10-year overall survival was 44% for the pelvic-only irradiation arm and 55% for the pelvic plus para-aortic irradiation arm; however, DFS was similar in both arms; 40% for the pelvic-only arm and 42% for the pelvic plus para-aortic arm. Locoregional failures were similar at 10 years for both arms (pelvic only, 35%; pelvic plus para-aortic, 31%). The cumulative incidence of Grade 4 and 5 toxicities at 10 years in the pelvic plus para-aortic arm was 8%, compared with 4% in the pelvic-only arm.

K. RTOG 90-01 (38,39) evaluated 380 surgically staged patients (IIb–IVA or Ib–IIa greater than 5 cm in size, or those with positive LN) and randomized them to whole pelvic and para-aortic radiotherapy with brachytherapy vs. whole pelvic radiotherapy and brachytherapy with concurrent cisplatin and 5-FU (75 mg/m^2/day 1 and 1000 mg/m^2/day days 2–5, every 21 days for 2 cycles). The RR was 0.48 for recurrence favoring cisplatin-based chemoradiotherapy. Total dosing was 85 Gy to point A. The patients in the chemotherapy arm had an improved 8 Y OS of 67% vs. 41%, and a DFS rate of 61% vs. 46%. The chemotherapy arm had a decreased local-regional recurrence rate of 18% vs. 35% and distant metastasis of 2% vs. 35%. The chemotherapy arm had a nonsignificant increase in para-aortic LN failures at 7% vs. 4%.

L. NCIC cervical cancer trial (40): This is the only trial to show no difference in survival with concurrent chemotherapy and radiation. 253 patients staged IB > 5 cm to IVA were included. This trial evaluated radiotherapy vs. weekly concurrent radiotherapy and cisplatin (40 mg/m^2) for 4 weeks to 6 weeks. Criticisms of this study were that patients had a lower hemoglobin level and longer treatment times. Whole pelvic radiotherapy was dosed at 45 Gy with LDR at 35 Gy $\times$ 1 or HDR at 8 Gy $\times$ 3 vs. the same radiotherapy doses with weekly cisplatin at 40 mg/m^2 $\times$ 6. The 5 YS was 62% vs. 58% NS.

M. GOG 169 (41) was a randomized phase III clinical trial with 264 eligible patients. It compared single-agent cisplatin at 50 mg/m^2 in patients with stage 4B, persistent, or recurrent cervical cancer to combination cisplatin and paclitaxel dosed at 50 mg/m^2 and 135 mg/m^2 every 21 days. The addition of paclitaxel improved the response rate (36% vs. 19%, $P = .002$) and progression-free survival (4.8 months vs. 2.8 months, $P = .001$), but did not impact the median overall survival (9.7 vs. 8.8 months, $P = $ NS).

N. GOG 179 (42) randomized patients with stage 4B, persistent, or recurrent cervical cancer to cisplatin 50 mg/m^2 q21d vs. topotecan 0.75 mg/m^2 D1,2,3 and cisplatin 50 mg/m^2 on D1 q21d. The PFS was 3 vs. 5 months, favoring the topotecan-cisplatin combination. The OS was 6.5 vs. 9.4 months, favoring the platinum doublet. The response rate was 17% for cisplatin alone vs. 27% for the combination. Febrile neutropenia occurred more often with the topotecan-cisplatin arm with 17% vs. 8% of patients having complications. Grade 3/4 neutropenia occurred in 70% of patients on the topotecan-cisplatin arm. QOL measures not significantly different between the 2 arms.

O. GOG 204 (43) evaluated 513 patients with Stage IVB or recurrent cervical cancer. Four platinum doublets were evaluated. The control arm was cisplatin-paclitaxel. The experimental-to-cisplatin-paclitaxel hazard ratios of death were 1.15 (95% CI, 0.79 to 1.67) for vinorelbine-cisplatin (VC), 1.32 (95% CI, 0.91 to 1.92) for gemcitabine-cisplatin (GC), and 1.26 (95% CI, 0.86 to 1.82) for topotecan-cisplatin (TC). The hazard ratios for progression-free survival (PFS) were 1.36 (95% CI,

0.97 to 1.90) for VC, 1.39 (95% CI, 0.99 to 1.96) for GC, and 1.27 (95% CI, 0.90 to 1.78) for TC. Response rates (RRs) for PC, VC, GC, and TC were 29.1%, 25.9%, 22.3%, and 23.4%, respectively.

P. Gemcitabine-cisplatin concurrent chemotherapy for locally advanced cervical cancer (44). 515 patients with Stage IIB to IVA disease were randomly assigned to arm A (cisplatin 40 mg/m² and gemcitabine 125 mg/m² weekly for 6 weeks with concurrent external beam radiotherapy dosed to 50.4 Gy in 28 fractions, followed by brachytherapy dosed to 30 to 35 Gy and then 2 additional 21-day cycles of cisplatin, 50 mg/m² on day 1, plus gemcitabine, 1000 mg/m² on days 1 and 8) or to arm B (cisplatin at 40 mg/m² weekly and concurrent external beam radiotherapy followed by brachytherapy). The PFS at 3 years was 74.4% in arm A vs. 65% in arm B. The OS (log-rank $P = .0224$; HR, 0.68; 95% CI, 0.49 to 0.95) and time to progressive disease (log-rank $P = .0012$; HR, 0.54; 95% CI, 0.37 to 0.79) were both better for arm A. Grade 3/4 toxicities were 86.5% in arm A vs. 46.3% in arm B. Problems with this study: the primary endpoint was changed mid-study to PFS; the sample size of approximately 500 evaluable patients was based on the original OS primary endpoint of 436 deaths out of 500 patients at an 80% power.

Q. GOG 191 (24) studied 109 eligible patients with Stage IIB to IVA with a hemoglobin < 14 g/dL who were assigned to concurrent weekly cisplatin and radiation with or without recombinant human erythropoietin (40,000 units SQ weekly) to keep the Hg level at standard levels of 10 g/dL vs. ≥ 12 g/dL. Thromboembolism (TE) occurred in 4 of 52 patients receiving chemotherapy and radiation compared to 11 of 57 patients treated with chemotherapy and radiation and erythropoietin, not all considered treatment related. No deaths occurred from TE. The study closed prematurely, with less than 25% of the planned accrual, due to potential concerns for thromboembolic events (TE) with erythropoietin.

REFERENCES

1. Massad LS. Assessing disease extent in women with bulky or clinically evident metastatic cervical cancer: yield of pretreatment studies. *Gynecol Oncol.* 2000;76(3):383–387.
2. Havrilesky LJ. FDG-PET for management of cervical and ovarian cancer. *Gynecol Oncol.* 2005;97(1):183–191.

3. Amit A. The role of hybrid PET/CT in the evaluation of patients with cervical cancer. *Gynecol Oncol.* 2006;100(1):65–69.
4. Landoni F. Class II vs. class III radical hysterectomy in stage IB–IIA cervical cancer: a prospective randomized study. *Gynecol Oncol.* 2001;80(1):3–12.
5. Landoni F. Randomised study of radical surgery vs. radiotherapy for stage Ib–IIa cervical cancer. *Lancet.* 1997;350(9077):535–540.
6. Wolf JK. Adenocarcinoma in situ of the cervix: significance of cone biopsy margins. *Obstet Gynecol.* 1996;88(1):82–86.
7. Greer BE. Stage IA2 squamous carcinoma of the cervix: difficult diagnosis and therapeutic dilemma. *Am J Obstet Gynecol.* 1990;162(6): 1409–1411.
8. Delgado G. Ovarian metastasis in stage IB carcinoma of the cervix: a Gynecologic Oncology Group study. *Gynecol Oncol.* 1992; 166(1):50–53.
9. Whitney CW. The abandoned radical hysterectomy: a Gynecologic Oncology Group study. *Gynecol Oncol.* 2000;79(3):350–356.
10. Cosin JA. Pretreatment surgical staging of patients with cervical carcinoma: the case for lymph node debulking. *Cancer.* 1998;82(11): 2241–2248.
11. Ziebarth AJ. Completed vs. aborted radical hysterectomy for node-positive stage IB cervical cancer in the modern era of chemo-radiation therapy. *Gynecol Oncol.* 2012;126(1):69–72.
12. Potter ME. Early invasive cervical cancer with pelvic lymph node involvement: to complete or not to complete radical hysterectomy? *Gynecol Oncol.* 1990;37(1):78–81.
13. Magrina JF. The prognostic significance of pelvic and aortic lymph node metastasis. *CME J Gynecol Oncol.* 2001;6(3):302–306.
14. Goff BA. Impact of surgical staging in women with locally advanced cervical cancer. *Gynecol Oncol.* 1999;74(3):436–442.
15. Smith KB. Postoperative radiotherapy for cervix cancer incidentally discovered after a simple hysterectomy for either benign conditions or noninvasive pathology. *Am J Clin Oncol.* 2010;33(3):229–232.
16. Rose PG. Impact of hydronephrosis on outcome of stage IIIB cervical cancer patients with disease limited to the pelvis, treated with radiation and concurrent chemotherapy: a Gynecologic Oncology Group study. *Gynecol Oncol.* 2010;117(2):270–275.
17. Piver MS. Five classes of extended hysterectomy for women with cervical cancer. *Obstet Gynecol.* 1974;44:265–272.
18. Boran N. Scalene lymph node dissection in locally advanced cervical carcinoma: is it reasonable or unnecessary? *Tumori.* 2003;89(2): 173–175.
19. Chambers SK. Sequelae of lateral ovarian transposition in irradiated cervical cancer patients. *Int J Radiat Oncol Biol Phys.* 1991;20(6): 1305–1308.
20. Sedlis A. A randomized trial of pelvic radiation therapy vs. no further therapy in selected patients with stage IB carcinoma of the cervix after

radical hysterectomy and pelvic lymphadenectomy: a Gynecologic Oncology Group study. *Gynecol Oncol.* 1999;73(2):177–183.

21. Delgado G. Prospective surgical-pathological study of disease free interval in patients with stage IB squamous cell carcinoma of the cervix: a Gynecologic Oncology Group study. *Gynecol Oncol.* 1990;38(3): 352–357.

22. Peters WA. Concurrent chemotherapy and pelvic radiation therapy compared with pelvic radiation therapy alone as adjuvant therapy after radical surgery in high-risk early-stage cancer of the cervix. *J Clin Oncol.* 2000;18(8):1606–1613.

23. Obermair A. Anemia before and during concurrent chemoradiotherapy in patients with cervical carcinoma: effect on progression-free survival. *Int J Gynecol Cancer.* 2003;13(5):633–639.

24. Thomas G. Phase III trial to evaluate the efficacy of maintaining hemoglobin levels above 12.0 g/dL with erythropoietin vs. above 10.0 g/dL without erythropoietin in anemic patients receiving concurrent radiation and cisplatin for cervical cancer. *Gynecol Oncol.* 2008; 108(2):317–325.

25. Long HJ III. Randomized phase III trial of cisplatin with or without topotecan in carcinoma of the uterine cervix: A Gynecologic Oncology Group study. *J Clin Oncol.* 2005;23(21):4626–4633.

26 Russell AH. Radical reirradiation for recurrent or second primary carcinoma of the female reproductive tract. *Gynecol Oncol.* 1987;27(2): 226–232.

27. Monk BJ. Open interstitial brachytherapy for the treatment of local-regional recurrences of uterine corpus and cervix cancer after primary surgery. *Gynecol Oncol.* 1994;52(2):222–228.

28. Delgado D. A prospective surgical pathological study of stage I squamous carcinoma of the cervix: a Gynecologic Oncology Group study. *Gynecol Oncol.* 1989;35(3):314–320.

29. Keys HM. Radiation therapy with and without extrafascial hysterectomy for bulky stage IB cervical carcinoma: a randomized trial of the Gynecologic Oncology Group. *Gynecol Oncol.* 2003;89(3):343–353.

30. Rotman M. A phase III randomized trial of postoperative pelvic irradiation in stage IB cervical carcinoma with poor prognostic features: a follow-up of a Gynecologic Oncology Group study. *Int J Radiat Oncol Biol Phys.* 2006;65(1):169–176.

31. Keys HM. Cisplatin, radiation, and adjuvant hysterectomy compared with radiation and adjuvant hysterectomy for bulky stage IB cervical carcinoma. *N Engl J Med.* 1999;340(15):1154–1161.

32. Whitney CW. Randomized comparison of fluorouracil plus cisplatin vs. hydroxyurea as an adjunct to radiation therapy in stage IIB–IVA carcinoma of the cervix with negative para-aortic lymph nodes: a Gynecologic Oncology Group and Southwest Oncology Group study. *J Clin Oncol.* 1999;17(5):1339–1348.

33. Rose PG. Concurrent cisplatin-based radiotherapy and chemotherapy for locally advanced cervical cancer. *N Engl J Med.* 1999;340(15): 1144–1153.
34. Monk BJ, Wang J, Im S. Rethinking the use of radiation and chemotherapy after radical hysterectomy: a clinical-pathologic analysis of a Gynecologic Oncology Group/Southwest Oncology Group/Radiation Therapy Oncology Group trial. *Gynecol Oncol.* 2005;96(3):721–728.
35. Varia MA. Cervical carcinoma metastatic to para-aortic nodes: extended field radiation therapy with concomitant 5-fluorouracil and cisplatin chemotherapy: a Gynecologic Oncology Group study. *Int J Radiat Oncol Biol Phys.* 1998;42(5):1015–1023.
36. Lanciano R. Randomized comparison of weekly cisplatin or protracted venous infusion of fluorouracil in combination with pelvic radiation in advanced cervix cancer: a Gynecologic Oncology Group study. *J Clin Oncol.* 2005;23(33):8289–8295.
37. Rotman M. Prophylactic extended-field irradiation of para-aortic lymph nodes in stages IIB and bulky IB and IIA cervical carcinomas. Ten-year treatment results of RTOG 79-20. *JAMA.* 1995;274(5):387–393.
38. Morris M. Pelvic radiation with concurrent chemotherapy compared with pelvic and para-aortic radiation in high-risk cervical cancer. *N Engl J Med.* 1999;340(15):1137–1143.
39. Eifel PJ. Pelvic irradiation with concurrent chemotherapy vs. pelvic and para-aortic irradiation for high-risk cervical cancer: an update of Radiation Therapy Oncology Group trial (RTOG) 90-01. *J Clin Oncol.* 2004;22(5):872–880.
40. Pearcey R. Phase III trial comparing radical radiotherapy with and without cisplatin chemotherapy in patients with advanced squamous cell cancer of the cervix. *J Clin Oncol.* 2002;20(4):966–972.
41. Moore DH. Phase III study of cisplatin with or without paclitaxel in stage IVB, recurrent, or persistent squamous cell carcinoma of the cervix: a Gynecologic Oncology Group study. *J Clin Oncol.* 2004;22(15): 3113–3119.
42. Long HJ III. Randomized phase III trial of cisplatin with or without topotecan in carcinoma of the uterine cervix: a Gynecologic Oncology Group study. *J Clin Oncol.* 2005;23(21):4626–4633.
43. Monk BJ. Phase III trial of four cisplatin-containing doublet combinations in stage IVB, recurrent, or persistent cervical carcinoma: a Gynecologic Oncology Group study. *J Clin Oncol.* 2009;27(28): 4649–4655.
44. Duenas-Gonzales A. Phase III, open-label, randomized study comparing concurrent gemcitabine plus cisplatin and radiation followed by adjuvant gemcitabine and cisplatin vs. concurrent cisplatin and radiation in patients with stage IIB to IVA carcinoma of the cervix. *J Clin Oncol.* 2011;29(13):1678–1685.

Ovarian Cancer

I. General Characteristics

A. One in 70 women will develop ovarian cancer in their lifetime. In 2013, 22,240 new cases are approximated, and 14,030 deaths. Ovarian cancer is most commonly found at Stage III and most women die from bowel obstruction.

B. Symptoms include abdominal fullness, dyspepsia, constipation, tenesmus, pelvic fullness or pressure, bloating, anorexia, and electrolyte abnormalities (hypercalcemia).

C. The route of spread for ovarian cancer is primarily transcoelomic. Cancer cells flake off the ovarian surface and implant throughout the abdomen and pelvis. Other routes of spread are lymphatic and hematogenous.

II. General Workup

A. The pretreatment workup includes a history and physical examination, lymph node (LN) survey, laboratory tests including a CBC, CMP, coagulation profile, CA-125, and other indicated tumor markers. A chest x-ray is recommended in addition to abdominal/pelvic imaging (CT/MRI). Colonoscopy and esophagoduodenoscopy can be considered based on symptoms.

III. General Treatment

A. Surgery usually consists of an exploratory laparotomy, abdominal cytology, hysterectomy, bilateral salpingo-oophorectomy, omentectomy, and cytoreduction.

B. Patients with evidence of up to Stage IIIB cancer should be surgically staged to include peritoneal biopsies and a pelvic and para-aortic LN dissection. Three-fourths of advanced-stage cancers will have positive retroperitoneal LN. LN drainage tends to follow the ovarian vessels. Dissection around the high precaval and para-aortic regions is important.

C. The definition of **complete debulking** is removal of all gross tumor to no residual visible disease (microscopic status). **Optimal debulking** is removal of all gross tumor to less than 1 cm visible macroscopic disease. **Suboptimal resection** is defined as remaining visible tumor with a diameter greater than 1 cm.

D. Surgical staging is often inadequate when performed by general surgeons (68%) or general gynecologists (48%), compared to gynecologic oncologists (3%).

IV. Histology

A. WHO classification of ovarian tumors:

1. Common epithelial

   Serous

   Mucinous

   Endometrioid

   Clear cell

   Brenner

   Mixed epithelial

   Undifferentiated

   Mixed mesodermal

   Unclassified

2. Sex cord stromal tumors

   Granulosa stromal cell

   Granulosa cell

   Thecoma-fibroma

   Androblastoma: Sertoli-Leydig cell tumors

   Well-differentiated Pick's adenoma (Sertoli cell tumor)

   Intermediate differentiation

   Poorly differentiated

   Heterologous elements

   Lipid cell tumors

   Gynandroblastoma

   Unclassified

3. Germ cell tumors

   Dysgerminoma

   Endodermal sinus tumor

   Embryonal carcinoma

   Polyembryoma

   Choriocarcinoma

   Teratoma

   Immature

   Mature: dermoid cyst

   Monodermal: carcinoid, struma ovari

   Mixed

   Gonadoblastoma

4. Soft tissue tumors

5. Unclassified

6. Metastatic secondary tumors: 5% to 6% of adnexal masses are metastases from the breast, gastrointestinal tract, or urinary tract.

V. General Staging

A. FIGO Staging

   Stage I: Growth limited to the ovaries

   Stage IA: Growth limited to one ovary, intact capsule, no tumor on external surface of ovary, no ascites

   Stage IB: Growth limited to both ovaries, no tumor on external surface, capsules intact, no ascites

   Stage IC: Tumor either Stage IA or Stage IB but with extension to ovarian surface or with ascites containing malignant cells or positive washings or rupture of the capsule

   Stage II: Growth involving one or both ovaries with pelvic extension

   Stage IIA: Extension or metastasis to uterus and/or tubes

   Stage IIB: Extension to other pelvic tissues

Stage IIC: Tumor either Stage IIA or IIB, tumor on the surface of the ovaries, and with ascites containing malignant cells or positive washings, or a ruptured capsule

Stage III: Tumor involving one or both ovaries with peritoneal implants outside the pelvis or positive retroperitoneal or inguinal LN. Superficial liver metastases are Stage III. Tumor appears limited to true pelvis but with histologically proven malignant extension to small bowel or omentum.

Stage IIIA: Tumor grossly limited to true pelvis but with histologically confirmed microscopic implants of abdominal peritoneal surfaces, negative LN

Stage IIIB: Tumor involving one or both ovaries with histologically confirmed implants of abdominal peritoneal surfaces none exceeding 2 cm in diameter, negative LN

Stage IIIC: Abdominal implants > 2 cm in diameter and/or positive retroperitoneal or inguinal LN

Stage IV: Growth involving one or both ovaries with distant metastases. If pleural effusion is present, thoracentesis must be performed for cytologic analysis, which must be positive with malignant cells. Parenchymal liver metastasis is inclusive of Stage IV disease.

B. AJCC Staging

T1: Tumor is limited to one or both ovaries

T1a: Tumor is limited to one ovary. The capsule, or outer wall of the tumor, is intact, there is no tumor on the ovarian surface, and there are no cancer cells in ascites or peritoneal lavage.

T1b: Tumor is limited to both ovaries. The capsule is intact, there is no tumor on the ovarian surface, and there are no cancer cells in ascites or peritoneal lavage.

T1c: Tumor is limited to one or both ovaries with any of the following: ruptured capsule, tumor on ovarian surface, or cancer cells in the ascites or peritoneal lavage.

T2: Tumor involves one or both ovaries with spread into the pelvis

T2a: Tumor has spread and/or attaches to the uterus and/or fallopian tubes.

T2b: Tumor has spread to other pelvic tissues. There are no cancer cells in ascites or peritoneal lavage.

T2c: Tumor has spread to pelvic tissues, with cancer cells in ascites or peritoneal lavage.

T3: Tumor involves one or both ovaries, with microscopically confirmed peritoneal metastasis outside the pelvis and/or metastasis to regional (nearby) LNs.

T3a: Microscopic peritoneal metastasis beyond the pelvis

T3b: Macroscopic peritoneal metastasis beyond the pelvis, 2 cm or less in greatest dimension

T3c: Peritoneal metastasis beyond the pelvis, more than 2 cm in greatest dimension

Lymph nodes (LNs)

NX: Not able to be assessed

N0: Regional LNs contain no metastases

N1: Evidence of LNs metastasis

Metastasis (M) is defined as follows:

MX: Not able to be assessed

M0: No distant metastases are found (this excludes peritoneal metastasis)

M1: Distant metastases are present

Stage grouping

Stage IA: T1a, N0, M0

Stage IB: T1b, N0, M0

Stage IC: T1c, N0, M0

Stage IIA: T2a, N0, M0

Stage IIB: T2b, N0, M0

Stage IIC: T2c, N0, M0

Stage IIIA: T3a, N0, M0

Stage IIIB: T3b, N0, M0

Stage IIIC: T3c, N0, M0, or T (any), N1, M0

Stage IV: T (any), N (any), M1

EPITHELIAL OVARIAN CANCER

I. Characteristics

A. Risk factors for epithelial ovarian cancer include age (median age of 61 years), low or nulliparity, infertility, and genetic risk. The *BRCA 1* and *2* genes are located on chromosome 17q21 and 13q12-13, respectively. Mutations in these genes can cause autosomal dominant inherited forms of familial cancer and yield a combined 80% overall risk of ovarian cancer; 11% to 25% of patients of serous ovarian cancers harbor one of these mutations. HNPCC (hereditary non-polyposis colon cancer) yields a 10% risk of ovarian cancer and can present with other cancers such as endometrial cancer (60% risk), colon cancer (60% risk), and urothelial cancers. The use of oral contraceptive pills and pregnancy reduce the overall genetic risk (relative risk = 0.66).

II. Workup: Workup follows the general preoperative/staging workup as described above.

III. Histology

Histologic Subtypes	Percent of Epithelial Ovarian Tumors	Percent Bilaterality
Serous	46%	73%
Mucinous	36%	47%
Endometrioid	8%	33%
Clear cell	3%	13%
Transitional	2%	
Mixed	3%	
Undifferentiated	2%	
Unclassified	1%	

A. Serous is the most common type of epithelial ovarian cancer. Serous cancers are graded in a 2-tiered fashion: low grade and high grade.

B. Clear cell carcinoma: These tumors are difficult to treat; 63% are refractory to primary platinum chemotherapy. There is an increased risk of DVT: 42% vs. 18% compared to serous histologies (1). The OS is approximately 12 months for patients with advanced-stage disease.

C. Mucinous tumors are often large and the serum CEA can be positive. They have a higher rate of discordance between frozen and final pathology at 34%: 11% were downgraded and 23% were upgraded. This is due in part to their larger size. LN metastases are rare in apparent Stage I cancers and an LND can potentially be omitted in these cases without adverse effect on PFS or OS (2). Appendectomy is still recommended to ensure primary tumor site identification.

D. The ovaries are "fertile soil" for metastatic disease. Metastatic disease can be distinguished from a primary ovarian tumor by the following: Metastatic tumors to the ovaries are bilateral in 77% of cases, and often smaller in size. Primary tumors are commonly larger than 17 cm and usually unilateral (bilateral only in 13%).

IV. Staging: Follows FIGO and AJCC staging protocols.

A. Upstaging based on LN metastasis has been reviewed in 14 studies. The mean incidence of LN metastases in clinical Stages I–II EOC was 14.2% (range 6.1%–29.6%) of which 7.1% were only in the para-aortic region, 2.9% only in the pelvic region, and 4.3% in both the para-aortic and pelvic regions. Grade 1 tumors had a mean incidence of LN metastases of 4.0%, Grade 2 tumors 16.8%, and Grade 3 tumors 20.0%. According to histological subtype, the highest incidence of LN metastases was found in the serous subtype (23.3%), the lowest in the mucinous subtype (2.6%). Patterns of LN metastases were largely independent of laterality: among those with unilateral lesions and positive nodes, 50% had ipsilateral LN involvement, 40% had bilateral involvement, and 7% to 13% had isolated contralateral LN positive (3).

V. Treatment: Treatment is usually primary surgery followed by adjuvant chemotherapy for all tumors staged greater than IA Grade 1. Neoadjuvant chemotherapy followed by surgery can be considered for patients who are poor surgical candidates or who have extensive disease that appears unresectable, or potentially not optimally debulkable. Treatment should start within 25 days of surgery.

A. Different models have attempted to stratify predictive values of various findings for optimal debulking (ascites, carcinomatosis, CA-125 level) but the proposed models usually fail with validation sets. False-positive criteria range from 10% to 68% for laboratory, clinical, or radiologic criteria. If there is progressive or refractory disease on chemotherapy, a change in chemotherapy regimen should be considered. If the tumor has regressed, it may be appropriate to surgically assess the patient and attempt debulking via laparoscopy or laparotomy.

B. Cytoreductive surgery for Stage IV ovarian cancer can be attempted with 30% achieving optimal cytoreduction; 30% of patients can be expected to have complications (mostly infectious or wound). The preoperative performance status should be 2 or lower. Bristow et al. (4) demonstrated that survival depended on location of the Stage IV disease: The median survival for patients with a pleural effusion was 19 months, lung metastasis was 12 months, parenchymal liver metastasis was 18 months, and other extraperitoneal sites was 26 months. If patients had liver metastasis and had optimal intra- and extrahepatic cytoreduction to < 1 cm, the median OS was 50 months; if there was optimal extrahepatic and suboptimal hepatic resection, the median OS was 27 months; and if there was suboptimal resection at all sites, there was an OS of 8 months.

C. Removal of LNs for advanced-stage disease has been studied (5); 427 patients with Stage II-B, III-C, or IV all underwent optimal surgery, including removal of bulky LNs greater than 1 cm in diameter. Intraoperative randomization was performed and the control arm completed optimal surgery, whereas the treatment arm underwent additional retroperitoneal lymphadenectomy to remove pelvic (at least 25 nodes) and para-aortic (at least 15 nodes) LNs. After surgery, all patients received platinum-based chemotherapy. The 5-year (Y) PFI was 31.2% for the LND group compared to 21.6% for those in the control arm. The LND group was more likely to require blood transfusions, had a longer surgery, and had more postoperative complications. At 68.4 months, 202 of the 427 patients had died. There was no difference in the risk of death: 48.5% of the LND group and 47% of the control group were alive 68.4 months after surgery.

D. If ovarian cancer is diagnosed incidentally after a TAH-BSO without staging, surgical staging should be considered. The risk of undiagnosed higher-stage disease is 22% to 29% (6); 4% to 25% of unstaged clinical Stage I ovarian cancers have positive LNs, and the incidence of isolated contralateral positive LNs ranges from 7% to 13%.

E. The timing of ovarian cyst rupture makes a difference. According to one study (7), preoperative cyst rupture had a larger influence on PFS than intraoperative cyst rupture. For preoperative cyst rupture, the HR for OS was 2.65 vs. 1.64 for intraoperative cyst rupture (8).

VI. Chemotherapy for epithelial ovarian cancer:

Platinum-sensitive and platinum-resistant disease. Platinum resistance is defined as disease recurrence less than 6 months after completion of first-line platinum-based chemotherapy. If recurrence occurs at less than 6 months, non-platinum-based salvage therapies should be used; if greater than 6 months pass between completion of first-line platinum-based chemotherapy and recurrence, re-attempts with platinum-based regimens should be used. Platinum resistance is defined as disease progression occurring 6 months after primary-based treatment. Platinum refractory patients have disease progression while on chemotherapy. Response rates for second-line chemotherapy depend on the time to recurrence after primary chemotherapy. The longer the interval from primary therapy, the better the response rate: 6 to 12 months, 27%; 13 to 24 months, 33%; > 24 months, 59%.

A. First-line chemotherapy involves platinum-based chemotherapy regimens with a taxane. Single-agent platinum regimens can be considered in older or compromised patients.

B. Second-line agents are used when cancer recurs after first-line therapy has been given.

C. Neoadjuvant chemotherapy is chemotherapy given prior to surgery. Surgery is usually attempted after 2 to 3 cycles of chemotherapy. This has been shown to reduce the radical nature of surgery with a decreased risk of colostomy and hemorrhage.

D. Consolidation: Chemotherapy that is used after primary or adjuvant chemotherapy to decrease the chance of cancer recurrence in patients with CCR. This is usually a short duration of treatment.

E. Maintenance: Chemotherapy that is used after primary or adjuvant chemotherapy to decrease the chance of cancer recurrence in patients with CCR. This is usually of a longer duration than consolidation therapy.

F. Intraperitoneal (IP) chemotherapy: Chemotherapy is administered directly into the abdominal cavity. IP chemotherapy using platinum and taxane regimens is indicated for optimally debulked patients Stage II or higher.

G. HIPEC (hyperthermic intraperitoneal chemotherapy): Heated cytotoxic regimens are administered at the time of primary or recurrent debulking surgery and circulated intraperitoneally for a specific amount of time.

VII. Treatment by Stage

A. Stage IA Grade 1 tumors: Surgery is definitive. If fertility is a concern, consider leaving the uterus and contralateral ovary.

   B. Stage IA, Grade 2 or 3 and Stage IB and IC, any grade: Primary treatment is surgery. If fertility is a concern, consider leaving the uterus and contralateral ovary. Adjuvant chemotherapy is platinum based with a taxane for 3 to 6 cycles.

   C. Stages II, III, IV: Primary treatment is surgery. Adjuvant chemotherapy is platinum based with a taxane for 6 cycles. This can be administered IV or IP. Consideration can be given to neoadjuvant chemotherapy for advanced-stage or medically compromised patients.

VIII. Second-look laparotomy is the pathological surgical assessment for residual disease after primary adjuvant chemotherapy in a patient with a clinical complete response. It is used to guide decisions for either continuing chemotherapy, changing chemotherapy, or discontinuing chemotherapy. It can also be used to guide treatment in patients who were suboptimally debulked, or who were primarily unstaged. Routine second-look laparotomy is not the current standard of care; 40% of second-look patients are pathologically positive, and of those who are negative, 50% will recur (9).

Second-Look Laparotomy Disease Status	5-Year Survival
No evidence of disease	50%
Microscopic	35%
Macroscopic	5%

IX. Recurrence: Most recurrences occur within the first 2 years. The risk of recurrence for a Grade 1, Stage I ovarian cancer is < 10%. The risk of recurrence for Stage 3 ovarian cancer is much higher, over 50%.

X. Secondary cytoreduction is the removal of gross recurrent disease after primary or secondary chemotherapy. There are some criteria attributed to Chi (10), which help stratify patients as appropriate surgical candidates. These are based on time, location, and number of recurrent tumor sites. If the recurrence occurs at greater than 30 months from primary chemotherapy, secondary cytoreduction can be attempted regardless of number of involved sites. If the interval is less than 30 months, and there are 1 to 2 sites of recurrence, cytoreduction can again be attempted. If there is carcinomatosis, ascites, or the patient is platinum refractory, it is often not wise to attempt secondary cytoreduction. For those who had less than 0.5 cm of residual disease after secondary cytoreduction, an improvement in OS to 56 months was seen vs. 27 months for those who were suboptimally debulked. The overall success at secondary optimal cytoreduction ranges between 24% and 84%.

XI. Cerebellar degeneration can occur from antibodies to ovarian cancer. This is called **paraneoplastic cerebellar degeneration.** The incidence is 2:1000 patients with gynecologic cancers. There are two main antibodies: the anti-Yo antibody reacts against the Purkinje cells and the anti-Hu antibody reacts against all neurons.

XII. Survival

    A. Relative Survival

2 Y	5 Y	10 Y (11)
65%	44%	36%

    B. 5-Year Survival by Stage

Stage	All Grades	Grade 1	Grade 2	Grade 3
Ia	85%	92.5%	86%	63%
Ib	69%	85%	90%	79%
Ic	59%	78%	49%	51%
IIa	62%	64%	65%	39%
IIb	51%	79%	43%	42%
IIc	43%	68%	46%	20%
IIIa	31%	58%	38%	20%
IIIb	38%	73%	42%	21%
IIIc	18%	46%	22%	14%
IV	8%	14%	8%	6%

    C. 5-Year Survival by Residual Disease

Residual Disease	5 YS
Microscopic	40% to 75%
Optimal	30% to 40%
Suboptimal	5%

XIII. Survival Care

    A. Follow-up:

        Every 3 months for 2 years

        Every 6 months up to 5 years

        Annually for subsequent visits

    B. At each visit:

        Physical and pelvic examination

        Symptom review

        Consider CA-125*

C. *Discussion should be held with the patient regarding following of tumor markers. Rustin demonstrated no improvement in survival when tumor markers were followed. Patients had a poorer quality of life with additional unsuccessful cycles of chemotherapy given based on laboratory data. Assessment of symptoms, along with physical examination, can guide the clinician regarding when to order lab tests, imaging, and when to initiate second-line chemotherapy (12).

D. CT imaging: CT cannot often detect subcentimeter disease.

XIV. Epithelial Ovarian Cancer Trials

A. Primary Adjuvant Chemotherapy Trials

1. ICON 1 (13): This trial evaluated 477 patients who had early ovarian cancer "staged" with hysterectomy, bilateral salpingo-oophorectomy, and recommended omentectomy. Eligibility was if the treating physician was uncertain as to if the patient required chemotherapy. 93% of patients were "Stage I." Patients were randomized between NFT and single-agent carboplatin (AUC 5), CAP, or another platinum regimen. Histology was: 32% serous, 15% clear cell, 23% mucinous. Most patients were apparent Stage I; however, there were 7% of patients with Stage II or III disease; 70% were Grade 2 or 3. At 51 months, the OS was 79% in the chemotherapy arm vs. 70% in the NFT arm. The 5 Y PFS was 73% in the chemotherapy group vs. 62% in the NFT group. For clinical Stage I disease that did not get staged, there was a 38% recurrence rate without further treatment and a 30% death rate. Chemotherapy had a HR of 0.66 for survival.

2. ACTION (14): This trial ran concurrently with ICON 1 but 30% of 448 patients were comprehensively staged. Patients were randomized to observation or to chemotherapy. Chemotherapy consisted of 4 to 6 cycles of single-agent platinum or a platinum-containing regimen. 40% of patients were Stage IA or IB and 60% had Grade 1 or Grade 2 disease. The 5 YS in the observation and adjuvant chemotherapy arms were 75% and 85%. Patients who received chemotherapy had a better RFS (HR 0.63). In nonoptimally staged patients, the adjuvant chemotherapy group had an improved OS and RFS (HR 1.75, HR 1.78). Among patients in the observation arm, optimal staging provided an improvement in OS and RFS (HR 2.31, HR 1.82). There was no benefit seen from adjuvant chemotherapy in the optimally staged patients. This suggests that in the suboptimally

staged group, there were undiagnosed higher-staged patients who benefited when given chemotherapy. A 10-year follow-up found support for most of the original conclusions, except that overall survival after optimal surgical staging was improved, now among patients who received adjuvant chemotherapy (HR of death 1.89). (15)

3. ICON 2 (16): This trial evaluated 1526 eligible surgically staged patients who needed primary adjuvant chemotherapy. Patients were staged I–IV and were randomized to single-agent platinum-based chemotherapy or CAP. This trial was stopped early due to the availability of taxanes. These patients were then grouped into the control arm of ICON 3 as their outcomes were statistically nonsignificant with an OS HR of 1.0. The median survival in both groups was 33 months and the 2 YS was 60% for both arms. CAP was more toxic.

4. ICON 3 (17): This trial evaluated 274 eligible surgically staged patients Stages I–IV, 20% of whom were Stages I and II. Patients were randomized between a paclitaxel/carboplatin doublet vs. the ICON 2 group of single-agent carboplatin or CAP. The OS was 36 months for carboplatin/paclitaxel and 35 months for the control groups of single-agent carboplatin and CAP. The PFS were 17 months vs. 16 months for the control arm. There were a lot of confounding factors in this study: A large number of patients were deemed to have recurrent disease based on elevated CA-125 levels prior to showing clinical recurrence. In addition, 30% of those who did not get paclitaxel as primary treatment received paclitaxel as second-line treatment.

5. ICON 4 (17): This trial evaluated 802 eligible patients with recurrent platinum-sensitive ovarian cancer 75% recurred more than 12 months following initial therapy. Patients were randomized to paclitaxel 175–185 mg/m^2 and cisplatin 50 mg/m^2 or carboplatinum AUC 5 vs. single-agent cisplatin 75 mg/m^2 or carboplatin AUC 5. The doublet therapy showed a statistically significant improvement over the single-agent group with a median PFS of 13 months vs. 10 months (HR 0.76, $P = .0004$). The doublet therapy showed an improvement in median survival by 5 months (29 months vs. 24 months; HR of 0.82, $P = 0.02$). This translated to a 2 YS of 57% vs. 50% and a 1 Y PFS of 50% vs. 40%. Criticisms of this trial were that 75% of patients were in a good prognosis group. This is essentially a trial of platinum-sensitive disease.

6. ICON 5/GOG 182 EORTC 55012 (18): This trial evaluated 4,312 surgically staged Stage III and IV patients for primary adjuvant therapy. The control arm was the doublet of carboplatin AUC 6 and paclitaxel 175 mg/m² administered for 8 cycles. The experimental arms consisted of carboplatin/paclitaxel/gemcitabine as sequential doublets or in triplicate, for a total of 8 cycles, or carboplatin/paclitaxel/topotecan as sequential doublets for a total of 8 cycles, and carboplatin/paclitaxel/liposomal doxorubicin as a triplicate regimen for 8 cycles. There was no difference in median PFS or OS with the PFS in the control arm being 16 months and the OS being 44 months, both in the optimally and suboptimally debulked patients. The median PFS for patients with suboptimal, gross optimal (< 1 cm residual), and microscopic residual disease were 13, 16, and 29 months respectively, and the median OS rates were 33, 40, and 68 months.

7. ICON 7 (19): This trial evaluated 1,528 eligible patients staged I to IV patients, of whom 26% were suboptimally debulked. The control arm was carboplatin AUC 5 or 6 and paclitaxel 175 mg/m² IV every 3 weeks for 6 cycles. The experimental arms consisted of carboplatin and paclitaxel with bevacizumab at 7.5 mg/kg IV every 3 weeks for 6 cycles, with bevacizumab continued for an additional 12 cycles or until progression of disease. The PFS was 20.3 months vs. 21.8 months with maintenance bevacizumab (HR = 0.81). The maximum effect was seen at 12 months corresponding with the end of bevacizumab treatment. At 42 months, the PFS was 22.4 months vs. 24.1 months with maintenance bevacizumab (P = .04). A high-risk, early-stage subgroup was identified (FIGO Stage I or IIA clear cell or Grade 3 tumors), as well as a high-risk subgroup for progression that included Stage IV or suboptimally debulked patients: These patients obtained a PFS benefit from bevacizumab of about 4 months (18.1 months vs. 14.5 months) and a respective median OS of 36.6 months vs. 28.8 months compared to standard therapy. Hypertension attributed to bevacizumab was seen in 18% of patients who received bevacizumab vs. 2% of patients in the control arm. Bowel perforation was seen in 10 patients in the bevacizumab group vs. 3 patients in the control arm. OS data is mature in 2014.

8. GOG 1 (20): 86 evaluable surgical Stage 1 patients were randomized to observation, pelvic radiation, or melphalan chemotherapy. Recurrence was 17% in the observation group, 30% in those radiated, and 6% in those who received

chemotherapy. Recurrence was related to grade: Grade 1, 11%; Grade 2, 22%; Grade 3, 27%.

9. GOG 111 (21). This trial evaluated 386 eligible suboptimally debulked stage III and IV patients. Patients with greater than 1 cm residual disease were randomly assigned to receive cisplatin 75 mg/m^2 and cyclophosphamide 750 mg/m^2 or cisplatin 75 mg/m^2 and 24-hour paclitaxel 135 mg/m^2. Overall response rates in the first arm was 73% compared to 60%. PFS was longer in the paclitaxel-containing arm at 17.9 months vs. 12.9 months. OS was longer in the paclitaxel arm at 37.5 months compared to 24.4 months.

10. OV-10 (22): This trial evaluated cyclophosphamide and cisplatin vs. 3-hour paclitaxel and cisplatin in 680 eligible patients with stage IIB, IIC, III, or IV disease, who were optimally and suboptimally debulked. The ORR was 58.6% in the cisplatin and paclitaxel arm vs. 44.7% in the cyclophosphamide and cisplatin arm. The PFS was 15.5 months vs. 11.5 months favoring the paclitaxel arm and the OS was 35.6 months vs. 25.8 months, again, all favoring paclitaxel.

11. GOG 132 (23): This trial evaluated 648 suboptimal Stage III and any Stage IV patients. There were 3 arms: a doublet of cisplatin and paclitaxel dosed at 75 mg/kg and 135 mg/kg; single-agent paclitaxel dosed at 200 mg/kg; single-agent cisplatin dosed at 100 mg/kg. The PFS, respectively, was 14 months, 11 months, and 16 months. The, OS respectively, was 26 months, 26 months, and 30 months. The response rate was, respectively, 67%, 67%, and 47%.

12. GOG 157 (24): This trial evaluated 3 vs. 6 cycles of paclitaxel and carboplatin in 427 eligible patients staged IAG3, IBG3, IC, and II. The primary endpoint was recurrence rate. 457 patients were registered, 213 in each arm. 70% were Stage I, 30% were Stage II, and there were 30% clear cell cancers in each arm. The recurrence rate was 27.4% for 3 cycles vs. 19% for 6 cycles (CI 0.53 to 1.13). The probability of surviving 5 years was 81% for 3 cycles vs. 83% for 6 cycles (CI 0.66 to 1.57). The HR for recurrence was 0.74, $P = .18$ (NS). Criticisms of the study were: insufficient power to detect a difference; and only 29% (126) of patients were staged appropriately. Chan updated the data in 2006 and found a benefit to 6 cycles of chemotherapy specifically for serous tumors with a 5 YS of 83% vs. 60% (HR=0.33, $P = .04$).

13. GOG 158 (25): This trial compared 792 optimally cytoreduced Stage III ovarian cancer patients to 24-hour paclitaxel and cisplatin vs. 3-hour paclitaxel and carboplatin. This was designed as a noninferiority study and there was provision for second-look laparotomy, which about 50% chose to do (Greer, subset analysis proved that second-look laparotomy was not beneficial). 85% were able to receive all 6 cycles. The PFS was 19 months for paclitaxel and cisplatin and 20 months for paclitaxel and carboplatin. The OS was 48 months for paclitaxel cisplatin and 57 months for paclitaxel carboplatin. The RR of recurrence was 0.88 (95% CI, 0.75 to 1.03), and the RR for the OS was 0.84 (95% CI, 0.7 to 1.02) favoring carboplatin and paclitaxel. The carboplatin arm had less myelotoxicity and electrolyte problems, with similar neurotoxicity.

14. GOG 218 (26): This randomized trial evaluated 1,873 staged III or IV suboptimally debulked patients with a control arm of carboplatin and paclitaxel. The investigational arms consisted of carboplatin and paclitaxel with either bevacizumab for 5 months during primary therapy or an extended dosing of bevacizumab after 6 initial cycles of carboplatin, paclitaxel and bevacizumab for a total of 18 cycles. The PFS was, respectively, 10.3, 11.2, and 14.1 months. The OS, respectively, was 39.9, 38.7, and 39.7 months. Maximum separation of the PFS occurred at 15 months and the curves merged 9 months later.

15. SCOTROC 1 (27): This trial evaluated 1,077 patients with stage IC to IV disease and randomized them to docetaxel 75 mg/m^2 vs. paclitaxel at 175 mg/m^2 each with carboplatin at an AUC of 5 for 6 cycles. The PFS was 15 months vs. 14.8 months. Docetaxel was found to not be inferior. The OS was 64.2% vs. 68.9% respectively.

B. Dose Density Trials

1. GOG 97 (28): This study investigated 4 cycles vs. 8 cycles of cyclophosphamide and cisplatin in 458 eligible patients. The 4-cycle regimen dosed the chemotherapy doublets at 1,000/100 mg/m^2 whereas the 8-cycle doublet dosed the chemotherapy at 500/50 mg/m^2 given every 3 weeks. This provided no difference in OS, and the total dosing was the same.

2. Fruscio weekly cisplatin (29): This trial evaluated 285 eligible patients and randomized them to weekly cisplatin at 50 mg/m^2 for 9 weeks vs. cisplatin at 75 mg/m^2 for 6 cycles every

3 weeks. At 16.8 years follow-up, no difference in PFS was seen (17.2 months vs. 18.1 months, HR = 1.08) and no difference in OS was seen (35 months vs. 32 months, HR = 0.97) for the dose dense weekly cisplatin vs. standard treatment.

3. The Scottish Dose Dense Trial (30): This trial evaluated 6 cycles of cyclophosphamide at 750 mg/m^2 and cisplatin at doses of either 50 mg/m^2 or 100 mg/m^2. The overall survival for the 100 mg/m^2 and 50 mg/m^2 patients was 32.4% and 26.6%, and the overall relative death rate was 0.68 ($P = .043$). From this trial the standard 75 mg/m^2 dose was chosen for its modest toxicity.

4. The Dutch/Danish Study (31): This trial randomized 222 patients between different doublet doses of carboplatin and cyclophosphamide. Carboplatin was dosed at an AUC of either 4 or 8 for six cycles in combination with cyclophosphamide at a constant dose of 500 mg/m^2. There was no difference in OS (2 YS 45%) or complete pathologic response (32 and 30%).

5. Gore et al. (32) randomized 227 patients to single-agent carboplatin at either an AUC of 6 for 6 courses or an AUC of 12 for 4 courses every 4 weeks. There was no difference in PFS or OS at 5 years at 31% and 34%, respectively. There was more toxicity in the AUC 12 arm.

6. GOG 134 (33): This trial included 271 eligible patients with persistent, recurrent or progressive disease who were evaluated with paclitaxel dosed at 135 mg/m^2/24 hr, paclitaxel at 175 mg/m^2/24 hr, or paclitaxel at 250 mg/m^2/24 hr. The 135 mg/m^2 arm was closed early. The partial and complete response to paclitaxel at 250 mg/m^2 (36%) was higher than those on 175 mg/m^2 (27%, $P = .027$). The median duration for OS was 13.1 months and 12.3 months for paclitaxel 175 mg/m^2 and 250 mg/m^2, respectively. Thus, paclitaxel exhibited a dose effect with regard to response rate, but there was no survival benefit.

7. European-Canadian randomized trial of paclitaxel in relapsed ovarian cancer (34): This trial evaluated infusion length of paclitaxel in recurrent ovarian cancer in 391 eligible patients. This was a 2 × 2 study design of 3-hour vs. 24-hour infusion and 135 mg/m^2 vs. 175 mg/m^2. The high-dose group had a longer PFS at 19 vs. 14 weeks ($P = .02$). The 175 mg/m^2 dose was found to have a better response rate at 19% vs. the 135 mg/m^2 dose with a response rate of 16% (NS). There was no difference in survival.

8. JGOG 3016 (35): This trial evaluated 631 Stage II, III, and IV patients. Carboplatin was dosed at an AUC of 6 and given every 3 weeks with either: weekly paclitaxel at 80 mg/m^2 or standard 3-week dosing at 180 mg/m^2. The median PFS was 28 months vs. 17.2 months. The HR for progression was 0.71, (CI 95%, 0.58 to 0.88) (P = .0015). The median OS was not yet reached. The 3-year overall survival was 72% versus 65% (P = .03), respectively. The 5 year OS data is 58.6% vs. 51.0%, respectively, with a hazard ratio of 0.79.

9. GOG 26FF (36): This phase II study evaluated single-agent paclitaxel at 170 mg/m^2 IV over 24hr q 3 weeks, in 43 refractory or platinum-resistant patients. The overall response rate was 37%. The median PFI was 4.2 months, the median survival was 16 months. PFS was 4 months.

C. **Intraperitoneal Trials**

1. GOG 104 (37): This trial evaluated 546 patients for primary adjuvant chemotherapy after "optimal" debulking to a size of less than 2 cm. IV cyclophosphamide was given for 6 cycles every 3 weeks with either intraperitoneal cisplatin or intravenous cisplatin (both dosed at 100 mg/m^2). The median OS was significant favoring the IP arm at 49 months vs. the IV group at 41 months. The HR for death was lower in the intraperitoneal group, 0.76; 95% CI, 0.61 to 0.96; P = .02.

2. GOG 114 (38): This trial evaluated 462 Stage III patients who were optimally debulked to less than 1 cm. Patients were randomized to IV cisplatin and cyclophosphamide every 3 weeks for 6 cycles vs. IV carboplatin at an AUC 9 for 2 cycles followed by IP cisplatin at 100 mg/m^2 with IV paclitaxel every 3 weeks for 6 cycles. Second-look laparotomy was optional. The PFS was 27.6 months vs. 22.5 months with P = .01, the OS was 63.2 months vs. 52.5 months with a P = 0.05, all favoring IP therapy.

3. GOG 172 (39): This trial evaluated 415 Stage III patients who were optimally debulked to less than 1 cm residual. Patients were randomized to either IV paclitaxel at 135 mg/m^2 over 24 hours, with cisplatin dosed at 75 mg/m^2 or to IP cisplatin on day 1 dosed at 100 mg/m^2 with IV paclitaxel at 135 mg/m^2 over 24 hours on day 2, and paclitaxel again on day 8 dosed

at 60 mg/m^2 IP. 64% had gross residual disease after primary surgery and 50% of patients chose a second-look surgery. 41% of the IV group vs. 57% of the IP group had a pathologic complete response at SLL. Only 42% of the IP group completed all IP cycles whereas 83% of the IV group received all 6 cycles. The PFS was 18 months for the IV arm vs. 24 months for the IP arm (P = .05). The OS was 50 months for the IV arm vs. 66 months for the IP arm with a 16-month survival advantage favoring IP therapy (P = .03). A 5.5 month PFS was seen. Patients with no visible residual disease did well with a 78-month median survival for those on the IV arm and the median survival has not been reached for the IP arm.

4. IP catheter outcomes GOG 172 (40): Of the 58% of patients not completing 6 IP cycles, one-third were catheter-related (catheter infection in 20 of 41 cases, blocked catheter in 10 of 41 cases). One-third were related to IP treatment (pain, bowel complications, patient refusal, other noncatheter infection). One-third of discontinuations were probably unrelated to the catheter (nausea, renal, metabolic). Left colon resection or colostomy related to a decreased ability to tolerate IP chemotherapy. Appendectomy, small bowel resection, or right colon surgery did not appear to affect IP tolerance. Optimal placement is use of a 9.6 F catheter through a separate incision (not the laparotomy incision), and tunneled at least 10 cm, with 10 cm length left in the peritoneal cavity. A waiting time of 24 hours post insertion before use was recommended to avoid leakage.

D. Maintenance/Consolidation Trials

1. GOG 178 (41): This trial evaluated consolidation therapy in 222 eligible Stage III and IV patients and randomized patients to 12 vs. 3 cycles of paclitaxel at 175 mg/m^2 months after completion of 6 cycles of platinum/paclitaxel with a clinical complete response. At 50% enrollment, the protocol dictated interim analysis. This showed an improvement in PFS favoring the 12 cycles with a HR of 2.31. The study was closed at this point. The PFS was 28 months vs. 21 months favoring 12 cycles (P = .002). Patients were allowed to crossover so all those on the 3-cycle arm could complete up to 12 cycles of therapy.

2. Follow-up study to GOG 178 (42): Criticisms cited from this study were the crossover may have masked a difference between study arms, there was insufficient power within the study, and treatment at relapse equalized outcomes. The PFS was 22 vs. 14 months favoring the 12-month paclitaxel. OS was 53 vs. 48 months (P = .34 NS).

3. A retrospective institutional evaluation (43) reviewed 59 eligible patients with a median follow-up of 51 months. The median time from CR to start of second-line chemotherapy was 21 months; the median time to the start of third-line agents was 43 months. Twelve months elapsed between completion of first-line therapy and recurrence in 50% of patients. Thus, a similar time frame of 40 months between clinical complete response and the start of third-line therapies exists, which is comparable to results in GOG 178.

4. GOG 175 (44): This trial evaluated 542 eligible patients who were staged IA or IB Grade 3 or clear cell, all Stage IC and all Stage II ovarian cancer. They were all given IV carboplatin AUC 6 and paclitaxel 175 mg/m^2 for 3 cycles followed by randomization to either observation or weekly paclitaxel for 24 weeks. The 5 Y recurrence probability rate was 23% for those observed, and 20% for those who received maintenance paclitaxel, HR = 0.8. The 5 YS was 85.4% vs. 86.2% (NS).

E. **Recurrent Disease Trials**

1. EORTC 55005: Gemcitabine-carboplatin vs. carboplatin (45): This trial evaluated platinum-sensitive relapsed ovarian cancer in 356 eligible patients. Single-agent carboplatin AUC 5 vs. carboplatin AUC 4 with gemcitabine dosed at 1000 mg/m^2 given days 1 and 8, every 21 days. The PFS was improved with the addition of gemcitabine (8.6 months vs. 5.8 months). The study was not powered to detect a difference in OS. The overall response rate was 47% with the addition of gemcitabine vs. 30% with single-agent carboplatin. 60% of patients recurred at greater than 12 months and 40% recurred between 6 months and 12 months.

2. A randomized phase III study of pegylated liposomal doxorubicin vs. topotecan in recurrent epithelial ovarian cancer (46): This trial evaluated 474 patients with recurrent disease and response to single-agent therapy. Liposomal doxorubicin was dosed at 50 mg/m^2 every 4 weeks, and topotecan was dosed at 1.5 mg/m^2/day for 5 days every 3 weeks. The median

survival for patients was 63 weeks for pegylated liposomal doxorubicin vs. 60 weeks for topotecan. For those patients who had platinum-sensitive disease there was a significant difference in time until progression: 108 weeks vs. 70 weeks, favoring pegylated liposomal doxorubicin, P = .017, HR = 1.432.

3. OCEANS (47): This trial evaluated 484 eligible patients receiving carboplatin AUC 4 and gemcitabine 1000 mg/m² D1 and 8 with or without the addition of bevacizumab at 15 mg/kg IV every 3 weeks in recurrent platinum-sensitive disease. Six cycles to 10 cycles were given showing an ORR of 78.5% vs. 57.4%, favoring the bevacizumab arm. The PFS demonstrated a HR of 0.48, favoring the bevacizumab arm, with months until progression of 12.4 vs. 8.4. The median OS was 35.2 months vs. 33.3 months (HR 1.027; 95% CI 0.792 to 1.331) favoring the bevacizumab arm. OS results were possibly confounded by extensive use of subsequent anticancer therapies.

4. CALYPSO EORTC 55051 (48): 976 patients with recurrent late relapsing platinum-sensitive ovarian cancer were treated with the doublets of carboplatin AUC 5 and liposomal doxorubicin dosed at 30 mg/m² every 4 weeks (CD) vs. the standard of carboplatin AUC 5 and paclitaxel 175 mg/m² for at least 6 cycles every 3 weeks (CP). 40% of patients had received two prior regimens before entering the study. A maximum of nine cycles were administered. The overall response rate was 63%, including 38% of patients who achieved a complete response. Patients in the CD arm had a better PFS of 11.3 months compared to the CP arm with 9.4 months (HR 0.82). Median survival times were 30.7 months and 33 months for the CD arm vs. the CP arm (NS). CD led to delayed progression but similar OS compared to CP in platinum-sensitive ovarian cancer.

5. DESKTOP I (Descriptive Evaluation of Preoperative Selection Criteria for Operability) (49): 267 platinum-sensitive recurrent ovarian cancer patients were retrospectively reviewed for predictability of secondary cytoreduction. Complete resection was associated with longer survival compared to any residual postoperative disease (45.2 vs. 19.7 months). Variables associated with complete resection were performance status, early-stage FIGO disease (I/II), residual disease left after primary surgery (none vs. any), absence of ascites, and less than 500 mL of ascites. A combination of PS, early FIGO stage, no residual

disease, and absent ascites predicted complete resection in 79% of patients.

6. DESKTOP II (50): This was a multicenter trial which evaluated 516 recurrent platinum-sensitive ovarian cancer patients. Patients were screened with the DESKTOP I prediction factors for operability for recurrent disease. 51% scored positive. The rate of complete resection was 76%, confirming score validity. 11% had second operations for complications.

F. Interval Debulking Trials

1. EORTC 44865 (51): This trial randomized 319 patients stage III and IV after suboptimal surgery to chemotherapy with cyclophosphamide and cisplatin for 6 cycles or to chemotherapy with cyclophosphamide and cisplatin for 3 cycles with interval debulking followed by 3 more cycles. The interval debulking group had a significantly better median PFS of 18 months vs. 13 months. The median OS was 26 months vs. 20 months, favoring the interval debulking group. The risk of death decreased by 33%, $P = .008$.

2. GOG 152 (52): This trial randomized 424 eligible patients stage III and IV after suboptimal surgery to chemotherapy with cisplatin and paclitaxel for 6 cycles or to chemotherapy for 3 cycles with interval debulking, followed by 3 more cycles of chemotherapy. The median PFS was 10.5 months vs. 10.7 months, the OS was 34 months in both groups. The RR for death = 0.99.

3. There were differences between the two interval debulking studies. Namely, there were more effective second-line therapies for the EORTC study, the chemotherapy regimens were different, residual disease was 5 cm or less for fewer than two-thirds of patients in GOG 152 vs. one-third of patients in the EORTC study, and generalists did a majority of the primary surgery in the EORTC study. Furthermore, residual disease after 3 cycles of chemotherapy was greater than 1 cm in 65% of patients in the EORTC study, thus there was an increased chance of good cytoreduction, vs. 45% who were converted to optimal debulking in the GOG study.

G. Neoadjuvant Therapy Trials

1. EORTC 55971 (53): This trial evaluated 632 eligible patients who were staged IIIC or IV. They were randomized to upfront debulking surgery vs. 3 cycles of neoadjuvant platinum-based

chemotherapy followed by interval surgery and subsequent chemotherapy. Inclusion criteria were biopsy-proven ovarian cancer, in combination with a pelvic mass, the presence of metastases of $\geq$ 2 cm outside the pelvis, and a CA-125/CEA ratio $\geq$ 25. The median follow-up was 4.8 years. Baseline characteristics for arms A and B were, respectively: median largest metastasis, 80/80 mm; FIGO Stage IIIc, 76%/76%. The largest residual tumor was $\leq$ 1 cm in 48% after PDS (arm A) and 83% after IDS (arm B). Complications of PDS and IDS were, respectively: postoperative mortality 2.7%/0.6%; sepsis 8%/2%; grade 3/4 hemorrhage 7%/4%. The PFS was 11 months in both arms (HR 0.99; CI 0.87 to 1.13). An OS of 29 and 30 months was seen for arms A and B (HR 0.98; CI: 0.85 to 1.14). Some critics suggest that the above OS is still less than the 36 months seen in the carboplatin/paclitaxel arm of GOG 111 evaluating suboptimally debulked ovarian cancer.

2. A meta-analysis (54) suggests that for each extra cycle of neoadjuvant chemotherapy, there is a 4.1-month decrease in survival. Within this meta-analysis, each 10% increase in cytoreduction yielded a 5.5% median increase in survival time, which equates to 3 months.

3. The impact of disease distribution in Stage III ovarian cancer patients was evaluated (55): 417 patients from 3 randomized GOG trials who were microscopically cytoreduced and given adjuvant IV platinum/paclitaxel were reviewed. Patients were divided into three groups based on preoperative disease burden: minimal disease (MD) was defined by pelvic tumor and retroperitoneal metastasis; abdominal peritoneal disease (APD) was considered disease limited to the pelvis, retroperitoneum, lower abdomen, and omentum; and upper abdominal disease (UAD) with disease affecting the diaphragm, spleen, liver, or pancreas. The median OS was: not reached in MD patients, 80 months in the APD, and 56 months in the UAD groups ($P < .05$). The 5 YS were: for MD, 67%; APD, 63%; and UAD, 45%. In multivariate analysis, the UAD group had a significantly worse prognosis than MD and APD both individually and combined (PFS HR 1.44; $P = .008$ and OS HR 1.77; $P = .0004$). Thus, it is suggested that there is a biological difference in ovarian cancer patients proportional to the amount of disease at presentation.

OVARIAN TUMORS OF LOW MALIGNANT POTENTIAL (LMP)

I. Characteristics

A. LMP tumors represent 5% to 15% of ovarian malignancies. The median age at diagnosis is 39 to 45 years old. 20% of these tumors are diagnosed at Stage III or IV. There are no known risk factors.

B. Clinical features include a mass, abdominal pain, bloating, abdominal distension, early satiety, dyspepsia, and an elevated CA-125.

C. The route of spread is often transcoelomic, and can be lymphatic.

D. Prognostic factors are stage, residual tumor, the presence of invasive implants, and micropapillary histology.

II. Histology

A. Pathologically, there is the absence of stromal invasion and the tumors have at least 2 of the following: nuclear atypia, mitotic activity, pseudostratification, and epithelial budding. There are two main histologic types: serous and mucinous. If foci are found of stromal invasion measuring 3 to 5 mm or 10 mm^2, the tumor is considered microinvasive. Outcomes for microinvasive tumors are usually favorable and parallel LMP tumors. If a mucinous borderline tumor is found to have 3 or more layers of epithelial cell stratification, it is considered a carcinoma.

B. Frozen section diagnosis of borderline tumors can be difficult. In one study of patients with a final diagnosis of LMP tumor, 10% were diagnosed as having invasive cancer and 25% were reported to have benign cystadenomas on intraoperative frozen section. Therefore, the sensitivity of the frozen section analysis for low malignant potential tumors was 65% (95% CI 55%, 75%) (56). Size greater than 8 cm, micropapillary, endometrioid, or clear cell carcinoma histologies can contribute to this difficulty.

C. The micropapillary subtype is a distinct entity and carries an adverse prognosis. *BRAF* mutations are commonly found in this subtype. The distinguishing architecture is a height-to-width ratio of 5:1. It is often associated with invasive implants. Micropapillary histology has a higher rate of recurrence at 26%.

D. Serous LMP tumors represent 62% of all LMP tumors; 30% are diagnosed as Stage I, and they are often bilateral. 10% to 20% have invasive implants.

E. Mucinous LMP tumors represent about 38% of LMP tumors and 80% to 90% are found as Stage I; 5% are bilateral. There is a greater malignant potential with these tumors than with the serous LMP tumors.

F. Invasive implants are a major factor in determining whether to treat with adjuvant therapies or not. The 7 Y OS for patients with noninvasive implants is 96%, and for those with invasive implants, 66%. The risk of invasive implants accompanies histology: for serous borderline tumors the risk is 6%, but increases to 49% with micropapillary tumors.

III. Workup: Workup is the same as for epithelial ovarian cancer.

IV. Staging: Staging is the same as for epithelial ovarian cancer. Contralateral ovarian and uterine conservation may be considered in patients considering future fertility.

V. Treatment

A. Treatment is primarily surgical and follows the same directives as those for malignant ovarian cancer: complete surgical staging with full cytoreduction to microscopic disease status.

B. Fertility sparing treatment is a reasonable option if desired. A cystectomy or USO can be performed with additional staging LN dissection, biopsies, and omentectomy. The recurrence rate overall is 12%. If a cystectomy is performed, the recurrence rate is 23%, compared to 8% with a USO. The median time to recurrence is 2.6 years after a cystectomy and 4.7 years after a USO.

C. If surgical staging is complete, there is data to suggest that repeat staging is not beneficial in this patient population, given that no micropapillary histology is present. One series (56) compared early-stage LMP tumors in 31 staged patients to 42 unstaged patients. The OS was similar in both groups. LN positivity made no difference in OS. Oftentimes endosalpingosis is seen in the LN.

D. Adjuvant chemotherapy should be considered if there are invasive implants. Treatment usually includes adjuvant chemotherapy that is platinum based. There is an average 25% response rate for LMP tumors to chemotherapy. At second look, the response to chemotherapy was 15% if noninvasive implants were present, vs. 57% if invasive implants were present, thus borderline tumors are not completely chemoresistant (57).

VI. Recurrence

A. Recurrence in a spared contralateral ovary can occur in 16% of patients, but is easily treated by resection of the ovary. There were no deaths in those managed conservatively.

B. Recurrent disease is often indolent. Recommended treatment is repeat cytoreduction. Overall, 5% to 10% recur. There is data to suggest that 73% recur as low-grade invasive cancers (58).

VII. Survival

A. The 10 YS by stage is:

Stage I: 99%

Stage II: 98%

Stage III: 96%

Stage IV: 77%

VIII. Survival Care: Follows the same pattern as that of epithelial ovarian cancer.

FALLOPIAN TUBE CANCER

I. Characteristics

A. The origin of ovarian cancer may be changing with recent developments. It may be that ovarian cancer is actually a metastatic primary fallopian tube cancer (PFTC). The incidence of PFTC is 0.41/100,000 women (59). Bilateral involvement is found in 5% to 30% of patients, and one-third of patients have LN metastasis at the time of staging. Route of spread is transcoelomic, lymphatic, and hematogenous.

B. Hu's criteria were established to assist in the definitive diagnosis of PFTC (60). This was further modified by Sedlis in 1978 (61) and the criteria is as follows: the main tumor is in the tube and arises from the endosalpinx; the pattern histologically reproduces the epithelium of fallopian tube mucosa and shows a papillary pattern; the transition between benign and malignant tubal epithelium should be demonstrable; and the ovaries and endometrium are normal or contain less tumor than the tube.

C. There is often a triad of symptoms: pelvic pain, a pelvic mass, and watery vaginal discharge (hydrops tubae profluens). This occurs in 11% of patients. A pelvic mass is diagnosed in 12% to 66% of patients.

II. **Workup:** Workup includes a history and physical examination with lab tests. Tumor markers including a CA-125 are drawn. An abnormal Pap smear has been found to be positive in 18% to 60% of patients. Imaging with ultrasound, CT, or MRI can be helpful.

III. **Histology:** 90% of tumors are serous, but other subtypes are found including endometrioid, transitional, and MMMT.

IV. **Staging:** Staging follows the same criteria as that for ovarian cancer.

V. **Treatment**

    A. Primary treatment is usually surgical.

    B. Surgery includes full staging with a TAH-BSO, LN dissection (if less than Stage IIIC), omentectomy, peritoneal biopsies, and debulking to microscopic residual disease.

    C. Chemotherapy follows the same principles as that of ovarian cancer with first-line platinum- and paclitaxel-based combination regimens.

    D. Treatment by stage and grade:

        Stage I Grade 1: Definitive surgery

        Stage I Grade 2 or 3: Surgery and adjuvant chemotherapy

        Stage II–IV: Surgery and adjuvant chemotherapy

VI. **Survival**

    A. 5-year survival by stage

        Stage I: 72%

        Stage II: 38%

        Stage III: 18%

        Stage IV: 0%

VII. **Survival care:** Follows the same principles as that of epithelial ovarian cancer.

PRIMARY PERITONEAL CANCER

I. Differentiation between primary peritoneal and primary ovarian carcinomas can be difficult. Pathological criteria are: the bulk of tumor is on the peritoneum rather than on the ovaries; normal-sized ovaries are present or the ovaries are enlarged by a benign process; tumor involves the ovaries to a depth that is less than 5 mm and is less than 5 mm wide; the tumor is serous by nature.

II. Primary peritoneal cancer can be considered an expression of hereditary breast and ovarian cancer syndromes. There is a 2% to 4.3% risk of primary peritoneal cancer after prophylactic oophorectomy in hereditary cancers.

III. Workup, staging, treatment, survival, and survival care follow the same principles as that of epithelial ovarian cancer.

GERM CELL TUMORS (GCT)

I. Characteristics

A. Germ cell tumors are hypothesized to arise from an unfertilized ovum. They represent 15% to 20% of ovarian cancers, and 70% of ovarian tumors in women less than 30 years of age. The median age at diagnosis is 19 years old, 30% are malignant, 60% to 75% are Stage I at diagnosis, and 25% to 30% are Stage III at diagnosis.

B. Clinical symptoms include a mass, abdominal distension, bloating, pelvic pressure, or pain. Pain can occur from mass effect, torsion, and/or hemorrhage.

C. Paraneoplastic syndromes are common: hyperthyroidism can occur from teratomatous thyroid tissue, hypertension from renin-producing teratomas, hypoglycemia from insulin production, as well as autoimmune hemolytic anemia from teratomas.

II. Workup

A. The pretreatment workup includes a physical examination, CXR, abdominal pelvic imaging to include pelvic ultrasound, CT, or MRI, serum tumor markers, and a karyotype in short or premenarchal females.

B. Serum tumor markers specific to histology include:

Dysgerminoma: hCG (5%), LDH

Endodermal sinus tumor: AFP, LDH

Immature teratoma: AFP, LDH

Embryonal carcinoma: hCG, AFP, LDH

Choriocarcinoma: hCG

Polyembryoma: hCG, AFP, LDH

Mixed: hCG, AFP, LDH

III. Staging

    A. Staging for GCT is per epithelial ovarian cancer FIGO and AJCC protocols.

    B. Inadequately staged patients can be managed in 2 ways: with surgical re-exploration and staging; or chemotherapy without re-exploration, especially if the histological subtype demands chemotherapy regardless of stage.

IV. Treatment

    A. Surgical exploration is advised if a mass greater than 2 cm is found in premenarchal girls, or a mass greater than 6 to 8 cm is found in adolescents or postmenopausal females. If tumor markers such as AFP or hCG are found elevated, and pregnancy is ruled out, exploration should also be considered. Surgical treatment includes: washings, a USO if fertility is desired along with staging biopsies, omentectomy, LN dissection, and debulking of disease. If fertility is not desired, a hysterectomy with BSO is indicated in addition to the above staging procedures.

    B. The role of optimal cytoreduction is also important with these tumors. In a study of 76 patients, a 28% recurrence rate was seen if they were completely resected, vs. a 68% recurrence rate if there was residual disease (62). In another study of patients treated with PVB, those with measurable disease had a 34% disease-free survival vs. 65% if optimally debulked (63).

    C. Adjuvant chemotherapy is recommended for all tumors except for Stage IA dysgerminomas and Stage IAG1 immature teratomas. Chemotherapy is recommended to be platinum based and consists of BEP for 3–4 cycles. Bleomycin should be eliminated for cycle 4, if given.

    D. The number of BEP cycles is debated. Three cycles are recommended for optimally debulked Stages 1 to 3 disease. Four cycles are given for suboptimally debulked disease or Stage 4 disease. If tumor markers are still elevated, chemotherapy should continue for 2 cycles past normalization of these markers.

V. Recurrence

    A. Recurrence is documented by physical examination, a rise in serum tumor markers, or imaging. 90% of relapses occur within 2 years.

B. Germ cell tumors are classified as platinum resistant if there is recurrence within 4 to 6 weeks. Patients with elevated tumor markers at presentation and who do not achieve a negative marker status at 4 cycles are considered to be failure of response. Salvage chemotherapy should be implemented.

C. Some clinicians have recommended salvage cytoreduction showing a 61% 5 YS if optimally salvaged vs. 14% 5 YS in those not secondarily optimally cytoreduced (64).

VI. Follow-Up

A. For nondysgerminomatous tumors, follow-up should occur every 3 months for the first 2 years, every 6 months up to 5 years.

B. For dysgerminomas, a 10-year follow-up is recommended. Serum hCG and AFP should be measured for all patients, even if not initially elevated. 10% to 20% of tumors do relapse.

VII. Histological Subtypes and Directed Therapies

A. Dysgerminomas represent 40% of GCT; 95% are found in Stage I. There is greater malignant potential if the tumor is larger than 10 cm, there is an elevated LDH, a high mitotic index, and necrosis. 5% of tumors produce hCG and PLAP, due to the presence of syncytiotrophoblastic tissue.

1. Adjuvant therapy is indicated for patients staged IB or greater. BEP for 3 to 4 cycles is the recommended regimen; alternatively radiotherapy can be considered.

2. It is important to check a karyotype because 15% of patients are intersex with XY gonadal dysgenesis. If this is found, a prophylactic bilateral gonadectomy should be considered because of the high risk for contralateral dysgerminoma. Gonadectomy should be performed before puberty except in females with testicular feminization. The gonads should be removed after puberty in these cases.

3. If a dysgerminoma is found incidentally after primary surgery, restaging can be considered but is not always indicated, if there is no bulky disease.

4. For Stage IA patients, there is a 20% recurrence rate. If patients were unstaged, consider surveillance, and salvage therapies initiated at recurrence. If there is recurrent disease, radiotherapy or chemotherapy can be administered.

B. Gonadoblastomas are rare benign germ cell tumors. These tumors have up to a 10% chance of malignant transformation. The gonads should be removed if a gonadoblastoma is found in a dysgenic gonad.

C. Endodermal sinus tumors represent 22% of GCT.

1. The histologic pearl is the presence of Schiller-Duval bodies. These are hyaline bodies that resemble the glomerulus in the kidney.

2. All patients require adjuvant postoperative chemotherapy, which should begin within 7 to 10 days of surgery due to rapid growth of disease. Recommended therapy is BEP for 3 to 4 cycles, or POMB-ACE every 3 weeks for 4 cycles. Survival is 2% to 10% without chemotherapy. This is the most virulent of the GCT.

D. Embryonal carcinoma is a rare tumor which occurs in younger patients. There are no trophoblastic tissues in this tumor. Adjuvant treatment should consist of BEP chemotherapy regardless of stage.

E. Choriocarcinoma is a rare tumor, especially the nongestational type. Adjuvant treatment should consist of BEP chemotherapy regardless of stage.

F. Polyembryoma is an extremely rare GCT with fewer than 40 cases reported in the literature. Embryoid bodies are seen at pathology. Adjuvant treatment consists of BEP chemotherapy regardless of stage.

G. Mixed GCT constitute 1% to 15% of all GCT. They most commonly consist of dysgerminomatous and endodermal sinus tumor components. Adjuvant treatment should consist of BEP chemotherapy regardless of stage.

H. Mature cystic teratoma, also known as a **dermoid**, represents 95% of ovarian teratomas. All 3 germ cell layers are represented. This tumor does not constitute a malignancy. It can present as a mass, and it can cause pain via torsion or rupture.

1. The tubercle of Rokitansky is a mural density seen on radiologic imaging.

2. Treatment is surgical with a cystectomy or USO.

3. Malignant degeneration can occur in 1–2% of MCTs. This is usually found in a focus of squamous cell carcinoma from skin lining the cyst. Intraoperative spill of sebaceous contents can cause a chemical peritonitis.

4. **Gliomatosis peritonei** is the presence of benign peritoneal implants of mature neuroglia. These implants usually undergo remission upon resection of the primary tumor.

I. **Immature teratomas (IT)** constitute 20% of GCTs. An IT is defined as the presence of any immature neural tissue. Immature neural tissue is seen as rosettes or neurotubules within the tumor.

1. The amount of immature tissue on one low-power slide determines the grade. The grading system for IT is: G1, < 1 low-power field (LPF 10x) of neural elements in any slide; G2, no greater than a total of 3 LPFs of neural elements in any slide; G3, greater than 3 LPFs full of neural elements in at least 1 slide.

2. Chemotherapy is indicated for all patients except Stage IA Grade 1. Recommended therapy is BEP every 3 weeks × 3 to 4 cycles.

3. A second-look laparotomy is recommended if there is residual tumor seen on imaging after completion of chemotherapy. This can remove chemoresistant disease or determine if there was conversion to mature teratoma.

VIII. **Germ Cell Tumor Trials**

A. GOG 10 (62): 76 patients with malignant germ cell tumors received VAC postoperatively; 54 patients were optimally debulked; 28% of these failed compared to 68% of those who were incompletely resected and failed. Therefore, PVB was trialed for those who were suboptimally resected.

B. GOG 45 (63): 97 eligible patients with Stage II to IV or recurrent disease were treated with 3 to 4 cycles of PVB. Of 35 patients with tumors other than dysgerminoma who had clinically measurable disease, 43% had a CR. The OS was 71% and the DFS was 51%.

C. GOG 78 (65): This study evaluated 93 eligible patients with surgically staged and resected germ cell tumors.

Three cycles of BEP were given as primary adjuvant therapy; 89 of the 93 patients were continuously disease free. At second-look laparotomy 2 patients were found to have foci of IT but remained CCR. Final conclusions were that 91 of 93 patients were progression free after surgery and 3 cycles of BEP. Patients with IT may benefit from secondary debulking if residual disease is identified.

D. GOG 90 (66): 20 patients with incompletely resected ovarian dysgerminoma were treated with cisplatin, bleomycin, and either vinblastine or etoposide. Consolidation chemotherapy with vincristine, dactinomycin, and cyclophosphamide (VAC) was included for some. Eleven patients had clinically measurable disease postoperatively, and 10 responded completely. Fourteen second-look procedures were done, and all were negative; 19 of 20 patients were disease-free with a median follow-up of 26 months.

E. GOG 116 (67): This study evaluated 39 eligible Stage IB–III completely resected dysgerminoma patients. Carboplatin and etoposide were used as primary adjuvant therapy. This doublet therapy was found to be well tolerated for those who needed to reduce chemotoxicity. Critics suggest the lack of bleomycin can contribute to an inferior outcome such as that seen in testes cancer (pharmacologic sanctuary), so the doublet should not be used without bleomycin in ovarian germ cell tumors.

F. A GOG assessment of SLL in GCT evaluated 117 patients from GOG studies 45, 78, and 90. Of the 45 patients treated with BEP after optimal debulking, 38 had a negative SLL. They concluded there was no need for SLL. A subgroup analysis suggested that SLL may be of value in approximately 33% of patients with suboptimal debulking for germ cell tumor with teratomatous elements. Of the 24 patients with teratoma in the primary tumor, 16 patients had bulky residual disease; 14 of 16 patients were disease free after secondary debulking.

IX. Chemotherapy Protocols for Ovarian GCT

Maximum dosing for bleomycin is 360 to 400 mg/m^2

BEP

> Bleomycin: 15 units/m²/week × 5; then on day 1 of course 4
>
> Etoposide: 100 mg/m²/day × 5 days every 3 weeks
>
> Cisplatin: 20 mg/m²/day × 5 days, or 100 mg/m²/day × 1 day every 3 weeks

VBP

> Vinblastine: 0.15 mg/kg on days 1 and 2 every 3 weeks
>
> Bleomycin: 15 units/m²/week × 5; then on day 1 of course 4
>
> Cisplatin: 100 mg/m² on day 1 every 3 weeks

VAC

> Vincristine: 1 to 1.5 mg/m² on day 1 every 4 weeks
>
> Actinomycin D: 0.5 mg/day × 5 days every 4 weeks
>
> Cyclophosphamide: 150 mg/m²/day every 4 weeks

POMB/ACE

> POMB
>
> Day 1: Vincristine 1 mg/m² IV; methotrexate 300 mg/m² 12-hour infusion
>
> Day 2: Bleomycin 15 mg IV 24-hour infusion; folinic acid rescue to start 24 hours after methotrexate 15 mg every 12 hours for 4 doses
>
> Day 3: Bleomycin 15 mg IV 24-hour infusion
>
> Day 4: Cisplatin 120 mg/m² IV 12-hour infusion with IVF and 3 g magnesium
>
> ACE
>
> Days 1 to 5: Etoposide 100 mg/m²/day
>
> Day 3, 4, 5: Actinomycin D 0.5 mg IV
>
> Day 5: Cyclophosphamide 500 mg/m² IV

OMB

> Day 1: Vincristine 1 mg/m² IV; methotrexate 300 mg/m² IV 12-hour infusion
>
> Day 2: Bleomycin 12 mg IV 24-hour infusion; folinic acid rescue to start 24 hours after start of methotrexate 15 mg every 12 hours IV for four doses
>
> Day 3: Bleomycin 15 mg IV 24-hour infusion

SEX CORD STROMAL TUMORS

 I. **Characteristics**: Sex cord stromal tumors represent 5% to 8% ovarian malignancies and 5% of childhood tumors. They are bilateral in 2% of patients. 85% of these tumors produce steroid hormones. The route of spread is transcoelomic, lymphatic, and hematogenous.

 II. **Workup:** The pretreatment workup includes serum hormonal evaluation (free testosterone, estradiol, 17-hydroxy-progesterone, serum cortisol, DHEAS, DHEA, AFP, LDH, inhibin A, inhibin B, and hCG), and imaging including CXR and ultrasound, CT, or MRI.

III. **Staging:** Staging is the same as epithelial ovarian cancer. There is data to suggest a primary LN dissection does not often yield positive results (68).

IV. **Treatment:** Surgical treatment is with washings, a USO if fertility is desired, along with staging biopsies, omentectomy, LN dissection, and debulking of disease. A D&C should be considered if fertility preservation is undertaken. If fertility is not desired, a hysterectomy with BSO is indicated.

 V. **Histology**

   A. **Granulosa-Stromal Cell Tumors**
      1. **Granulosa cell tumors**
         Granulosa cell tumors represent 1% to 2% of ovarian tumors.

         a. These tumors tend to produce high levels of estrogen that can cause the re-feminization of postmenopausal patients, and isosexual precious puberty in prepubertal girls. Patients may experience associated vaginal bleeding, with up to 50% of patients having endometrial hyperplasia and up to 5% with a concordant uterine cancer.

         b. The histologic pearls are the presence of Call-Exner bodies and coffee bean nuclei.

         c. Most granulosa tumors are of the adult type (95%) and the rest are of the juvenile type.

         d. The juvenile type is relatively benign in early stages but can be aggressive in advanced stages. Associated syndromes are Ollier's disease (enchondromatosis) and Maffucci's syndrome (hemangiomas and sarcomas). The OS for Stage I juvenile tumors is 97% vs. 23% for Stage III/IV. There are no Call-Exner bodies in the juvenile type.

    e. It is important to check a serum estradiol ($>$ 30 pg/mL in a postmenopausal woman is abnormal) and both the alpha and beta inhibin levels.

    f. Treatment is surgical with comprehensive staging.

    g. Adjuvant chemotherapy is considered for Stage IC and higher. Recurrence is often indolent at 5 to 20 years.

    h. Prognostic factors for adverse outcomes are: size greater than 10 cm, rupture, greater than 2 mitosis/10 HPF, LVSI, and nuclear atypia.

    i. For recurrent or metastatic disease, patients can be retreated with BEP or other regimens to possibly include platinum with paclitaxel, high-dose progestins, GnRH analogs, or radiotherapy. One study demonstrated a 43% CCR with radiotherapy in patients with measurable disease (69).

2. Thecomas

Thecomas represent 1% of ovarian tumors and are bilateral in 3%. They are benign tumors. They can produce estrogen.

3. Fibroma-fibrosarcoma

Fibromas are the most common sex cord stromal tumor and 10% are bilateral. They are benign tumors. They occasionally secrete estrogen. They have an association with Meigs syndrome, which is the presence of an adnexal fibroma, ascites, and a pleural effusion.

B. Sertoli-Stromal Cell Tumors (Androblastomas) This tumor is diagnosed at a median age of 30 years old. This tumor can cause virilization. It is important to follow the serum AFP and testosterone. Adjuvant chemotherapy is recommended if the tumor contains heterologous elements or is poorly differentiated. Recurrance is usually within the first 2 years.

1. Sertoli cell tumor

Sertoli cell tumor is also called a Pick's adenoma.

    a. It produces estrogen in 65% of patients and can also produce androgens. It rarely produces hyperaldosteronism with associated hyperkalemia and hypertension.

    b. The histologic pearl is the Pick's body.

    c. There is an increased risk of malignancy if hemorrhage, necrosis, a high mitotic count, or poor differentiation is present.

2. Leydig cell tumors

Leydig cell tumors produce androgens in 80% and estrogen in 10% of patients; 2.5% are malignant. They usually present after the age of 50 years and are associated with thyroid disease.

3. Sertoli-Leydig cell tumor

Sertoli-Leydig cell tumors can cause virilization in one-half to two-thirds of patients. Most tumors produce testosterone and this can cause menstrual irregularities.

    a. The histologic pearl is the crystals of Reinke.

    b. 97% are found at Stage I, and less than 20% are malignant.

    c. For those that are malignant: 10% are Grade 2 and 60% are Grade 3. Malignant tumors tend to have more necrosis, are larger, and hemorrhage more frequently.

    d. Adjuvant chemotherapy should consist of BEP if malignant.

C. Gynandroblastoma tumors

Gynandroblastoma tumors can produce androgens and estrogens. These tumors can have both granulosa and Sertoli-Leydig components.

D. Sex cord tumor with annular tubules

1. Sex cord tumors with annular tubules can produce estrogen. Two-thirds are bilateral.

    a. These tumors can be associated with Peutz-Jeghers (PJ) syndrome and are benign when they have this association. PJ syndrome has an associated 15% risk of cervical adenocarcinoma (adenoma malignum) and hysterectomy should be considered after fertility is concluded.

    b. If patients are not diagnosed with PJ syndrome, these tumors are considered malignant. Treatment for non-PJ syndrome patients is surgical with a USO, LN dissection, and staging. A D&C, ECC, and colposcopy should be performed if fertility is desired, and a TAH-BSO otherwise.

E. Unclassified

1. Lipid cell tumors

Lipid cell tumors can be virilizing and produce Cushing's syndrome. They produce estrogen, progesterone, and testosterone.

a. They are malignant in 20% of cases. Indications of malignancy are: pleomorphism, necrosis, a high mitotic count, and a size greater than 8 cm.

b. Adjuvant BEP chemotherapy is recommended if found to be malignant.

2. Sex cord tumors not otherwise specified

Sex cord tumors not otherwise specified produce hormones and up to 17% of patients have Cushing's disease.

a. 43% of these tumors are malignant. Malignant tumors contain fibrothecomatous and/or granulosa cell-like proliferation as well as areas of tubular differentiation.

b. Adjuvant BEP chemotherapy is recommended if malignant.

VI. 5 Y Survival

A. Dysgerminoma

Stage I: 90% to 95%

All stages: 60% to 90%

B. Endodermal sinus tumor

Stage I and II: 90%

Stage III and IV: 50%

C. Immature teratoma

Stage I: 90% to 95%

All stages: 70% to 80%

Grade 1: 82%

Grade 2: 62%

Grade 3: 30%

D. Embryonal carcinoma

All stages: 39%

E. Choriocarcinoma: Poor

F. Polyembryoma: Poor

G. Mixed: Depends on tumor composition

H. Granulosa cell:

Stages I, II: 85% to 95%

Stages III, IV: 55% to 60%

I. Sertoli-Leydig:

Grade 3: Poor survival

VII. Sex Cord Stromal Tumor Trials

A. GOG 115 (70): This study evaluated 57 eligible patients who had incompletely resected Stage II–IV ovarian stromal malignancies. BEP was used as first-line therapy dosed at 20 units/m^2 IV push day 1 every 3 weeks × 4 cycles. The endpoint was negative second-look laparotomy: 37% had negative findings. Patients with measurable disease had the highest risk of progression and death. BEP was found to be active in stromal tumors.

REFERENCES

1. Duska LR, Garrett L, Henretta M, et al. When "never-events" occur despite adherence to clinical guidelines: the case of venous thromboembolism in clear cell cancer of the ovary compared with other epithelial histologic subtypes. *Gynecol Oncol.* 2010;116(3):374–377.
2. Schmeler KM, Tao X, Frumovitz M, et al. Prevalence of LN metastasis in primary mucinous carcinoma of the ovary. *Obstet Gynecol.* 2010;116(2, pt. 1):269–273.
3. Powless CA, Aletti GD, Bakkum-Gamez JN, et al. Risk factors for LN metastasis in apparent early-stage epithelial ovarian cancer: implications for surgical staging. *Gynecol Oncol.* 2011;122(3):536–540.
4. Bristow RE, Montz FJ, Lagasse LD, et al. Survival impact of surgical cytoreduction in stage IV epithelial ovarian cancer. *Gynecol Oncol.* 1999;72(3):278–287.
5. Panici PB, Maggioni A, Hacker N, et al. Systematic aortic and pelvic lymphadenectomy versus resection of bulky nodes only in optimally debulked advanced ovarian cancer: a randomized clinical trial. *J Natl Cancer Inst.* 2005;97(8):560–566.
6. Garcia-Soto AE, Boren T, Wingo SN, et al. Is comprehensive surgical staging needed for thorough evaluation of early-stage ovarian carcinoma? *Am J Obstet Gynecol.* 2012;206(3):242.e1–242.e5.
7. Vergote I, De Brabanter J, Fyles A, et al. Prognostic importance of degree of differentiation and cyst rupture in stage I invasive epithelial ovarian carcinoma. *Lancet.* 2001;357(9251):176–182.

8. Van Le L. Stage IC ovarian cancer: the clinical significance of intraoperative rupture. *Obstet Gynecol.* 2009;113(1):4–5.

9. Greer BE, Bundy BN, Ozols RF, et al. Implications of second-look laparotomy in the context of optimally resected stage III ovarian cancer: a non-randomized comparison using an explanatory analysis: a Gynecologic Oncology Group study. *Gynecol Oncol.* 2005;99(1):71–79.

10. Chi DS, McCaughty K, Diaz JP, et al. Guidelines and selection criteria for secondary cytoreductive surgery in patients with recurrent, platinum-sensitive epithelial ovarian carcinoma. *Cancer.* 2006;106(9):1933–1939.

11. Baldwin LA, Huang B, Miller RW, et al. Ten-year relative survival for epithelial ovarian cancer. *Obstet Gynecol.* 2012;120(3):612–618.

12. Rustin GJ, van der Burg ME, Griffin CL, et al. Early versus delayed treatment of relapsed ovarian cancer (MRC OV05/EORTC 55955): a randomised trial. MRC OV05; EORTC 55955 investigators. *Lancet.* 2010;376(9747):1155–1163.

13. Colombo N, Guthrie D, Chiari S, et al. International Collaborative Ovarian Neoplasm trial 1: a randomized trial of adjuvant chemotherapy in women with early-stage ovarian cancer. *J Natl Cancer Inst.* 2003;95(2):125–132.

14. Trimbos JB, Vergote I, Bolis G, et al. Impact of adjuvant chemotherapy and surgical staging in early-stage ovarian carcinoma: European Organisation for Research and Treatment of Cancer-Adjuvant ChemoTherapy in Ovarian Neoplasm trial. *J Natl Cancer Inst.* 2003;95(2):113–125.

15. Baptist Trimbos, Petra Timmers, Sergio Pecorelli, Corneel Coens, Koen Ven, Maria van der Burg, and Antonio Casado. Surgical Staging and Treatment of Early Ovarian Cancer: Long-term Analysis From a Randomized Trial PMCID: PMC2911043 doi: 10.1093/jnci/djq149 *J Natl Cancer Inst.* 2010 July 7; 102(13): 982–987.

16. ICON2: randomised trial of single-agent carboplatin against three-drug combination of CAP (cyclophosphamide, doxorubicin, and cisplatin) in women with ovarian cancer. ICON Collaborators. International Collaborative Ovarian Neoplasm Study. *Lancet.* 1998;352(9140): 1571–1576.

17. Parmar MK, Ledermann JA, Colombo N, et al. Paclitaxel plus platinum-based chemotherapy versus conventional platinum-based chemotherapy in women with relapsed ovarian cancer: the ICON4/AGO-OVAR-2.2 trial. *Lancet.* 2003;361(9375):2099–2106.

18. Bookman MA, Brady MF, McGuire WP, et al. Evaluation of new platinum-based treatment regimens in advanced-stage ovarian cancer: a phase III trial of the Gynecologic Cancer InterGroup (GCIG). *J Clin Oncol.* 2009;27:1419–1425.

19. Perren TJ, Swart AM, Pfisterer J, et al. A phase 3 trial of bevacizumab in ovarian cancer. *N Engl J Med.* 2011;365(26):2484–2496. Erratum in: *N Engl J Med.* 2012;366(3):284.

20. Hreshchyshyn MM, Park RC, Blessing JA, et al. The role of adjuvant therapy in stage I ovarian cancer. *Am J Obstet Gynecol.* 1980;138(2): 139–145.

21. McGuire WP, Hoskins WJ, Brady MF, et al. Cyclophosphamide and cis-platin compared with paclitaxel and cisplatin in patients with stage III and stage IV ovarian cancer. *N Engl J Med.* 1996;334(1):1–6.

22. Piccart MJ, Bertelsen K, James K, et al. Randomized intergroup trial of cisplatin-paclitaxel versus cisplatin-cyclophosphamide in women with advanced epithelial ovarian cancer: three-year results. *J Natl Cancer Inst.* 2000;92(9):699–708.

23. Muggia FM, Braly PS, Brady MF, et al. Phase III randomized study of cisplatin versus paclitaxel versus cisplatin and paclitaxel in patients with suboptimal stage III or IV ovarian cancer: a Gynecologic Oncology Group study. *J Clin Oncol.* 2000;18(1):106–115.

24. Bell J, Brady MF, Young RC, et al. Randomized phase III trial of three versus six cycles of adjuvant carboplatin and paclitaxel in early stage epithelial ovarian carcinoma: a Gynecologic Oncology Group study. *Gynecol Oncol.* 2006;102(3):432–439.

25. Ozols RF, Bundy BN, Greer BE, et al. Phase III trial of carboplatin and paclitaxel compared with cisplatin and paclitaxel in patients with opti-mally resected stage III ovarian cancer: a Gynecologic Oncology Group study. *J Clin Oncol.* 2003;21(17):3194–3200.

26. Burger RA, Brady MF, Bookman MA, et al. Incorporation of bevaci-zumab in the primary treatment of ovarian cancer. *N Engl J Med.* 2011;365(26):2473–2483.

27. Vasey PA, Jayson GC, Gordon A, et al. Phase III randomized trial of docetaxel-carboplatin versus paclitaxel-carboplatin as first-line chem-otherapy for ovarian carcinoma. *J Natl Cancer Inst.* 2004;96(22): 1682–1691.

28. McGuire WP, Hoskins WJ, Brady MF, et al. Assessment of dose-intensive therapy in suboptimally debulked ovarian cancer: a Gynecologic Oncology Group study. *J Clin Oncol.* 1995;13(7):1589–1599.

29. Fruscio R, Garbi A, Parma G, et al. Randomized phase III clinical trial evaluating weekly cisplatin for advanced epithelial ovarian cancer. *J Natl Cancer Inst.* 2011;103(4):347–351.

30. Kaye SB, Paul J, Cassidy J, et al. Mature results of a randomized trial of two doses of cisplatin for the treatment of ovarian cancer. Scottish Gynecology Cancer Trials Group. *J Clin Oncol.* 1996;14(7):2113–2119.

31. Jakobsen A, Bertelsen K, Andersen JE, et al. Dose-effect study of carbo-platin in ovarian cancer: a Danish Ovarian Cancer Group study. *J Clin Oncol.* 1997;15(1):193–198.

32. Gore M, Mainwaring P, A'Hern R, et al. Randomized trial of dose-intensity with single-agent carboplatin in patients with epithelial ovar-ian cancer. London Gynaecological Oncology Group. *J Clin Oncol.* 1998;16(7):2426–2434.

33. Omura GA, Brady MF, Look KY, et al. Phase III trial of paclitaxel at two dose levels, the higher dose accompanied by filgrastim at two dose levels in platinum-pretreated epithelial ovarian cancer: an intergroup study. *J Clin Oncol.* 2003;21(15):2843–2848.

34. Eisenhauer EA, ten Bokkel Huinink WW, Swenerton KD, et al. European-Canadian randomized trial of paclitaxel in relapsed ovarian cancer: high-dose versus low-dose and long versus short infusion. *J Clin Oncol.* 1994;12(12):2654–2666.

35. Katsumata N, Yasuda M, Takahashi F, et al. Dose-dense paclitaxel once a week in combination with carboplatin every 3 weeks for advanced ovarian cancer: a phase 3, open-label, randomised controlled trial. *Lancet.* 2009;374(9698):1331–1338.

36. Thigpen JT, Blessing JA, Ball H, et al. Phase II trial of paclitaxel in patients with progressive ovarian carcinoma after platinum-based chemotherapy: a Gynecologic Oncology Group study. *J Clin Oncol.* 1994;12(9):1748–1753.

37. Alberts DS, Liu PY, Hannigan EV, et al. Intraperitoneal cisplatin plus intravenous cyclophosphamide versus intravenous cisplatin plus intravenous cyclophosphamide for stage III ovarian cancer. *N Engl J Med.* 1996;335(26):1950–1955.

38. Markman M, Bundy BN, Alberts DS, et al. Phase III trial of standard-dose intravenous cisplatin plus paclitaxel versus moderately high-dose carboplatin followed by intravenous paclitaxel and intraperitoneal cisplatin in small-volume stage III ovarian carcinoma: an intergroup study of the Gynecologic Oncology Group, Southwestern Oncology Group, and Eastern Cooperative Oncology Group. *J Clin Oncol.* 2001;19(4):1001–1007.

39. Armstrong DK, Bundy B, Wenzel L, et al. Intraperitoneal cisplatin and paclitaxel in ovarian cancer. *N Engl J Med.* 2006;354(1):34–43.

40. Walker JL, Armstrong DK, Huang HQ, et al. Intraperitoneal catheter outcomes in a phase III trial of intravenous versus intraperitoneal chemotherapy in optimal stage III ovarian and primary peritoneal cancer: a Gynecologic Oncology Group study. *Gynecol Oncol.* 2006;100(1):27–32.

41. Markman M, Liu PY, Wilczynski S, et al. Phase III randomized trial of 12 versus 3 months of maintenance paclitaxel in patients with advanced ovarian cancer after complete response to platinum and paclitaxel-based chemotherapy: a Southwest Oncology Group and Gynecologic Oncology Group trial. *J Clin Oncol.* 2003;21(13):2460–2465.

42. Markman M, Liu PY, Moon J, et al. Impact on survival of 12 versus 3 monthly cycles of paclitaxel (175 mg/m^2) administered to patients with advanced ovarian cancer who attained a complete response to primary platinum-paclitaxel: follow-up of a Southwest Oncology Group and Gynecologic Oncology Group phase 3 trial. *Gynecol Oncol.* 2009;114(2):195–198.

43. McMeekin DS, Tillmanns T, Chaudry T, et al. Timing isn't everything: an analysis of when to start salvage chemotherapy in ovarian cancer. *Gynecol Oncol.* 2004;95(1):157–164.

44. Mannel RS, Brady MF, Kohn EC, et al. A randomized phase III trial of IV carboplatin and paclitaxel × 3 courses followed by observation versus weekly maintenance low-dose paclitaxel in patients with early-stage

ovarian carcinoma: a Gynecologic Oncology Group study. *Gynecol Oncol.* 2011;122(1):89–94.

45. Pfisterer J, Plante M, Vergote I, et al. Gemcitabine plus carboplatin compared with carboplatin in patients with platinum-sensitive recurrent ovarian cancer: an intergroup trial of the AGO-OVAR, the NCIC CTG, and the EORTC GCG. *J Clin Oncol.* 2006;24(29):4699–4707.

46. Gordon AN, Tonda M, Sun S, et al. Long-term survival advantage for women treated with pegylated liposomal doxorubicin compared with topotecan in a phase 3 randomized study of recurrent and refractory epithelial ovarian cancer. *Gynecol Oncol.* 2004;95(1):1–8.

47. Aghajanian C, Blank SV, Goff BA, et al. OCEANS: a randomized, double-blind, placebo-controlled phase III trial of chemotherapy with or without bevacizumab in patients with platinum-sensitive recurrent epithelial ovarian, primary peritoneal, or fallopian tube cancer. *J Clin Oncol.* 2012;30(17):2039–2045.

48. Pujade-Lauraine E, Wagner U, Aavall-Lundqvist E, et al. Pegylated liposomal doxorubicin and carboplatin compared with paclitaxel and carboplatin for patients with platinum-sensitive ovarian cancer in late relapse. *J Clin Oncol.* 2010;28(20):3323–3329.

49. Harter P, du Bois A, Hahmann M, et al. Surgery in recurrent ovarian cancer: the Arbeitsgemeinschaft Gynaekologische Onkologie (AGO) DESKTOP OVAR trial. *Ann Surg Oncol.* 2006;13(12):1702–1710.

50. Harter P, Sehouli J, Reuss A, et al. Prospective validation study of a predictive score for operability of recurrent ovarian cancer: the Multicenter Intergroup Study DESKTOP II. A project of the AGO Kommission OVAR, AGO Study Group, NOGGO, AGO-Austria, and MITO. *Int J Gynecl Cancer.* 2011;21(2):289–295.

51. van der Burg ME, van Lent M, Buyse M, et al. The effect of debulking surgery after induction chemotherapy on the prognosis in advanced epithelial ovarian cancer. Gynecological Cancer Cooperative Group of the European Organization for Research and Treatment of Cancer. *N Engl J Med.* 1995;332(10):629–634.

52. Rose PG, Nerenstone S, Brady MF, et al. Secondary surgical cytoreduction for advanced ovarian carcinoma. *N Engl J Med.* 2004;351(24):2489–2497.

53. Vergote I, Tropé CG, Amant F, et al. Neoadjuvant chemotherapy or primary surgery in stage IIIC or IV ovarian cancer. *N Engl J Med.* 2010;363(10):943–953.

54. Bristow RE, Tomacruz RS, Armstrong DK, et al. Survival effect of maximal cytoreductive surgery for advanced ovarian carcinoma during the platinum era: a meta-analysis. *J Clin Oncol.* 2002;20(5):1248–1259.

55. Hamilton CA, Miller A, Miller C, et al. The impact of disease distribution on survival in patients with stage III epithelial ovarian cancer cytoreduced to microscopic residual: a Gynecologic Oncology Group study. *Gynecol Oncol.* 2011;122(3):521–526.

56. Winter WE III, Kucera PR, Rodgers W, et al. Surgical staging in patients with ovarian tumors of low malignant potential. *Obstet Gynecol.* 2002;100:671–676.

57. Gershenson DM, Silva EG, Tortolero-Luna G, et al. Serous borderline tumors of the ovary with noninvasive peritoneal implants. *Cancer.* 1998;83(10):2157–2163.
58. Crispens MA, Bodurka D, Deavers M, et al. Response and survival in patients with progressive or recurrent serous ovarian tumors of low malignant potential. *Obstet Gynecol.* 2002;99(1):3–10.
59. Stewart SL, Wike JM, Foster SL, et al. The incidence of primary fallopian tube cancer in the United States. *Gynecol Oncol.* 2007;107(3):392–397.
60. Hu CY, Taymour ML, Hertig AT. Primary carcinoma of the fallopian tube. *Am J Obstet Gynaecol* 1950; 59:58–67.
61. Sedlis A. Carcinoma of the fallopian tube. *Surg Clin North Am* 1978;58:121–129.
62. Slayton RE, Park RC, Silverberg SG, et al. Vincristine, dactinomycin, and cyclophosphamide in the treatment of malignant germ cell tumors of the ovary. A Gynecologic Oncology Group study (a final report). *Cancer.* 1985;56(2):243–248.
63. Williams SD, Blessing JA, Moore DH. Cisplatin, vinblastine, and bleomycin in advanced and recurrent ovarian germ-cell tumors: a trial of the Gynecologic Oncology Group. *Ann Intern Med.* 1989;111(1):22–27.
64. Li J, Yang W, Wu X. Prognostic factors and role of salvage surgery in chemorefractory ovarian germ cell malignancies: a study in Chinese patients. *Gynecol Oncol.* 2007;105(3):769–775.
65. Williams S, Blessing JA, Liao SY, et al. Adjuvant therapy of ovarian germ cell tumors with cisplatin, etoposide, and bleomycin: a trial of the Gynecologic Oncology Group. *J Clin Oncol.* 1994;12(4):701–706.
66. Williams SD, Blessing JA, Hatch KD, et al. Chemotherapy of advanced dysgerminoma: trials of the Gynecologic Oncology Group. *J Clin Oncol.* 1991;9(11):1950–1955.
67. Williams SD, Kauderer J, Burnett AF, et al. Adjuvant therapy of completely resected dysgerminoma with carboplatin and etoposide: a trial of the Gynecologic Oncology Group. *Gynecol Oncol.* 2004;95(3):496–499.
68. Brown J, Sood AK, Deavers MT, et al. Patterns of metastasis in sex cord-stromal tumors of the ovary: can routine staging lymphadenectomy be omitted? *Gynecol Oncol.* 2009;113(1):86–90.
69. Wolf JK, Mullen J, Eifel PJ, Burke TW, Levenback C, Gershenson DM. Radiation treatment of advanced or recurrent granulosa cell tumor of the ovary. *Gynecol Oncol* 1999;73(1):35–41.
70. Homesley HD, Bundy BN, Hurteau JA, et al. Bleomycin, etoposide, and cisplatin combination therapy of ovarian granulosa cell tumors and other stromal malignancies: a Gynecologic Oncology Group study. *Gynecol Oncol.* 1999;72(2):131–137.
71. Kleppe M, Wang T, Van Gorp T, Slangen BF, Kruse AJ, Kruitwagen RF. Lymph node metastasis in stages I and II ovarian cancer: a review. *Gynecol Oncol.* 2011;123(3):610–614. doi: 10.1016/j.ygyno.2011.09.013. Epub 2011 Oct 6.

Uterine Cancer

I. Characteristics

A. Uterine corpus cancer is the most common female gynecologic cancer in the United States with an estimated 49,560 cases and 8,190 deaths in the United States in 2013. Currently, endometrial adenocarcinoma is the most common malignancy of the female genital tract and ranks as the fourth most common cancer in females.

B. Risk factors for endometrial cancer include the triad of obesity, diabetes, and hypertension. Other risk factors are a prolonged exposure to estrogens, nulliparity, early menarche, late menopause, and unopposed estrogen hormone therapy.

C. Most women present with abnormal uterine bleeding. Of those postmenopausal women who do present with bleeding, 10% result in a diagnosis of uterine cancer.

D. Other presenting signs and symptoms can be menorrhagia, intermenstrual bleeding, pain, pyometria, hematometria, and an abnormal Pap smear.

E. Hyperplasia and cellular atypia, alone or combined, have known rates for progression to uterine cancer (1).

Type of Hyperplasia	Total Cases	Persisted (%)	Progressed (%)	Mean Years Follow-Up
Simple	93	19	1	15.2
Complex	29	17	3	13.5
Atypical simple	23	23	8	11.4
Atypical complex	45	14	29	11.4

1. According to one collaborative study, a diagnosis of complex atypical hyperplasia was associated with a 43% chance of concurrent endometrial cancer. Of these specimens, 31% had myometrial invasion, and 10% had greater than 50% myometrial invasion (2).

II. **Prognostic factors**: Stage is the most important prognostic factor. Other factors include: depth of myometrial invasion, LVSI, grade, histology, tumor size, patient age, hormone receptor status.

III. **Pretreatment Workup**

A. Workup for abnormal bleeding begins with history and physical examination. Evaluation involves endometrial biopsy (EMB) with endocervical curettage or D&C. Pelvic ultrasound and Pap smear may also be performed, but are insufficient modalities used alone for persistent abnormal bleeding.

B. An endometrial stripe thickness that is 5 mm or greater in a postmenopausal patient is abnormal and biopsy should be performed. The accuracy of EMB and D&C are relatively the same, between 91% and 99%, when compared with final pathology (2).

C. Women with the following should be ruled out for cancer via biopsy: postmenopausal women with bleeding; postmenopausal patients with pyometria; asymptotic postmenopausal women with endometrial cells on Pap smear (especially if atypical); perimenopausal patients with intermenstrual bleeding or increasingly heavy periods; premenopausal patients with abnormal uterine bleeding, particularly if there is a history of anovulation.

D. In women over the age of 35 years with abnormal bleeding, an endometrial biopsy should be performed. 25% of cancers occur in premenopausal women and 5% occur in women less than 40 years of age.

E. The pretreatment workup for uterine cancer includes a chest x-ray, and abdominal-pelvic imaging. This can be with a pelvic ultrasound, CT, or MRI. Lab tests include a CBC, CMP, and CA-125 (which can predict lymph node [LN] metastasis).

IV. Histology

A. Epidemiological and clinical studies suggest that endometrial cancers be separated into two groups by histologic appearance and behavior:

    1. Type I tumors are the most common. The main risk factor in type I carcinomas is hyperestrogenism. These tend to be hormonally responsive and have an 83% all stage 5-year survival (YS). These cancers typically have a favorable prognosis with appropriate therapy.

        a. The most common type I cancer is endometrioid adenocarcinoma, which occurs in 75% of cases.

        b. Adenosquamous carcinoma is diagnosed in 18% to 25% of uterine cancers. The behavior is similar to that of endometrioid cancer.

        c. Villoglandular carcinoma occurs in 6% of uterine cancers. This subtype is distinguished by delicate fibrovascular cores. It is usually of low grade and is more differentiated than endometrioid adenocarcinoma.

        d. Secretory carcinoma occurs in 2% of uterine cancers and appears as a well-differentiated glandular pattern with intracytoplasmic vacuoles containing glycogen, similar to secretory endometrium. It is usually Grade 1.

        e. Mucinous carcinoma is diagnosed in 5% of cases and mucin is present as the major cellular component. There are columnar cells that are basally oriented or pseudostratified. It is necessary to rule out other cancers such as colon, mucinous ovarian, and primary endocervical cancers. It has the same prognosis as endometrioid cancer.

        f. Squamous carcinoma is associated with cervical stenosis, pyometria, and chronic inflammation. It is important to rule out a primary cervical cancer origin. It has a poorer prognosis.

    2. Type II cancers are poorly differentiated tumors, and are histologically represented by the serous and clear cell histologies. Type II tumors are more biologically aggressive and have a 53% all Stage 5 YS. Type II tumors account for 15% of uterine carcinomas, but represent 50% of all relapses. These type II tumors are classified as high risk, high grade, and are unresponsive to hormonal therapy.

a. Serous uterine carcinoma is diagnosed in 10% to 15% of endometrial cancers. If there is 10% or less serous components, it is called a mixed tumor. This subtype resembles serous carcinoma of the ovary. It is often found at an advanced stage. The depth of invasion is often not predictive of LN metastasis, and extrauterine disease is found in 60% of tumors. If the cancer is identified in a polyp without other evidence of uterine disease, 38% of patients will be found to have extrauterine spread. Intraperitoneal spread is common even when myometrial invasion is minimal. When comprehensively staged, 70% of patients are found to have advanced-stage disease: 25% of apparent Stage I cancers (3) have omental metastasis and 25% of patients have upper abdominal disease (4). Microscopically, there are fibrous papillary fronds, picket fencing of the terminal cells, LVSI is common, and psammoma bodies are often present. It is high grade by definition.

b. Clear cell carcinoma is diagnosed in 5% of uterine cancers. It also is an aggressive tumor. The cells contain a large amount of glycogen and when processed for histology, the glycogen in the cells give an appearance of cellular clearing and nuclear hobnailing.

3. Mixed Müllerian mesodermal tumors (MMMT) (carcinosarcoma) are now thought to be metaplastic epithelial (or carcinomatous) cancers. These tumors tend to occur in older women with a median age of 65 to 75 years old. Other characteristics include obesity, nulliparity, and diabetes. Tumor can be seen via speculum examination in 50% of women. Pathologically, there is a mixture of carcinomatous and sarcomatous tissues. The carcinomatous component is most commonly endometrioid, but can be of serous or clear cell histology. The sarcomatous/nonepithelial component is commonly an endometrial stromal sarcoma, but can be leiomyosarcoma, rhabdosarcoma, or chondrosarcoma. The presence or absence of heterologous elements is not predictive of outcome. Studies have shown similar allelic losses present in both the carcinomatous and sarcomatous areas of MMMTs in multiple patients. This suggests a late divergence in phenotype and a common abnormal clone for the entire cancer.

V. Staging

A. Staging is surgical. In 1989 the staging was changed from clinical to surgical. Surgical staging was further revised in 2009.

1. FIGO

   a. Surgical

   Stage I: Disease confined to the uterus

   - Stage IA: Limited to the endometrium or less than one-half the myometrium
   - Stage IB: Invasion more than one-half the myometrium

   Stage II: Extension to the cervix but not outside the uterus

   - Cervical stromal involvement

   Stage III: Extension outside the uterus but disease confined to the true pelvis

   - Stage IIIA: Tumor invades the serosa or adnexa
   - Stage IIIB: Vaginal metastasis, parametrial extension, pelvic extension
   - Stage IIIC: Lymph node (LN) metastasis

     Pelvic LN metastasis

     Para-aortic LN metastasis

   Stage IV: Metastasis to adjacent pelvic organs or distant metastasis

   - Stage IVA: Invasion of bowel or bladder mucosa
   - Stage IVB: Distant metastasis, including intra-abdominal metastasis (omentum or peritoneum) and/or inguinal LNs

   b. Clinical staging can be used for patients who are not surgical candidates.

   Stage I:

   - Stage IA: Uterus sounds to less than 8 cm
   - Stage IB: Uterus sounds to more than 8 cm

   Stage II: Carcinoma involving the corpus and the cervix but not outside the uterus

   Stage III: Carcinoma extending outside the uterus but not outside the true pelvis

   Stage IV: Carcinoma extending outside the true pelvis or obviously involving the mucosa of the bladder or rectum

   - IVA: Spread to the bladder or rectum
   - IVB: Spread to distant organs

2. AJCC Uterine Cancer Staging

   a. Tumor

   TX: Cannot be assessed

   T0: No evidence of tumor

   Tis: Carcinoma in situ

   T1: Tumor confined to corpus uteri

   - T1A: Tumor limited to the endometrium or invades less than one-half of myometrium

   - T1B: Tumor invades more than one-half of myometrium

   T2: Tumor invades the cervix but does not extend beyond the uterus

   T3: Local and/or regional spread of the tumor

   - T3A: Tumor involves the serosa and/or adnexa

   - T3B: Vaginal involvement: direct extension or metastasis, parametrial involvement, pelvic peritoneal involvement

   T4A: Tumor invades bladder or bowel mucosa

   b. Nodes

   NX: Cannot be assessed

   N0: No evidence of LN metastasis

   N1: (IIIC): Evidence of LN metastasis pelvic and/or para-aortic

   - a. Pelvic LN involvement

   - b. Para-aortic LN involvement

   c. Metastasis

   MX: Cannot be assessed

   M0: No evidence of distant metastasis

   M1: (IVB) Evidence of distant metastasis

   d. TNM Stage Grouping

   Stage 0: TisN0M0

   Stage 1: T1N0M0

   - 1A: T1aN0M0

   - 1B: T1bN0M0

   - 1C: T1cN0M0

Stage 2: T2N0M0

- 2A: T2aN0M0
- 2B: T2bN0M0

Stage 3: T3N0M0

- 3A: T3aN0M0
- 3B: T3bN0M0
- 3C1: TAnyN1M0
- 3C2: TAnyN2M0

Stage 4:

- 4A: T4AnyNM0
- 4B: AnyTAnyNM1

VI. Grade is specified as a 3-tiered system: Grade 1 tumors are highly differentiated, with < 5% of the tumor containing solid areas; Grade 2 tumors are moderately differentiated with 6% to 50% solid areas; Grade 3 tumors are poorly differentiated carcinomas with > 50% of the tumor containing solid components. If nuclear atypia is present at a higher degree than stated histological grade, the overall grade is increased by one degree.

VII. Treatment

A. Treatment is surgical with pelvic washings, hysterectomy, bilateral salpingo-oophorectomy, LN dissection, omentectomy (especially for serous or clear cell histologies), peritoneal biopsies (specifically for serous or clear cell histologies), and surgical debulking of extrauterine/metastatic disease.

B. Lymph Node Dissection

1. The boundaries for the pelvic LN dissection are the following: the distal half of the common iliac vessels, the anterior and medial aspect of the external iliac vessels, the ureter medially, the circumflex iliac vein distally, and the obturator nerve inferiorly. The para-aortic LN boundaries are the following: the fat pads over and lateral to the great vessels, the inferior mesenteric artery superiorly, and the mid common iliac vessels inferiorly. For a high para-aortic dissection, the LNs up to the renal vessels are removed lateral and anterior to the great vessels.

2. There is much controversy to the benefit and/or extent of a LN dissection. LN dissection has been shown not to increase the duration of surgery significantly. Some practitioners perform a LN dissection based on tumor risk factors. Others recommend a comprehensive LN dissection for all surgical candidates. Others have provided data that show that an LN dissection is not therapeutic but can provide staging information to guide adjuvant therapies.

3. For those who choose a selective LN dissection, the Mayo criteria is often employed to determine if a patient is low risk for LN metastasis. The Mayo criteria are: Grade 1 or 2 disease, tumor size that is 2 cm or less, and ≤ 50% myometrial invasion. If all these criteria are met, patients have a < 5% chance of positive LNs (5). Frozen section should be employed for this decision analysis. The accuracy of frozen section decreases with grade: 87% accurate with Grade 1, 65% with Grade 2, only 31% with Grade 3 (6). Doering et al. correlated visual inspection with frozen section and found 91% accuracy (7), and Franchi et al. supported this data with 85% accuracy and 72% sensitivity (8).

4. For those who perform comprehensive LN dissection, the following benefits are cited: there may be a therapeutic benefit with removal of micrometastasis; there is a 22% chance of extrauterine disease found with surgical staging; and 20% of tumors are upgraded at final pathology. Data has shown that removing nodes provides a survival benefit (9,10). An improvement in survival from 72% to 88% has been reported for patients undergoing lymphadenectomy with more than 11 LNs removed (11). Using SEER data, Chan et al. showed that in patients staged IB Grade 3 and above, more than 20 LNs removed was found to provide the best OS (12). In low-risk patients, there was no association with LN count and survival. The PORTEC 1 trial subset of Stage IC Grade 3 (unstaged) patients who were treated with pelvic radiotherapy had a 5 YS of only 58%. Most recurrences were distant (13). In contrast, Stage IIIC patients staged and treated have a 5 YS of 57% to 72% (14,15).

5. In some instances, lymph node dissection is not performed. This can occur when cancer is found incidentally after hysterectomy. Postoperative pathological review can risk stratify patients for possible post hoc staging. There can be

intraoperative complications that prevent full staging; or the patient may be medically intolerant of the procedure. Body habitus may also prohibit adequate staging: in the Lap-2 data, 50% of patients with a BMI > 40 were not able to have a para-aortic LND performed (16). For those who support no LN dissection, data from 2 randomized studies are commonly used.

   a. The CONSORT Bendetti Panici study evaluated 514 eligible clinical stage I uterine cancer patients who were randomized to lymphadenectomy compared to those who did not have a lymphadenectomy. Patients were randomly assigned to systematic pelvic LN dissection vs. no LN dissection. Researchers found that early and late postoperative complications were higher in the systematic LN dissection group. LN dissection improved staging as more patients were found to have an advanced stage (13.3% vs. 3.2%). However, the 5-year disease-free survival and OS were similar (81% vs. 86% in the lymphadenectomy arm and 82% vs. 90% in the nonlymphadenectomy arm) (17).

   b. The ASTEC Bendetti Panici study (18,19) evaluated 1,408 women with clinical Stage I endometrial cancer and randomized them to standard surgery (hysterectomy, bilateral salpingo-oophorectomy, washings with para-aortic LN palpation) or standard surgery plus lymphadenectomy. The primary outcome for this study was overall survival. The hazard ratio for death was higher in those who underwent comprehensive staging with LND, 1.16 ($P = .3$, CI 0.87 to 1.54). The absolute difference in 5-year OS was 1%.

C. Based on a surgical/pathological review, in patients thought to have disease confined to the uterus, extrauterine disease has been found in 22% of patients, LN metastasis has been found to occur in 9% to 13% of patients, and isolated para-aortic LNs have been found in 2% of patients. The rate of positive para-aortic LNs is approximately half the rate of positive pelvic LNs. For those who were identified with positive para-aortic LNs, 47 of 48 patients had one or more of the following: grossly positive pelvic LN; grossly positive adnexal metastasis; or outer one-third myometrial invasion (20). Omental metastasis has been found in up to 8% of patients.

GOG 33: Clinical Stage I: Frequency of Nodal Metastasis Among Risk Factors (%)

Risk Factor	Pelvic	Para-Aortic
Grade		
1	3	2
2	9	5
3	18	11
Depth of myometrial invasion		
Superficial	5	3
Middle	6	1
Deep	25	17
Site of disease		
Fundus	8	4
Cervix	16	14
Lymphovascular space invasion		
Negative	7	9
Positive	27	19

D. If gross cervical involvement is seen at diagnosis, preoperative radiation followed by an adjuvant simple hysterectomy can be considered. A radical hysterectomy as primary treatment can also be considered.

   1. There is data to suggest that performing a radical hysterectomy, based on a positive endocervical curettage only commonly shows no evidence of cancer on final pathology and may be overtreatment (21).

   2. If gross parametrial involvement is identified by physical examination or preoperative imaging, primary radiotherapy with dosing analogous to that for cervical cancer (80 Gy) can be considered, followed by a simple hysterectomy, with or without chemotherapy.

   3. There is data to suggest that the incidence of omental metastasis is 6% to 8% and is associated with grade of disease, extrauterine involvement, LN metastasis, deep myometrial invasion, and positive cytology.

E. Adjuvant treatment is commonly recommended in patients with endometrial cancer. Treatment is based on stage and risk factors. Early-stage disease is defined as Stages I and II. Advanced stage is defined as Stages III and IV.

   1. High intermediate risk early-stage disease is often treated with adjuvant radiation therapy. High intermediate risk is classified by two different studies. PORTEC 1: An intermediate high-risk subgroup was identified: patient age older than 60 years, depth of invasion greater than half myometrial thickness, or Grade 2 or 3 tumor. GOG 99 stratified patients by age and risk factors. If a patient fell into any of the following groups, they were considered high intermediate risk (HIR): patients age $\geq$ 70 years with 1 risk factor, age 50 to 69 years with 2 risk factors, and any age with all 3. The risk factors were: outer one-third myometrial invasion, Grade 2 or 3 tumor, and lymphovascular space invasion.

2. High-risk early-stage disease is defined variably. Stage I and II serous, clear cell, and variably Grade 3 cancers put patients into the high-risk early-stage disease category. There is data to show that (old) Stage 1CG3 tumors had a 58% 5 YS, so some clinicians recommend chemotherapy and radiation for these high risk patients.

3. Advanced-stage endometrial cancer. For advanced-stage disease (Stages III/IV) treatment is primarily surgical with comprehensive staging and cytoreduction to microscopic status if possible. Adjuvant therapy is commonly multimodal including both radiation and chemotherapy, and can include hormonal therapies.

   a. There is literature to support cytoreduction in advanced metastatic uterine cancer.

      i. Greer (22) treated 31 patients with Stage IVB disease with whole abdominal radiation. Those with a residual < 2 cm had a corrected 5 YS of 80% and an absolute 5 YS of 63%, whereas there were no survivors in the group with residual > 2 cm.

      ii. Goff evaluated patients with Stage IV disease. Those who were cytoreduced had a longer median survival of 18 months compared to an 8-month survival in those who were not able to be cytoreduced (23).

      iii. Bristow reviewed 65 patients with Stage IVB endometrial cancer who underwent cytoreduction. Optimal cytoreduction (residual tumor $\leq$ 1 cm in maximal diameter) was accomplished in 55%. The median survival rate of patients who underwent optimal surgery was 34 months vs. 11 months for patients with > 1 cm residual disease. Furthermore, patients with microscopic residual tumor survived significantly longer (median survival 46 months) compared to patients optimally cytoreduced but with macroscopic disease (24).

iv. Shih (25) also suggested optimal cytoreduction for Stage IV uterine cancer patients. Median survival: The median PFS was 40.3 months for patients with microscopic disease, 11 months for patients with any residual disease, and 2.2 months for patients who did not have attempted cytoreduction. The median OS was 42.2 months for patients with microscopic disease, 19 months for patients with any residual disease, and 2.2 months for patients that did not have attempted cytoreduction.

4. Type II cancers

a. Early-stage type II cancers (serous or clear cell histology). There is data to support platinum-based chemotherapy in addition to radiotherapy for patients staged 1A or above (26). Stage IA patients with no residual cancer in the hysterectomy specimen had no recurrences whether they received adjuvant therapy or not. 77% of Stage IB patients not treated with adjuvant chemotherapy recurred vs. no recurrences in the treated group; 20% of Stage IC patients who received chemotherapy recurred vs. 80% who did not. Recurrences tended to occur at the vaginal cuff in patients not treated with brachytherapy, thus brachytherapy in combination with chemotherapy was recommended for all patients staged IA (with residual) or higher.

b. Maximal cytoreduction for Stage IV serous uterine cancer can offer an improvement in survival. Bristow showed that patients with optimal cytoreduction had a median survival of 26.2 months vs. 9.6 months in patients with suboptimal surgery. Patients with microscopic residual tumor had a significantly longer median survival of 30.4 months vs. those with 0.1 to 1 cm residual disease who had a median survival of 20.5 months. A 41-month vs. a 34-month vs. an 11-month OS was observed for those patients who were microscopically cytoreduced, optimally cytoreduced to < 1 cm, or suboptimally cytoreduced (24).

5. MMMT (carcinosarcoma) used to be classified as a uterine sarcoma. Recent data have suggested an improvement in survival

with surgical cytoreduction (27). An adjuvant radiation trial from the EORTC evaluated a subset of carcinosarcoma patients and found a trend toward improvement in local control with whole pelvic radiotherapy, but there was no improvement in survival (28). Chemotherapy in combination with radiation has been shown to be effective in treatment of MMMTs. Ifosfamide and paclitaxel have been shown to produce a RR of 45% (29).

VIII. Recurrence: Recurrent disease can be broken into local recurrence or distant recurrence. A full metastatic workup should be performed with a physical examination; imaging of the chest, abdomen, and pelvis; lab tests for baseline organ function; and possibly PET imaging. Patients who were previously radiated in the pelvis tend to fail distantly at 70%, only 16% recur vaginally, and 14% recur in the pelvis. Patients without prior pelvic radiation tend to fail vaginally at 50%, 21% fail in the pelvis, and 30% distantly.

  A. If the recurrence is vaginal, radiation therapy can be administered. Prior radiotherapy does affect response. In the PORTEC 1 trial, data on relapsed patients showed a 5 YS of 65% if patients had no prior adjuvant radiation, vs. 19% if they had prior radiation. If there was a pelvic recurrence, the 5 YS was 0. The treatment of recurrence is whole pelvic radiotherapy in combination with brachytherapy dosed to 75 to 80 Gy. There is data to support surgical cytoreduction of vaginal lesions to < 2 cm. This is associated with an improvement in OS to 43 months vs. 10 months with cytoreduction (30).

  B. For extra-pelvic recurrences, chemotherapy with or without volume directed radiotherapy can be administered. Different regimens have been used. CAP: cyclophosphamide (500 mg/m^2), doxorubicin (40 mg/m^2), and cisplatin (70 mg/m^2), given every 4 weeks; single-agent paclitaxel has shown a 36% response rate (paclitaxel 250 mg/m^2 as 24-hr infusion); combination paclitaxel (175 mg/m^2), carboplatin AUC 6, and amifostine has shown a 40% response rate with an 8% complete response (31).

  C. Hormonal therapies, specifically progestins, have also been used. Medroxyprogesterone acetate (MPA) at a dose of 200 mg/day had a better response rate than 1000 mg/day in the GOG 81 study. The overall response rate was 25%, and there was a higher response in estrogen receptor and progesterone receptor positive patients. Megace has also been used at a dose of 80 to 160 mg twice daily with an 18% to 34% response rate (32). For those patients who are estrogen receptor positive on immunohistochemistry, tamoxifen or an aromatase inhibiter can be considered. If the patient is *Her-2/neu* positive, herceptin was found to have a 13% response rate in a phase II trial (GOG 181B) (33).

IX. **Postoperative hormonal replacement therapy,** namely estrogen, has been studied for quality of life and recurrence. GOG 137 (34) evaluated estrogen HRT given to women with a history of uterine cancer. There was no increased risk of recurrence identified (the relative risk was 1.27—the CI crossed 1.0).

X. 5% to 10% of women with a uterine cancer may have a **synchronous ovarian neoplasm**. Up to 25% of women under 40 years old can have this concurrent diagnosis. Concordant endometrioid histology in both the uterus and ovary are present 45% to 86% of the time. There is concordant grade in 69% of patients. Empirical criteria favoring metastatic uterine cancer over a synchronous ovarian tumor are: multinodular ovarian involvement, deep myometrial invasion, LVSI, bilateral ovarian involvement, and visualization of intratubal transit. Surgical staging or adjuvant recommendations are based on the worst-case scenario: i.e., if the ovarian tumor is Grade 3 and the uterine tumor a Grade 1, chemotherapy would commonly be recommended.

XI. **Survival**

   A. 5-Year Survival (35)

   Stage I: 78% to 90%

   Stage II: 74%

   Stage III: 36% to 56%

   Stage IV: 21% to 22%

XII. **Follow-Up**

   A. Every 3 months for the first 2 years

   Every 6 months for the next 3 years

   Then annual examinations thereafter

   B. Physical and pelvic examination should occur at each visit. Pap smears have not been found to increase the detection of recurrence, nor has annual chest x-ray. CA-125 can be drawn if it was initially elevated.

XIII. Adjuvant treatment of postmenopausal women with hormone receptor positive **breast cancer** has been **tamoxifen**. There are known gynecologic side effects from this medication. Aromatase inhibitors have been evaluated as crossover or primary therapy in some women, replacing tamoxifen treatment. Gynecologic side effects of tamoxifen can be vaginal bleeding, growth of uterine polyps in 8% to 36% of women, endometrial hyperplasia in 2% to 20%, and endometrial cancer ranging from 0% to 8%. The annual risk of cancer after 5 years of exposure is 6 cases per 1,000. Ultrasound diagnoses an endometrial stripe that is greater than 5 mm in 50% of patients on tamoxifen; but endometrial stripes up to 8 mm can be considered normal in these patients. A routine annual EMB is not recommended unless these women are symptomatic with postmenopausal bleeding of significant atypical discharge.

NOTABLE STUDIES IN UTERINE CANCER

I. High-Risk Early-Stage Disease Adjuvant Therapy Studies

A. Aalders studied 540 patients with Stage I endometrial cancer status post total abdominal hysterectomy and bilateral salpingo-oophorectomy, but who were not surgically staged. All received brachytherapy and were randomized to whole pelvic radiotherapy or no further treatment. There was no improvement in overall survival. The 5 YS was 89% in the EBRT arm vs. 91% in the NFT (NS). Vaginal and pelvic recurrences were 6.9% in the NFT arm vs. 1.9% if given external beam pelvic radiotherapy. Distant metastasis occurred more often in the radiotherapy arm. In the subset of patients with Stage IC Grade 3 disease, there were fewer recurrences in the EBRT arm, 18% vs. 7% (36).

B. PORTEC 1 (37,38): 715 eligible patients underwent total abdominal hysterectomy and bilateral salpingo-oophorectomy without surgical staging or lymphadenectomy. Patients were included if they had either: Grade 1 disease with > 50% invasion, Grade 2 with any invasion, or Grade 3 with < 50% invasion. Less than 2% of histologies were other than endometrioid. Patients were randomized to no additional therapy vs. whole pelvic radiation to 46 Gy. The 5-year (Y) recurrence rate was 4% vs. 14%, favoring radiotherapy ($P < .001$) and the 5 YS was 81% vs. 85% (NS). Distant metastasis was similar at 7% and 8%. The 8 Y RFS was 68% for both groups. The 8 Y OS survival was 71% in the radiation group and 77% in the control group (NS) due to salvage of relapse in the NFT arm (85% of vaginal recurrences were salvageable). A high intermediate-risk subgroup was identified: patient age older than 60 years, depth of invasion greater than half myometrial thickness, or Grade 2 or 3 tumor. In this high intermediate-risk group, the recurrence rate was 23% vs. 5%, favoring radiation. 73% of recurrences were in the vagina. Survival after recurrence was better for the control group rather than radiotherapy group. For the pelvic recurrence patients, 51% were salvaged if they had not received radiation, vs. 19% if they had received adjuvant radiation. Stage IB Grade 3 patients had higher rates of distant metastasis (15%). A subgroup of patients staged IC Grade 3 were not randomized but all received whole pelvic radiation. These patients all had a 5 YS of 58%.

C. Systemic pelvic lymphadenectomy randomized trial/CONSORT study (18): 514 eligible patients underwent hysterectomy with BSO and were randomized to systemic pelvic LND or no LND. LND improved surgical staging with 13.3% vs 3.2% of patients identified with LN metastasis. At 49 months of follow-up, the 5 Y DFS and OS were 81% and 85.9% in the LND arm and 81.7% and 90% in the no LND arm. There was no improvement in DFS or OS with LND. Researchers found the rate of recurrence in LN beds was 1.5% in each arm; therefore, LN basins were not where patients recurred.

D. GOG 99 (39): 392 eligible patients with type I cancers staged IB, IC, IIA, and occult IIB were evaluated. All were surgically staged with total abdominal hysterectomy, bilateral salpingo-oophorectomy, pelvic and para-aortic LN dissection. 75% of patients had endometrioid histology, 80% had Grade 1 or 2 tumors, 25% had lymphovascular space invasion, and 10% were Stage II. Patients were randomized to whole pelvic radiotherapy to 50.4 Gy without brachytherapy or no further therapy. Median follow-up was 68 months. The overall recurrence rate was 12% in the no further treatment (NFT) group and decreased to 3% with radiation. The OS was 86% in the NFT group vs. 92% in the radiotherapy arm (NS). A high intermediate risk (HIR) group was identified, which accounted for 132 patients (one-third of those enrolled) and two-thirds of the study-related deaths. This HIR group included patients age $\geq$ 70 years with one risk factor, age 50 to 69 years with 2 risk factors, and any age with all 3. The risk factors were: outer one-third myometrial invasion,

Grade 2 or 3 tumor, and lymphovascular space invasion. For this subgroup, the recurrence rate was reduced with adjuvant radiation from 26% to 6%. The major difference was the vaginal vault recurrences: 13 recurred vaginally in the NFT vs. 2 recurred in the radiation arm, and of these 2, both had refused radiation. 5% in each group had distant metastasis.

E. PORTEC 2 (40): This study evaluated 427 patients with Stage I or Stage IIA endometrial carcinoma with HIR factors. Patients were randomized to pelvic radiotherapy (46 Gy) or vaginal brachytherapy (21 Gy high-dose rate or 30 Gy low-dose rate). The 5-year vaginal recurrence rate was 1.8% for vaginal brachytherapy vs. 1.6% for pelvic radiotherapy. The 5-year rates of locoregional relapse were 5.1% for vaginal brachytherapy and 2.1% for pelvic radiotherapy. There were no differences in overall or disease-free survival.

F. Japanese Gynecologic Oncology Group-2033 (41): This study evaluated patients with Stage IC to Stage IIIC endometrial carcinoma with < 50% myometrial invasion who were randomized to whole pelvic radiation vs. cyclophosphamide (333 mg/m^2), doxorubicin (40 mg/m^2), and cisplatin (50 mg/m^2) (CAP chemotherapy) every 4 weeks for 3 or more courses. The 5-year PFS was nearly the same at 83.5% in the pelvic radiation group and 81.8% in the CAP group. The 5 Y OS was 85% in the radiation group vs. 87% in the chemotherapy group (NS). A subgroup of HIR patients—who were defined as having (a) Stage IC disease in patients over 70 years of age or having Grade 3 tumor or (b) Stage II or Stage IIIA (positive cytology) with > 50% myometrial invasion—were found to have significantly better outcomes with chemotherapy: the PFS for the radiation arm was 66% vs. 84% for the chemotherapy arm, and the OS was 74% in the radiation group vs. 90% in the chemotherapy group.

G. SEPAL study: Cohorts from two different Japanese gynecologic oncology teams totaling 671 patients were retrospectively analyzed with respect to the use of PA LND. Routine PA LND was practiced standardly at one facility and not at the other. Both facilities offered systemic PLND. A median PLND count was 34 in the PLND group vs. 59 in the combined PA and PLND group. Patients at intermediate or high risk of recurrence were offered adjuvant chemotherapy and radiation therapy. The OS was longer in the combination PA and PLND group with a HR of 0.53. The risk of death was reduced independent of adjuvant therapies so it was recommended that a combined PA and PLND be performed for all intermediate and high risk patients (42).

Advanced and Recurrent Endometrial Cancer Studies

A. GOG 28 (43): Evaluated melphalan, 5-FU, and Megace vs. doxorubicin, 5-FU and cyclophosphamide. The ORR in those with measurable disease was 38% in both groups; 36% of each group had stable disease, and only 26.4% progressed on treatment. The OS was 10.6 vs. 10.1 months respectively (both NS).

B. GOG 48 (44): This study evaluated 356 eligible patients and compared doxorubicin to the doublet of doxorubicin and cyclophosphamide. All patients had received prior therapy with progestins subsequent to progression of disease. A response rate of 22% vs. 32% was found and an OS of 6.8 vs. 7.6 months was identified with a 17% reduction in the rate of death.

C. GOG 94 (45,46): This trial evaluated 77 Stage III/IV type I and 103 type II endometrial cancers. A subgroup (phase II study) of patients with Stage I/II serous and clear cell uterine cancer patients were also evaluated. Treatment was WAR. The 3 Y recurrence-free survival was 29% and 27% for the type I and type II cancers, respectively. The OS were 31% and 35%, respectively. The 5 Y progression-free survival (PFS) for the phase II trial was 54%. The OS was 34%. This led to the development of GOG 122.

D. GOG 107 (47): This study evaluated doxorubicin 60 mg/m^2 vs. doxorubicin 60 mg/m^2 and cisplatin 50 mg/m^2 every 3 weeks in 281 eligible patients with Stage III/IV or recurrent endometrial cancer. The overall response rate was 25% vs. 42%. The median PFS was 3.8 vs. 5.7 months, and the median OS was 9.2 vs. 9 months for doxorubicin alone vs. the doublet, respectively. The doublet improved RR and PFS with little impact on OS.

E. GOG 122 (48): This trial randomized 400 patients with Stage III, IV, and recurrent disease to whole abdominal radiotherapy vs. doxorubicin 60 mg/m^2 and cisplatin 50 mg/m^2 (AP) for 7 cycles plus an additional 8th cycle of cisplatin alone every 3 weeks. 85% of patients had a pelvic LND, and 75% had a PA LND. Radiation was dosed at 45 Gy total (30 Gy WAR + 15 Gy boost to the PA LN and to the pelvis). 85% had microscopic residual disease, 25% were Stage IV, 50% were Stage IIIC. The PFS HR was 0.71 favoring AP demonstrating a 12% decrease in recurrence at 5 years with chemotherapy. The OS HR was 0.68 favoring chemotherapy. A 13% increase in OS was seen at 5 years in the chemotherapy arm. The 5 YS was 53% with chemotherapy vs. 42% with radiation.

F. GOG 139 (49): This trial evaluated a possible circadian difference in the administration of doxorubicin and cisplatin in 342 patients with stages III, IV, and recurrent disease. No benefit was found to timing the administration of chemotherapy based on increased glutathione levels early in the morning. The RR was 46% vs. 49%. The PFS was 6.5 months for the standard timed therapy and 5.9 months for the circadian timed therapy. The OS was 11.2 for standard vs. 13.2 months for the circadian therapy (both NS).

G. GOG 163 (50): Compared doxorubicin and paclitaxel vs. doxorubicin and cisplatin. There was no difference in PFS or OS in either group. The RR was 40% vs. 43%; the PFS was 7.2 vs. 6 months; and the OS was 12.6 vs. 13.6 months (NS).

H. GOG 177 (51): This study looked at the combination of paclitaxel 160 mg/m^2, doxorubicin 45 mg/m^2, and cisplatin 50 mg/m^2 (TAP) with G-CSF support vs. the doublet of doxorubicin 60 mg/m^2 and cisplatin 50 mg/m^2 (AP): 273 patients with stage III, IV, or recurrent disease were treated every 3 weeks for 7 cycles or until progression; 50% of patients on both arms received all cycles of therapy. There was a 22% CR in the TAP arm vs. a 7% CR on the AP arm and a PR of 36% vs. 27%. The overall response rates were 57% vs. 34%, the PFS was 8.3 vs. 5.3 months, and the median OS was 15.3 vs. 12.1 months, all favoring TAP.

I. GOG 184 (52): In this study, 552 eligible patients with Stages III and IV disease were randomized to receive chemotherapy consisting of the triplet of cisplatin 50 mg/m^2, doxorubicin 45 mg/m^2, and paclitaxel 160 mg/m^2 (TAP) vs. the doublet of cisplatin and doxorubicin (AP) at the same dosing for 6 cycles after volume directed radiation. 80% completed 6 cycles of chemotherapy. No difference in OS was found. The PFS was 64% for the TAP vs. 62% for the AP arm. A subgroup analysis found that TAP was associated with a 50% reduction in recurrence or death if there was gross residual disease.

J. GOG 209 (53): This noninferiority trial compared carboplatin AUC 6 and paclitaxel 175 mg/m^2 given every 3 weeks for 7 cycles to paclitaxel 160 mg/m^2, doxorubicin 45 mg/m^2, and cisplatin 50 mg/m^2 (TAP) with G-CSF support every 3 weeks for 7 cycles in 1,312 patients with metastatic or recurrent endometrial cancer. Patients were allowed to receive volume directed radiation. A 14-month RFS was found in each arm, with an OS of 32 months vs. 38 months, respectively. The neurotoxicity was 26% vs. 19% favoring carboplatin and paclitaxel, thus this regimen is not inferior to TAP.

K. Mundt et al. (54) found evidence to support the continued use of locoregional radiation in combination with chemotherapy for high-risk Stage III/IV patients. Patients were reviewed retrospectively. Patients treated with doxorubicin and platinum chemotherapy alone were found to have a 67% incidence of recurrence; 31% relapsed in the pelvis, vagina, or both, making the case for multimodality therapy.

L. GOG 129F: Single-agent paclitaxel was evaluated in a phase II trial for patients with persistent or recurrent endometrial cancer (55). Paclitaxel was dosed at 200 mg/m^2, and 175 mg/m^2 for patients with prior pelvic radiation therapy, every 3 weeks. A 27.3% overall RR was seen in 44 patients.

M. GOG 139S (56): This study evaluated histology among different uterine cancer studies totaling 1,203 patients from 4 randomized trials. The response with different combinations of doxorubicin, cisplatin, and paclitaxel was not associated with histology except for the clear cell subtype (ORR for type I was 44%; type II serous, 44%; type II clear cell, 32%). A main predictor of OS was histology with the type II tumors having a HR of 1.2 for serous and 1.5 for clear cell carcinoma. The breakdown of histology by GOG study is: GOG 122 had 50% endometrioid, 20% serous, 5% clear cell, and 10% mixed histologies, 80% were Grade 2, 3; GOG 177 had 15% and 19% serous in each arm; GOG 184 had 13% serous in each arm; GOG 99: none.

MMMT-Carcinosarcoma Trials

A. GOG 150 (57): This trial evaluated 206 patients with Stage I to IV optimally debulked carcinosarcoma, and randomized them to WAR with a pelvic boost vs. ifosfamide with mesna and cisplatin. The recurrence rate was 58% in the WAR arm vs. 52% in chemotherapy arm, NS. There was a significant survival benefit to chemotherapy (HR 0.67) with a 5 YS of 47% vs. 37%. Recurrence was vaginal in 3.8% of patients who received WAR compared to 9.9% in the chemotherapy arm. The final recommendation was that chemotherapy and vaginal brachytherapy may be the best combination for carcinosarcoma.

B. GOG 161 (58): This trial evaluated 179 patients with stage III/IV, persistent, or recurrent disease. Ifosfamide/mesna dosed at 1.6 gm/m² IV daily for 3 days plus and paclitaxel 135 mg/m² every 3 weeks was compared to ifosfamide/mesna 2 g/m² IV daily for 3 days every 3 weeks up to 8 cycles. A higher RR of 45% was seen with the doublet compared to 29% with the single agent. The PFS was found to be significant at 5.8 vs. 3.6 months, as was the OS of 13.5 vs. 8.4 months, both favoring the doublet.

UTERINE SARCOMAS

I. Characteristics

A. Sarcomas arise from the mesodermal tissues of the body. In gynecology, they most commonly originate in the uterus.

B. These tumors comprise 3% of all uterine cancers, have a 3% risk of adnexal metastasis, and represent 3.3 cases per 100,000 women.

C. Clinically patients can present with postcoital bleeding, intermenstrual bleeding, an enlarged uterus, or the cancer can mimic a prolapsed fibroid on examination.

D. The main risk factor is a history of prior pelvic radiation.

E. The route of spread can be lymphatic, peritoneal, or hematogenous.

II. Pretreatment workup includes an EMB or D&C, a CXR, CT of the abdomen and pelvis, and consideration of a chest CT if there is a confirmed diagnosis. 19% of patients with leiomyosarcoma have lung metastasis. Routine preoperative lab tests are important.

III. Staging is surgical. This includes hysterectomy, bilateral salpingo-oophorectomy, exploration of the abdomen and pelvis, possible LND, biopsy of any suspicious extrauterine lesions, and omentectomy. Staging was updated in 2009. It differentiates leiomyosarcomas from endometrial stromal sarcoma (ESS) and adenosarcomas (AS).

A. FIGO staging for leiomyosarcomas

Stage I: Tumor limited to uterus

- IA: < 5 cm
- IB: > 5 cm

Stage II: Tumor extends to the pelvis

- IIA: Adnexal involvement
- IIB: Tumor extends to extrauterine pelvic tissue

Stage III: Tumor invades abdominal tissues (not just protruding into the abdomen)

- IIIA: One site
- IIIB: More than one site
- IIIC: Metastasis to pelvic and/or para-aortic LNs

Stage IV:

- IVA: Tumor invades bladder and/or rectum
- IVB: Distant metastasis

B. FIGO staging for endometrial stromal sarcoma (ESS) and adeno-sarcoma (AS)

Stage I: Tumor limited to uterus

- IA: Tumor limited to endometrium/endocervix with no myometrial invasion
- IB: Less than or equal to half myometrial invasion
- IC: More than half myometrial invasion

Stage II: Tumor extends to the pelvis

- IIA: Adnexal involvement
- IIB: Tumor extends to extrauterine pelvic tissue

Stage III: Tumor invades abdominal tissues (not just protruding into the abdomen)

IIIA: One site

IIIB: More than one site

IIIC: Metastasis to pelvic and/or para-aortic LNs

Stage IV:

- IVA: Tumor invades bladder and/or rectum
- IVB: Distant metastasis

IV. There are four main histologic types of sarcoma: leiomyosarcoma, endometrial stromal sarcoma, undifferentiated sarcoma, and adenosarcoma.

    A. Leiomyosarcoma (LMS) is the most common uterine sarcoma. It originates from the uterine smooth muscle. It represents 40% of uterine sarcomas. It can present at any age but most commonly arises in women aged 45 to 55 years old. Only 15% are diagnosed preoperatively with an EMB or D&C. For diagnosis, it is necessary to demonstrate coagulative necrosis. One or both of the following are also necessary: cellular atypia, or more than 10 mitosis/HPF. The rate of ovarian metastasis is 3% (59) and the rate of LN metastasis is 6.6% to 11% (60, 61). LND has not shown to be of benefit for staging as up to 70% of women with positive LN already have extrauterine disease (62).

        1. If a LMS is found incidentally after hysterectomy, a second staging surgery should be considered if there was morcellation of the uterus; a supracervical hysterectomy was performed initially (in these cases, the cervix should be removed on reoperation), or there was no evaluation of the abdomen or pelvis. A second staging surgery for a LN dissection or BSO has not been found to be beneficial (63).

        2. Adjuvant therapy is considered based on stage. For Stages I and II: no further therapy vs. pelvic radiotherapy for local control can be offered. For Stages III and IV: chemotherapy with or without pelvic radiotherapy can be offered. Chemotherapy can consist of single-agent doxorubicin with a RR of 25%, single-agent ifosfamide with a RR of 17%, combination ifosfamide and doxorubicin with a RR of 30%, or combination gemcitabine and docetaxel with a RR of 53%. Aromatase inhibitors can be considered if the tumor is ER positive.

        3. For isolated lung recurrences, thoracotomy with resection can yield a survival benefit. The 5 YS was 43% in one series (64).

    B. Endometrial stromal sarcoma (ESS) is commonly diagnosed in women aged 42 to 53 years old. This tumor represents about 8% of uterine sarcomas and arises from the stromal cells between the endometrial glandular cells. It is by definition a low-grade tumor, meaning fewer than 10 mitoses/HPF. It cannot be diagnosed by D&C. Final pathology needs to document LVSI and invasion. If one of these two components is absent, then the diagnosis is an endometrial stromal nodule. There is a 20% risk of pelvic LN metastasis, so consideration for a LND should be entertained. Removal of the ovaries is recommended as these are hormone-dependent cancers and can respond to endogenous estrogen. Stage is the most important prognostic factor.

1. Adjuvant therapy is considered based on stage. For Stages I and II, consider observation vs. pelvic radiotherapy. 20% of recurrences have been documented in the pelvis.

2. For Stage III or Stage IV, consider hormonal therapy with Megace (40 mg to 160 mg daily), with or without radiotherapy. An 88% RR with a 50% CR has been seen (65). ERT may increase the chance of recurrence. There is data to show that 33.3% of recurrences are pelvic only, if no adjuvant radiation was given. For recurrent disease, a 33% response rate was seen with ifosfamide and doxorubicin. Aromotase inhibitors can also be considered in these tumors.

C. Undifferentiated sarcoma (the former term for high-grade ESS) is a high-grade lesion, meaning there are more than 10 mitoses/HPF. This is an aggressive tumor and it responds poorly to treatment. Stage is the most important prognostic factor. Radiotherapy is not recommended for undifferentiated sarcomas. Chemotherapy should be considered with a single agent or combination agents including doxorubicin, ifosfamide, cisplatin, and docetaxel.

D. Adenosarcoma represents 1% of uterine sarcomas. The median age of diagnosis is 50 years old. Abnormal bleeding is common and speculum examination can visualize tumor in 50% of cases. These are low-grade malignancies, but 20% can recur more than 5 years after surgery. There is an increased risk of recurrence if deep myometrial invasion is present. A subset, adenosarcoma with sarcomatous overgrowth, have a poor prognosis. 20% of patients in this subset can have pelvic LN metastasis, so a LN dissection should be considered.

V. **Prognostic factors:** Stage is the most important prognostic factor; the depth of myometrial invasion, LVSI, grade, histology, tumor size, patient age, and hormone receptor status can all affect outcome.

VI. **Follow-Up**

A. Every 3 months for the first 2 years

Every 6 months for the next 3 years

Then annual examinations thereafter

B. Physical and pelvic examination should occur at each visit. Pap smears have not been found to increase the detection of recurrence, nor has annual chest x-ray. CA-125 can be drawn if it was initially elevated.

REFERENCES

1. Kurman RJ, Kaminski PF, Norris HJ. The behavior of endometrial hyperplasia. A long-term study of "untreated" hyperplasia in 170 patients. *Cancer.* 1985;56(2):403–412.
2. Trimble CL, Kauderer J, Zaino R, et al. Concurrent endometrial carcinoma in women with a biopsy diagnosis of atypical endometrial hyperplasia: a Gynecologic Oncology Group study. *Cancer.* 2006;106(4): 812–819.
3. Chan JK, Loizzi V, Youssef M, et al. Significance of comprehensive surgical staging in noninvasive papillary serous carcinoma of the endometrium. *Gynecol Oncol.* 2003;90(1):181–185.
4. Geisler JP, Geisler HE, Melton ME, et al. What staging surgery should be performed on patients with uterine papillary serous carcinoma? *Gynecol Oncol.* 1999;74(3):465–467.
5. Mariani A, Webb MJ, Keeney GL, et al. Low-risk corpus cancer: is lymphadenectomy or radiotherapy necessary? *Am J Obstet Gynecol.* 2000; 182(6):1506–1519.
6. Goff BA, Rice LW. Assessment of depth of myometrial invasion in endometrial adenocarcinoma. *Gynecol Oncol.* 1990;38(1):46–48.
7. Doering DL, Barnhill DR, Weiser EB, et al. Intraoperative evaluation of depth of myometrial invasion in stage I endometrial adenocarcinoma. *Obstet Gynecol.* 1989;74(6):930–933.
8. Franchi M, Ghezzi F, Melpignano M, et al. Clinical value of intraoperative gross examination in endometrial cancer. *Gynecol Oncol.* 2000;76(3):357–361.
9. Cragun JM, Havrilesky LJ, Calingaert B, et al. Retrospective analysis of selective lymphadenectomy in apparent early-stage endometrial cancer. *J Clin Oncol.* 2005;23:3668–3675.
10. Chan JK, Cheung MK, Huh WK, et al. Therapeutic role of lymph node resection in endometrioid corpus cancer: a study of 12,333 patients. *Cancer.* 2006;107(8):1823–1830.
11. Kilgore LC, Partridge EE, Alvarez RD, et al. Adenocarcinoma of the endometrium: survival comparisons of patients with and without pelvic node sampling. *Gynecol Oncol.* 1995;56:29–33.
12. Chan JK, Kapp DS, Cheung MK, et al. The impact of the absolute number and ratio of positive lymph nodes on survival of endometrioid uterine cancer patients. *Br J Cancer.* 2007;97(5):605–611.
13. Creutzberg CL, van Putten WL, Wárlám-Rodenhuis CC, et al. Outcome of high-risk stage IC, grade 3, compared with stage I endometrial car-

cinoma patients: the Postoperative Radiation Therapy in Endometrial Carcinoma Trial. *J Clin Oncol.* 2004;22(7):1234–1241.

14. Nelson G, Randall M, Sutton G, et al. FIGO stage IIIC endometrial carcinoma with metastases confined to pelvic lymph nodes: analysis of treatment outcomes, prognostic variables, and failure patterns following adjuvant radiation therapy. *Gynecol Oncol.* 1999;75(2):211–214.

15. Ayhan A, Taskiran C, Celik C, et al. Surgical stage III endometrial cancer: analysis of treatment outcomes, prognostic factors and failure patterns. *Eur J Gynaecol Oncol.* 2002;23(6):553–556.

16. Walker JL, Piedmonte MR, Spirtos NM, et al. Laparoscopy compared with laparotomy for comprehensive surgical staging of uterine cancer: Gynecologic Oncology Group study LAP-2. *J Clin Oncol.* 2009;27(32):5331–5336.

17. Benedetti Panici P, Basile S, Maneschi F, et al. Systematic pelvic lymphadenectomy vs. no lymphadenectomy in early-stage endometrial carcinoma: randomized clinical trial. *J Natl Cancer Inst.* 2008; 100(23):1707–1716.

18. ASTEC/EN.5 Study Group; Blake P, Swart AM, Orton J, et al. Adjuvant external beam radiotherapy in the treatment of endometrial cancer (MRC ASTEC and NCIC CTG EN.5 randomised trials): pooled trial results, systematic review, and meta-analysis. *Lancet.* 2009;373(9658):137–148.

19. Kitchener H, Swart AM, Qian Q, et al; ASTEC study group. Efficacy of systemic pelvic lymphadenectomy in endometrial cancer (MRC ASTEC trail): a randomised study. *Lancet.* 2009;373(9658):125–136.

20. Morrow CP, Bundy BN, Kurman RJ, et al. Relationship between surgical-pathological risk factors and outcome in clinical stage I and II carcinoma of the endometrium: a Gynecologic Oncology Group study. *Gynecol Oncol.* 1991;40(1):55–65.

21. Disaia PJ. Predicting parametrial involvement in endometrial cancer: is this the end for radical hysterectomies in stage II endometrial cancers? *Obstet Gynecol.* 2011;116(5):1016–1017.

22. Greer BE, Hamberger AD. Treatment of intraperitoneal metastatic adenocarcinoma of the endometrium by the whole-abdomen moving-strip technique and pelvic boost irradiation. *Gynecol Oncol.* 1983; 16(3):365–373.

23. Goff BA, Kato D, Schmidt RA, et al. Uterine papillary serous carcinoma: patterns of metastatic spread. *Gynecol Oncol.* 1994;54(3):264–268.

24. Bristow RE, Duska LR, Montz FJ. The role of cytoreductive surgery in the management of stage IV uterine papillary serous carcinoma. *Gynecol Oncol.* 2001;81(1):92–99.

25. Shih KK, Yun E, Gardner GJ, et al. Surgical cytoreduction in stage IV endometrioid endometrial carcinoma. *Gynecol Oncol.* 2011;122(3): 608–611.

26. Kelly MG, O'Malley DM, Hui P, et al. Improved survival in surgical stage I patients with uterine papillary serous carcinoma (UPSC)

treated with adjuvant platinum-based chemotherapy. *Gynecol Oncol.* 2005;98(3):353–359.

27. Tanner EJ, Leitao MM Jr, Garg K, et al. The role of cytoreductive surgery for newly diagnosed advanced-stage uterine carcinosarcoma. *Gynecol Oncol.* 2011;123(3):548–552.

28. Reed NS, Mangioni C, Malmstrom H, et al. First results of a randomized trial comparing radiotherapy versus observation postoperatively in patients with uterine sarcomas. An EORTC-GCG study. *Int J Gynecol Cancer.* 2003;13:4.

29. Homesley HD, Filiaci V, Markman M. Phase III trial of ifosfamide with or without paclitaxel in advanced uterine carcinosarcoma: a Gynecologic Oncology Group Study. *J Clin Oncol.* 2007; 25(5):526–531.

30. Awtrey CS, Cadungog MG, Leitao MM, et al. Surgical resection of recurrent endometrial carcinoma. *Gynecol Oncol.* 2006;102(3): 480–488.

31. Scudder SA, Liu PY, Wilczynski SP, et al. Paclitaxel and carboplatin with amifostine in advanced, recurrent, or refractory endometrial adenocarcinoma: a phase II study of the Southwest Oncology Group. *Gynecol Oncol.* 2005;96(3):610–615.

32. Thigpen JT, Brady MF, Alvarez RD, et al. Oral medroxyprogesterone acetate in the treatment of advanced or recurrent endometrial carcinoma: a dose-response study by the Gynecologic Oncology Group. *J Clin Oncol.* 1999;17(6):1736–1744.

33. Fleming GF, Sill MW, Darcy KM, et al. Phase II trial of trastuzumab in women with advanced or recurrent, HER2-positive endometrial carcinoma: a Gynecologic Oncology Group study. *Gynecol Oncol.* 2010;116(1):15–20.

34. Barakat RR, Bundy BN, Spirtos NM, et al. Randomized double-blind trial of estrogen replacement therapy versus placebo in stage I or II endometrial cancer: a Gynecologic Oncology Group study. *J Clin Oncol.* 2006;24:587–592.

35. Lewin SN, Herzog TJ, Barrena Medel NI, et al. Comparative performance of the 2009 International Federation of Gynecology and Obstetrics' staging system for uterine corpus cancer. *Obstet Gynecol.* 2010;116(5): 1141–1149.

36. Aalders J, Abeler V, Kolstad P, et al. Postoperative external irradiation and prognostic parameters in stage I endometrial carcinoma: clinical and histopathologic study of 540 patients. *Obstet Gynecol.* 1980;56(4): 419–427.

37. Creutzberg CL, van Putten WL, Koper PC, et al. Surgery and postoperative radiotherapy versus surgery alone for patients with stage-1 endometrial carcinoma: multicentre randomised trial. PORTEC Study Group. Postoperative Radiation Therapy in Endometrial Carcinoma. *Lancet.* 2000;355(9213):1404–1411.

38. Creutzberg CL, Nout RA, Lybeert ML, et al. Fifteen-year radiotherapy outcomes of the randomized PORTEC-1 trial for endometrial carcinoma. *Int J Radiat Oncol Biol Phys.* 2011;81(4):e631–e638.

39. Keys HM, Roberts JA, Brunetto VL, et al. A phase III trial of surgery with or without adjunctive external pelvic radiation therapy in intermediate risk endometrial adenocarcinoma: a Gynecologic Oncology Group study. *Gynecol Oncol.* 2004;92(3):744–751.

40. Nout RA, Smit VT, Putter H, et al. Vaginal brachytherapy versus pelvic external beam radiotherapy for patients with endometrial cancer of high-intermediate risk (PORTEC-2): an open-label, non-inferiority, randomised trial. *Lancet.* 2010;375(9717):816–823.

41. Susumu N, Sagae S, Udagawa Y, et al. Randomized phase III trial of pelvic radiotherapy versus cisplatin-based combined chemotherapy in patients with intermediate- and high-risk endometrial cancer: a Japanese Gynecologic Oncology Group study. *Gynecol Oncol.* 2008;108(1): 226–233.

42. Todo Y, Kato H, Kaneuchi M et al. Survival effect of para-aortic lymphadenectomy in endometrial cancer (SEPAL study): a retrospective cohort analysis. *Lancet.* 2010;375(9721):1165–1172.

43. Cohen CJ, Bruckner HW, Deppe G, et al. Multidrug treatment of advanced and recurrent endometrial carcinoma: a Gynecologic Oncology Group study. *Obstet Gynecol.* 1984;63(5):719–726.

44. Thigpen JT, Blessing JA, DiSaia PJ, et al. A randomized comparison of doxorubicin alone versus doxorubicin plus cyclophosphamide in the management of advanced or recurrent endometrial carcinoma: a Gynecologic Oncology Group study. *J Clin Oncol.* 1994;12(7):1408–1414.

45. Sutton G, Axelrod JH, Bundy BN, et al. Adjuvant whole abdominal irradiation in clinical stages I and II papillary serous or clear cell carcinoma of the endometrium: a phase II study of the Gynecologic Oncology Group. *Gynecol Oncol.* 2006;100(2):349–354.

46. Sutton G, Axelrod JH, Bundy BN, et al. Whole abdominal radiotherapy in the adjuvant treatment of patients with stage III and IV endometrial cancer: a Gynecologic Oncology Group study. *Gynecol Oncol.* 2005;97:755–763.

47. Thigpen JT, Brady MF, Homesley HD, et al. Phase III trial of doxorubicin with or without cisplatin in advanced endometrial carcinoma: a Gynecologic Oncology Group study. *J Clin Oncol.* 2004;22(19):3902–3908.

48. Randall ME, Filiaci VL, Muss H, et al. Randomized phase III trial of whole-abdominal irradiation versus doxorubicin and cisplatin chemotherapy in advanced endometrial carcinoma: a Gynecologic Oncology Group study. *J Clin Oncol.* 2006;24(1):36–44.

49. Gallion HH, Brunetto VL, Cibull M, et al. Randomized phase III trial of standard timed doxorubicin plus cisplatin versus circadian timed doxorubicin plus cisplatin in stage III and IV or recurrent endome-

trial carcinoma: a Gynecologic Oncology Group study. *J Clin Oncol.* 2003;21(20):3808–3813.

50. Fleming GF, Filiaci VL, Bentley RC, et al. Phase III randomized trial of doxorubicin + cisplatin versus doxorubicin + 24-h paclitaxel + filgrastim in endometrial carcinoma: a Gynecologic Oncology Group study. *Ann Oncol.* 2004;15(8):1173–1178.

51. Fleming GF, Brunetto VL, Cella D, et al. Phase III trial of doxorubicin plus cisplatin with or without paclitaxel plus filgrastim in advanced endometrial carcinoma: a Gynecologic Oncology Group study. *J Clin Oncol.* 2004;22(11):2159–2166.

52. Homesley HD, Filiaci V, Gibbons SK, et al. A randomized phase III trial in advanced endometrial carcinoma of surgery and volume directed radiation followed by cisplatin and doxorubicin with or without paclitaxel: a Gynecologic Oncology Group study. *Gynecol Oncol.* 2009;112:543–552.

53. Miller D, Filiaci V, Fleming G, et al. Randomized phase III noninferiority trial of first line chemotherapy for metastatic or recurrent endometrial carcinoma: a Gynecology Oncology Group study. *Gynecol Oncol.* 2012;125:771–773.

54. Mundt AJ, McBride R, Rotmensch J, et al. Significant pelvic recurrence in high-risk pathologic stage I–IV endometrial carcinoma patients after adjuvant chemotherapy alone: implications for adjuvant radiation therapy. *Int J Radiat Oncol Biol Phys.* 2001;50(5):1145–1153.

55. Lincoln S, Blessing JA, Lee RB, et al. Activity of paclitaxel as second-line chemotherapy in endometrial carcinoma: a Gynecologic Oncology Group study. *Gynecol Oncol.* 2003;88(3):277–281.

56. McMeekin DS, Filiaci VL, Thigpen JT, et al. The relationship between histology and outcome in advanced and recurrent endometrial cancer patients participating in first-line chemotherapy trials: a Gynecologic Oncology Group study. *Gynecol Oncol.* 2007;106(1):16–22.

57. Wolfson AH, Brady MF, Rocereto T, et al. A gynecologic oncology group randomized phase III trial of whole abdominal irradiation (WAI) vs. cisplatin-ifosfamide and mesna (CIM) as post-surgical therapy in stage I–IV carcinosarcoma (CS) of the uterus. *Gynecol Oncol.* 2007;107(2):177–185.

58. Homesley HD, Filiaci V, Markman M, et al. Phase III trial of ifosfamide with or without paclitaxel in advanced uterine carcinosarcoma: a Gynecologic Oncology Group study. *J Clin Oncol.* 2007;25(5):526–531.

59. Leitao MM, Sonoda Y, Brennan MF, et al. Incidence of lymph node and ovarian metastasis in leiomyosarcoma of the uterus. *Gynecol Oncol.* 2003;91(1):209–212.

60. Giuntoli RL II, Metzinger DS, DiMarco CS, et al. Retrospective review of 208 patients with leiomyosarcoma of the uterus: prognostic indicators, surgical management, and adjuvant therapy. *Gynecol Oncol.* 2003;89(3):460–469.

61. Kapp DS, Shin JY, Chan JK. Prognostic factors and survival in 1396 patients with uterine leiomyosarcoma: emphasis on impact of lymphadenectomy and oophorectomy. *Cancer.* 2008;112(4):820–830.
62. Goff BA, Rice LW, Fleischhaker D, et al. Uterine leiomyosarcoma and endometrial stromal sarcoma: lymph node metastases and sites of recurrence. *Gynecol Oncol.* 1993;50(1):105–109.
63. O'Cearbhaill R, Hensley ML. Optimal management of uterine leiomyosarcoma. *Expert Rev Anticancer Ther.* 2010;10(2):153–169.
64. Levenback C, Rubin SC, McCormack PM, et al. Resection of pulmonary metastases from uterine sarcomas. *Gynecol Oncol.* 1992;45(2):202–205.
65. Chu MC, Mor G, Lim C, et al. Low-grade endometrial stromal sarcoma: hormonal aspects. *Gynecol Oncol.* 2003;90(1):170–176.

Vulvar Cancer

I. Characteristics

A. Vulvar cancer represents 3% to 5% of all female genital cancers and 1% of all malignancies in women. In 2013, there are 4,700 new cases and 990 deaths predicted. The average age at diagnosis is 65 years old, although it is trending toward a younger age.

B. Clinical features include pruritus, ulceration, or a mass. The most common location of lesions are the labia majora (40%), the labia minora (20%), periclitoral region (10%), and perineal area (15%). The route of spread is either by direct extension, lymphatic embolization to the groin nodes, or lymphatic or hematogenous spread to distant sites.

C. Risk factors are multifactorial: age > 70 years old, lower socioeconomic status, hypertension, diabetes, prior lower genital tract dysplasia or cancer, immunosuppression, and HPV infection are known to increase the risk of vulvar cancer. VIN is the precancerous state and 76% of patients with VIN3 are HPV positive. There is about a 23% rate of subclinical invasive disease in VIN3.

D. Groin LN metastasis: Subclinical LN metastasis can occur in 10% to 36% of normally palpated groins (2). Clinical staging clearly under-stages patients. On the contrary, 20% of palpably enlarged LNs are pathologically negative; 28% of patients with positive groin LNs will have positive pelvic LNs.

E. The risk for nodal metastasis is related to both depth of invasion and tumor size. The risk of positive LNs with 1 mm DOI is minimal at < 1%. For a DOI of 2 mm, the risk is 7% to 8%. For a DOI of 3 mm, the risk is 12% to 17%. For a DOI of 5 mm, there is a 15% to 17% risk of LN metastasis. The risk of LN metastasis by lesion size is significant: for a size of 0 to 1 cm, there is a 7.7% risk of positive LNs; for a 2-cm lesion, the risk is 22%; for a 3-cm lesion, the risk is 27%; and for a 5-cm lesion, the risk is 35% to 40% (3).

II. Workup

A. Pretreatment workup includes a physical exam with careful evaluation of the vagina and cervix. 5% of invasive lesions are multifocal. Biopsy for diagnosis should occur at the center of any suspicious area.

B. Imaging with CT, MRI, or PET can be obtained if positive groin or pelvic LNs are suspected. Chest x-ray should be obtained, as well as standard lab tests. Proctoscopy can be helpful if there is a large lesion impinging on the posterior perineal triangle or anus.

C. If the groin lymph nodes appear positive, FNA can be considered prior to a groin LN dissection. If cytology from the FNA is positive, then aggressive surgical removal of bulky LNs should be considered because the usual doses of external beam radiation are not adequate to control large volume disease. There is no need to perform a complete LN dissection in light of bulky LNs; instead, remove the bulky disease and mark the area with hemoclips prior to radiotherapy. If the LNs are fixed and unresectable, consider neoadjuvant chemotherapy and radiation.

D. The workup for melanoma is CT of the chest/abdomen/pelvis, MRI of the brain, LDH, and baseline PET. *BRAFV600E* gene mutation information should be obtained via immunohistochemistry on the tumor.

III. Histology

A. Squamous cell carcinoma represents 85% of all vulvar cancers.

B. Malignant melanoma represents 5% of vulvar cancers. There are 4 histologic subtypes of melanoma: superficial spreading, lentigo, acral, and nodular.

C. Other types are basal cell carcinoma, adenocarcinoma, sarcoma, and verrucous carcinoma.

D. Vulvar Paget's disease has cutaneous and noncutaneous (bladder/colorectal) subtypes. Underlying invasive adenocarcinoma is present in 4% to 17% of cases; 30% to 42% of patients may have or will later develop an adenocarcinoma at another nonvulvar location such as the breast, rectum, colon, or uterus.

E. Grading: GOG grading in vulvar cancer is slightly different than for other tumors. G1 tumors are well differentiated, G2 tumors are composed of less than one-third of G3 cells. G3 tumors are composed of greater than one-third yet less than one-half of G3 cells. G4 tumors have greater than one-half of the tumor composed of G3 cells.

F. The depth of invasion is measured from the epithelial-stromal junction of the adjacent most superficial dermal papilla to the deepest point of invasion.

IV. **Staging**: Vulvar cancer is staged surgically.

  A. FIGO 2009 staging is as follows:

  Stage I:

  - IA: Lesions ≤ 2 cm in size, confined to the vulva or perineum and with stromal invasion ≤ 1.0 mm, no nodal metastasis
  - IB: Lesions < 2 cm in size or with stromal invasion < 1.0 mm, confined to the vulva or perineum, with negative nodes

  Stage 2: Any sized lesion involving the lower one-third of the vagina, urethra, or anus

  Stage 3: Positive LN

  - 3A: 1 LN with metastasis greater than 5 mm or 1 to 2 LNs with metastasis less than 5 mm each
  - 3B: 2 LNs with metastasis greater than 5 mm or 3+ LNs each with metastasis less than 5 mm
  - 3C: Extracapsular involvement of any number of LNs

  Stage 4:

  - 4A:
    - 4A1: upper two-thirds involvement of the vagina, urethra, or anus
    - 4A2: fixed or ulcerated LN
  - 4B: distant metastases including pelvic LN

  B. AJCC Staging Vulvar Cancer

  1. Primary Tumor (T):

  - TX: Primary tumor cannot be assessed
  - T0: No evidence of primary tumor
  - T1:
    - T1a: Lesion less than 2 cm in size, confined to the vulva or perineum and with stromal invasion ≤ 1.0 mm

- T1b: Lesions > 2 cm in size or any size with stromal invasion > 1.0 mm, confined to the vulva or perineum

- T2: Tumor of any size with extension to adjacent perineal structures: lower/distal one-third urethra, lower/distal one-third vagina, anal involvement

- T3: Tumor of any size with extension to any of the following: upper/proximal two-thirds urethra, upper/proximal two-thirds vagina, bladder mucosa, rectal mucosa, or fixed to pelvic bone

2. Regional LNs (N):
   - NX: Regional LN cannot be assessed
   - N0: No regional LN metastasis
   - N1: 1 or 2 regional LNs with the following features
     - N1a: 1 or 2 LNs metastases each 5 mm or less
     - N1b: 1 LN metastasis 5 mm or greater
   - N2: Regional LN metastasis with the following features:
     - N2a: 3 or more LNs metastases each less than 5 mm
     - N2b: 2 or more LNs metastases 5 mm or greater
     - N2c: LN metastasis with extracapsular spread
   - N3: Fixed or ulcerated regional LN metastasis

3. Distant metastasis (M):
   - M0: No distant metastasis
   - M1: Distant metastasis (including pelvic LN metastasis)

4. TNM Stage Grouping
   - Stage I:
     - Stage IA: T1a N0 M0
     - Stage IB: T1b N0 M0
   - Stage II: T2 N0 M0
   - Stage III:
     - Stage IIIA: T1, T2 N1a, N1b M0
     - Stage IIIB: T1, T2 N2a, N2b M0
     - Stage IIIC: T1, T2 N2c M0
   - Stage IV:
     - Stage IVA: T1, T2 N3 M0

- T3 any N M0
- Stage IVB: Any T any N M1

C. Melanoma is surgically staged in a similar fashion. There are a few different methods of staging. Stage is the most important prognostic factor. Breslow's staging is used by the AJCC because it is more reproducible and better for ulcerated lesions.

1. Stage:

Stage	Clark's Level	Chung's Level	Breslow's Level/Depth
I	Intraepithelial	Intraepithelial	< 0.76 mm
II	Papillary dermis	< 1 mm from granular layer	0.76–1.5 mm
III	Fills dermal papillae	1.1–2 mm from granular layer	1.51–2.25 mm
IV	Reticular layer	> 2 mm from granular layer	2.266–3 mm
V	Subcutaneous fat	Subcutaneous fat	> 3 mm

2. Chung's staging has replaced Clark's staging because it does not take into account that vulvar skin is non-hair-bearing and contains less subcutaneous tissue.

3. Melanoma AJCC Staging

a. Primary tumor (T):

- TX: Primary tumor cannot be assessed
- T0: No evidence of primary tumor
- T1: Melanomas < 1.0 mm in thickness
  - T1a: without ulceration and mitoses < $1/mm^2$
  - T1b: with ulceration or mitoses > $1/mm^2$
- T2: Melanomas 1.01 to 2.0 mm
  - T2a: without ulceration
  - T2b: with ulceration
- T3: Melanomas 2.01 to 4.0 mm
  - T3a: without ulceration
  - T3b: with ulceration
- T4: Melanomas > 4.0 mm

- T4a: without ulceration
- T4b: with ulceration

b. Regional LN (N):

- Nx: Regional LN cannot be assessed
- N0: No regional LN metastasis
- N1: 1 node
  - N1a: micrometastasis*
  - N1b: macrometastasis**
- N2: 2 to 3 nodes
  - N2a: micrometastasis*
  - N2b: macrometastasis**
  - N2c: in transit metastasis *without* metastatic nodes
  - N3: 4 or more metastatic nodes, or matted nodes, or in transit metastases/satellite(s) *with* metastatic node(s)

*Micrometastases are diagnosed after sentinel LN biopsy and completion lymphadenectomy (if performed).

**Macrometastases are defined as clinically detectable nodal metastases confirmed by therapeutic lymphadenectomy or when nodal metastasis exhibits gross extracapsular extension.

c. Metastasis (M):

- M0: No distant metastasis (no pathologic M0; use clinical M to complete stage group)
  - M1a: Metastases to skin, subcutaneous tissues, or distant LNs
  - M1b: Metastases to lung
  - M1c: Metastases to all other visceral sites or distant metastases to any site combined with an elevated serum LDH

d. TNM Stage Grouping

- Stage I:
  - Stage IA: T1a N0 M0
  - Stage IB: T1b N0 M0
    T2a N0 M0

- Stage II
  - Stage IIA: T2b N0 M0
    T3a N0 M0
  - Stage IIB: T3b N0 M0
    T4a N0 M0
  - Stage IIC: T4b N0 M0
- Stage III
  - Stage IIIA: T1 – 4a N1a M0
    T1 – 4a N2a M0
  - Stage IIIB: T1 – 4b N1a M0

    T1 – 4b N2a M0

    T1 – 4a N1b M0

    T1 – 4a N2b M0

    T1 – 4a N2c M0
  - Stage IIIC: T1 – 4b N1b M0

    T1 – 4b N2b M0

    T1 – 4b N2c M0

    Any T N3 M0
  - Stage IV: Any T Any N M1

V. Treatment

A. Management of squamous cell and adenocarcinomas is wide radical excision (radical hemi/vulvectomy) with a 2-cm gross margin and groin LN dissection. For lesions that invade less than a depth of 1 mm, a groin LND can be omitted. If the lesion is lateral (more than 1 cm from the midline), dissection of the contralateral groin can be omitted. If the lesion is midline, or within 1 cm of a midline structure, a bilateral groin LN dissection should be performed. For T4 lesions, a radical vulvectomy with bilateral groin LN dissection or a pelvic exenteration can be considered. Neoadjuvant combination chemotherapy and radiation therapy should also be considered for these advanced-stage patients.

B. The femoral triangle is anatomically bordered by the inguinal ligament superiorly, the sartorius muscle laterally, and the adductor longus muscle medially. The incision site for the groin LND starts 2 cm below a line drawn between the ASIS and the pubic tubercle. The skin flap is preserved. The upper flap is dissected toward the inguinal ligament. The LN-bearing tissue, which is attached to the inguinal ligament, is removed, and the superficial epigastric and superficial circumflex vessels should to be ligated. The lower flap is then dissected. The saphenous vein, which runs through the medial aspect of the triangle, should be conserved, and its tributaries ligated.

C. If an **ipsilateral groin LN** is found to be positive at final pathology for a unilateral tumor, management of the contralateral groin should be considered. Options include dissection of the contralateral groin, adjuvant bilateral groin and pelvic radiation, or a combination of contralateral groin LN dissection and if negative, unilateral groin/pelvic radiation.

D. The risk of contralateral positive LN with a negative ipsilateral groin LN dissection is between 0.4% and 2.6%. GOG 74 demonstrated a 2.4% risk of isolated contralateral positive LNs in tumors 2 cm or less in size. If the DOI was less than 5 mm, contralateral LN metastasis occurred in 1.2% (4). Contralateral positive LNs have been found in 0.9% of patients if the tumor was less than 2 cm wide (5). In another study, a 1.8% rate of positive contralateral LNs was demonstrated if the ipsilateral groin LNs were found to be negative. In no patients were contralateral positive groin LNs found if the tumor was less than 2 cm wide and invasion was less than 5 mm (6).

E. Sentinel groin LN dissection can potentially decrease the extent and complication rate of the groin LN dissection. The combined sequenced injection of Technetium-99m (^{99m}Tc) radiolabeled albumin and blue dye to the primary tumor, followed by intraoperative scintillation, has proven sensitive and specific enough for sentinel node identification. If frozen section is positive for LN metastasis, a complete groin LND should be performed.

F. There is a relationship between margin status and recurrence. Heaps et al. (7) reported on margin status: if there was less than 8 mm of fixed tumor-free tissue at resection, 13 of 23 patients recurred locally, whereas if the margins were greater than 8 mm, only 8 of 112 patients recurred. Thus, for positive or close margins, adjuvant radiation therapy to vulva can decrease the local recurrence rate. Those treated with adjuvant radiation therapy had a 44% recurrence rate vs. those observed who had a 75% recurrent rate (8). Tumor thickness greater than 5 mm, or LVSI, may also be indications for adjuvant local radiation.

G. Adjuvant groin and whole pelvic radiation therapy is indicated for FIGO Stages 3B, 3C, and 4A. Concurrent radiosensitizing cisplatin chemotherapy should be considered, following cervical cancer protocols, as the power for a randomized trial in vulvar cancer will not likely be achieved.

H. Basal cell carcinomas are rarely metastatic. Treatment is with excisional biopsy to include a minimum margin of 1 cm.

I. Verrucous carcinoma is locally invasive and rarely metastasizes. Treatment is wide radical excision. Radiation therapy is commonly avoided.

J. Vulvar sarcomas are also treated with wide radical excision. Combination chemotherapy and radiation may assist in disease management.

K. Vulvar melanoma patients should undergo a wide radical excision with bilateral groin LND.

   1. There is data to suggest that radical surgery vs. wide local excision yields no difference in overall survival (9).

   2. LN dissection in vulvar melanoma is of prognostic indication only, it is not therapeutic. Removal of enlarged nodes is adequate treatment.

   3. Margins: The surgically desired margin for in situ disease is 0.5 mm; for a 1-mm thick tumor, a 1-cm margin; for a 1.01- to 2-mm thick lesion, a 1- to 2-cm margin; for 2.01- to 4-mm thick lesions, a 2-cm margin; and for a lesion greater than 4-mm thick, a 2-cm margin.

   4. Most failures are distant.

   5. AJCC stage is the most important prognostic factor.

   6. Adjuvant therapy for vulvar melanoma can be single-agent chemotherapy including dacarbazine, temozolomide, cisplatin, vinblastine, or paclitaxel. Combination chemotherapy can consist of cisplatin and paclitaxel.

   7. Biological agents can be used with standard cytotoxic drugs or alone. Biologicals include ipilimumab, alpha-interferon, and vemurafenib.

L. Paget's disease:

1. For noncutaneous vulvar Paget's disease, there is no benefit to an extensive resection or deep vulvectomy.

2. For cutaneous vulvar Paget's, a simple wide resection is recommended, with a 1-cm clinically negative margin. The risk of recurrence is 34% at 3 years. Frozen section of the margins has not been found to be better than visual inspection (false-negative rate 35%–38%). Permanent section margin status also did not predict recurrence: with 33% recurrence if negative margins vs. 40% recurrence if positive margins (10).

M. There are complications of a radical vulvectomy and groin LN dissection. The wound infection rate is 29%. The wound breakdown rate is 38% for triple incision surgery vs. 68% for en-bloc resection. Lymphedema occurs at a rate of 7% to 19%. Lymphocysts occur at a rate of 7% to 28%. Cellulitis or lymphangitis can occur due to beta streptococcus. Prophylactic antibiotics are warranted in patients with chronic lymphedema and if prone to cellulitis. Nerve injuries or paresthesias can also occur.

VI. Recurrence

A. The risk for local recurrence is close surgical margins. There is data to support that an 8-mm fixed margin (a 1-cm fresh margin) is adequate to diminish local recurrence from 50% if margins were less than 8 mm, to 0% if margins were greater than 8 mm. Surgical margins of 2 cm are still recommended, but if anatomy does not permit, a 1-cm margin can be adequate (7). Farias-Eisner et al. (11) looked at radical local excision and LND for Stages I and II vulvar cancers, and found that radical local excision had the same survival as those treated more radically, and LN status had the largest impact on survival (98% OS if negative nodes were identified vs. 45% if positive nodes were found).

B. For local recurrence, a radical wide local excision should be preformed with additional radiotherapy given, if not done previously. Concurrent cisplatin chemotherapy should be considered.

C. Isolated perineal recurrences can be cured 75% of the time with surgery. If the recurrence is regional, a pelvic exenteration can be considered.

D. If distant metastases are identified on comprehensive workup, palliative chemotherapy and/or radiation therapy should be considered.

E. For LN recurrence in melanoma, pathology should be confirmed via biopsy, and imaging should also be obtained with PET/CT or CT of the chest/abdomen/pelvis. If the LN recurrence is in the groin, the entire LN basin should be dissected if not previously performed, and the enlarged LN should be resected. If a prior LN dissection was performed, removal of the node itself is adequate. If the disease is completely resected, radiation, alpha interferon, and/or a clinical trial can be offered. If the disease is unresectable, systemic therapy, radiation, or a clinical trial can be offered. If there are clinically positive superficial LNs or there are 3 or greater positive LNs, iliac and obturator LN dissection should be considered.

VII. Survival: The 2-year survival (YS) for patients with positive groin LN is 68%, and for those with positive pelvic LN is 23%.

    A. 5-year survival

        Stage I: 95%

        Stage II: 75% to 85%

        Stage III: 55%

        Stage IVA: 20%

        Stage IVB: 5%

VIII. Follow-up

    A. Every 3 months for the first 2 years

        Every 6 months for the next 3 years

        Annual visits thereafter

NOTABLE STUDIES

    A. GOG 36 (12,13): This surgical pathology study evaluated 637 patients with vulvar cancer, all of whom had tumors of less than 5 mm DOI. Risk factors for local recurrence and LN metastasis were studied. Multivariate risk factors that were predictive of groin LN metastasis were: tumor size < 2 cm (18.9% + LN); > 2 cm (41.6% + LN). Independent predictors of groin LN metastasis were: tumor grade, LVSI, depth of invasion, age, and fixed or ulcerated LN. A clinically negative groin examination had a false-negative rate of 23.9%. Those patients in

GOG 36 who were identified with positive groin LNs were randomized to GOG 37.

B. GOG 37 (14): This study identified 114 patients with positive groin LNs after a radical vulvectomy and bilateral groin LND, and randomized them to an ipsilateral pelvic LN dissection or to groin and pelvic radiation therapy. The radiation was dosed at 45 to 50 Gy. 5% recurred in the radiation group, and 24% recurred in the pelvic LND group. The 2 YS was 68% for those treated with groin and pelvic radiotherapy vs. 54% for those who received the pelvic LN dissection. The number of positive LNs influenced survival: 1 positive LN yielded an 80% OS, whereas 4 or more positive LNs had a 27% OS. The incidence of positive pelvic LNs if groin LNs were positive was 28%. There was a 9% incidence of local vulvar recurrence in both arms.

C. Follow-up to GOG 37 (15): The 6 YS for patients who received radiation was 61% vs. 41% for those who received pelvic LN dissection. The 6 YS for cancer-related deaths was 51% vs. 29% for the pelvic radiation vs. pelvic LND groups, respectively, HR = 0.49. Poor prognostic factors were clinically suspicious or fixed LNs, or > 2 positive groin LNs. A ratio of 20% positive LNs to total LNs was associated with contralateral metastasis, relapse, and cancer-related death.

D. GOG 74 (4,16): This study surgically evaluated the outcomes of 143 patients with early-stage vulvar tumors who underwent a superficial groin LN dissection with a modified radical vulvectomy. Overall, 7% developed isolated groin recurrences, and of those with a groin recurrence, 91.7% died. The median time to recurrence in the vulva was 35.9 months, and 7 months for recurrence in the groin. The median survival time after recurrence was 52.4 months for vulvar recurrence and 9.4 months for groin recurrence. This study is criticized for a high number of grade 3 tumors (28%) and that of the 9 groin recurrences, 3 were in an undissected groin (patients who refused groin dissection).

E. GOG 88 (17): Because patients in GOG 37 with positive groin LNs had favorable outcomes with radiotherapy, the question as to whether a groin LND was necessary if prophylactic radiation was administered was investigated. This study evaluated 50 patients after a radical vulvectomy and randomized them to prophylactic groin radiation or to groin LND. In this study, 0 out of 25 patients recurred if a LN dissection was performed, followed by radiation for positive LN (of which 20% were indeed positive), vs. an 18.5% recurrence if prophylactic groin radiation was administered to an undissected groin with therefore an unknown LN status. Criticisms of this study were (18): underdosing of the groins as the dose prescription point was to 3 cm and upon review, the average vessel depth was 6.1 cm (range 2 to 18.6 cm) with an average BMI of 25.6.

F. GOG 101 (19): This study evaluated 73 patients with T3 or T4 disease treated with neoadjuvant chemotherapy and radiation therapy. The radiation dose was 47.6 Gy given in 1.7 Gy fractions as a hyperfractionated split dose regimen with 2 concurrent cycles of cisplatin and 5-FU. 69 of 71 women were converted to a resectable status, with 68 patients keeping urinary and fecal capacity. 47% (33 of 71) had a CCR and 70% of these were CPR. 2.8% remained unresectable. There was a 55% OS. A companion study to GOG 101 (20) was done for patients with unresectable positive groin LNs (N2/3 nodes); 38 of 40 patients became resectable, with 15 of 37 patients having a CPR. Overall, 29 of 38 patients had local control of their disease. 19 patients recurred: 9 locally and 8 distant.

G. GOG 205 (21): This study evaluated 58 patients with T3 or T4 disease treated with neoadjuvant chemotherapy and radiation therapy. Radiation therapy was dosed at 57.6 Gy with concurrent weekly cisplatin dosed at 40 mg/m². Surgical resection followed for residual tumor (or biopsy to confirm CCR). 64% of patients had a CCR (37 of 58) and 78% of these had a CPR. In this study there was no hyperfractionation, no midtreatment break, and no 5-FU. Management of the groin LNs in these studies was standardized. Clinically negative or resectable groin LNs underwent groin LN dissection prior to neoadjuvant therapy. If there were unresectable groin LNs, the groin dissection was performed after neoadjuvant therapy.

H. GOG 173 (22): In this study, 452 eligible patients with a tumor size ≥ 2 cm, ≤ 6 cm, and with at least 1-mm invasion underwent radical vulvectomy with groin lymphatic mapping. 772 groin dissections were performed. A sentinel lymph node (SLN) was identified in 418 of 452 patients. LN metastases were found in 132 of 418 patients (31.6%). The SLN was positive in 121 of 418 patients. 11 patients with a negative SLN were found to have positive LNs identified on final complete dissection pathology. The sensitivity of SLNB was 91.7%. In patients with tumors < 4 cm, the false-negative rate was 2%.

I. DiSaia et al. (23) recommended omitting the deep LND to decrease morbidity without compromising survival. 50 Stage I patients with negative superficial nodes were retrospectively reviewed. No deep LND was performed. There were no recurrences after 12 months.

J. GROINSS V (24): This study evaluated 403 patients. 623 groin dissections were performed. All tumors were squamous and less than 4 cm in size. A radical vulvectomy and sentinal groin LND were performed in all patients. Follow-up was 35 months. A combination of radioactive tracer and blue dye was used. Of 259 patients with unifocal vulvar disease and a negative sentinel node (median follow-up time, 35 months), 6 had groin recurrences diagnosed, for a false-negative rate of 2.3%. The 3 YS rate was 97%. The short-term morbidity was decreased in the SLN patients compared with those patients with a positive sentinel node who underwent a complete inguinofemoral lymphadenectomy. Wound breakdown in the groin was 11.7% vs. 34.0%, and cellulitis occurred at 4.5% vs. 21.3%. The long-term morbidity was also less with recurrent erysipelas occurring at a rate of 0.4% vs. 16.2%, and lymphedema of the legs seen in 1.9% vs. 25.2% of patients.

K. Vemurafenib (25) is an antibody against the *BRAF* receptor. The V600E mutation occurs in some melanomas and constitutively activates the *BRAF* gene. In a randomized trial of 675 untreated metastatic melanoma patients Stage IIIc or IV, who were *BRAF* V600E positive, vemurafenib was compared to dacarbazine. Vemurafenib was dosed at 960 mg orally twice daily and dacarbazine at 1000 mg/m^2 intravenously every 3 weeks. The 6-month overall survival was 84% in the vemurafenib group and 64% in the dacarbazine group. Response rates were 48% for vemurafenib and 5% for dacarbazine.

REFERENCES

1. Modesitt SC, Waters AB, Walton L, et al. Vulvar intraepithelial neoplasia III: occult cancer and the impact of margin status on recurrence. *Obstet Gynecol.* 1998;92(6):962–966.
2. Iversen T, Aalders JG, Christensen A, et al. Squamous cell carcinoma of the vulva: a review of 424 patients, 1956–1974. *Gynecol Oncol.* 1980;9(3):271–279.

3. Gonzalez Bosquet J, Kinney WK, Russell AH, et al. Risk of occult inguinofemoral lymph node metastasis from squamous carcinoma of the vulva. *Int J Radiat Oncol Biol Phys.* 2003;57(2):419–424.
4. Stehman FB, Bundy BN, Dvoretsky PM, et al. Early stage I carcinoma of the vulva treated with ipsilateral superficial inguinal lymphadenectomy and modified radical hemivulvectomy: a prospective study of the Gynecologic Oncology Group. *Obstet Gynecol.* 1992;79(4):490–497.
5. de Hullu JA, van der Zee AG. Surgery and radiotherapy in vulvar cancer. *Crit Rev Oncol Hematol.* 2006;60(1):38–58.
6. Gonzalez Bosquet J, Magrina JF, Magtibay PM, et al. Patterns of inguinal groin metastases in squamous cell carcinoma of the vulva. *Gynecol Oncol.* 2007;105(3):742–746.
7. Heaps JM, Fu YS, Montz FJ, et al. Surgical-pathologic variables predictive of local recurrence in squamous cell carcinoma of the vulva. *Gynecol Oncol.* 1990;38(3):309–314.
8. Faul CM, Mirmow D, Huang Q, et al. Adjuvant radiation for vulvar carcinoma: improved local control. *Int J Radiat Oncol Biol Phys.* 1997;38(2):381–389.
9. Trimble EL, Lewis JL Jr, Williams LL, et al. Management of vulvar melanoma. *Gynecol Oncol.* 1992;45(3):254–258.
10. Fishman DA, Chambers SK, Schwartz PE, et al. Extramammary Paget's disease of the vulva. *Gynecol Oncol.* 1995;56(2):266–270.
11. Farias-Eisner R, Cirisano FD, Grouse D, et al. Conservative and individualized surgery for early squamous carcinoma of the vulva: the treatment of choice for stage I and II (T1-2N0-1M0) disease. *Gynecol Oncol.* 1994;53(1):55–58.
12. Homesley HD, Bundy BN, Sedlis A, et al. Assessment of current International Federation of Gynecology and Obstetrics staging of vulvar carcinoma relative to prognostic factors for survival (a Gynecologic Oncology Group study). *Am J Obstet Gynecol.* 1991;164(4):997–1003; discussion 1003–1004.
13. Homesley HD, Bundy BN, Sedlis A, et al. Prognostic factors for groin node metastasis in squamous cell carcinoma of the vulva (a Gynecologic Oncology Group study). *Gynecol Oncol.* 1993;49(3):279–283.
14. Homesley HD, Bundy BN, Sedlis A, et al. Radiation therapy versus pelvic node resection for carcinoma of the vulva with positive groin nodes. *Obstet Gynecol.* 1986;68(6):733–740.
15. Kunos C, Simpkins F, Gibbons H, et al. Radiation therapy compared with pelvic node resection for node-positive vulvar cancer: a randomized controlled trial. *Obstet Gynecol.* 2009;114(3):537–546.
16. Stehman FB, Bundy BN, Ball H, et al. Sites of failure and times to failure in carcinoma of the vulva treated conservatively: a Gynecologic Oncology Group study. *Am J Obstet Gynecol.* 1996;174(4):1128–1132; discussion 1132–1133.

17. Stehman FB, Bundy BN, Thomas G, et al. Groin dissection versus groin radiation in carcinoma of the vulva: a Gynecologic Oncology Group study. *Int J Radiat Oncol Biol Phys.* 1992;24(2):389–396.

18. Koh WJ, Chiu M, Stelzer KJ, et al. Femoral vessel depth and the implications for groin node radiation. *Int J Radiat Oncol Biol Phys.* 1993;27(4):969–974.

19. Moore DH, Thomas GM, Montana GS, et al. Preoperative chemoradiation for advanced vulvar cancer: a phase II study of the Gynecologic Oncology Group. *Int J Radiat Oncol Biol Phys.* 1998;42(1):79–85.

20. Montana GS, Thomas GM, Moore DH, et al. Preoperative chemo-radiation for carcinoma of the vulva with N2/N3 nodes: a Gynecologic Oncology Group study. *Int J Radiat Oncol Biol Phys.* 2000;48(4):1007–1013.

21. Moore DH, Ali S, Koh WJ, et al. A phase II trial of radiation therapy and weekly cisplatin chemotherapy for the treatment of locally-advanced squamous cell carcinoma of the vulva: a Gynecologic Oncology Group study. *Gynecol Oncol.* 2012;124(3):529–533.

22. Levenback CF, Ali S, Coleman RL, et al. Lymphatic mapping and sentinel lymph node biopsy in women with squamous cell carcinoma of the vulva: a Gynecologic Oncology Group study. *J Clin Oncol.* 2012;30(31):3786–3791.

23. DiSaia PJ, Creasman WT, Rich WM. An alternate approach to early cancer of the vulva. *Am J Obstet Gynecol.* 1979;133(7):825–832.

24. van der Zee AG, Oonk MH, de Hullu JA, et al. Sentinel node dissection is safe in the treatment of early-stage vulvar cancer. *J Clin Oncol.* 2008;26(6):884–889.

25. Chapman PB, Hauschild A, Robert C, et al. Improved survival with vemurafenib in melanoma with BRAF V600E mutation. *N Engl J Med.* 2011;364(26):2507–2516.

Vaginal Cancer

I. Characteristics

A. Vaginal cancer represents 1% to 2% of all female genital tract malignancies. The median age at diagnosis is 60 years old. Most vaginal cancers are metastatic lesions from other sites, including the cervix, uterus, breast, gestational trophoblastic disease, and the GI tract. Primary vaginal cancers are commonly found in the upper one-third of the vagina, often in the posterior fornix. There are 2,890 new cases and 840 deaths estimated for 2013.

B. Symptoms include vaginal discharge, vaginal bleeding, tenesmus, pelvic pain, bladder irritation, and pelvic fullness.

C. If the patient has a history of uterine, cervical, or vulvar cancer, the vaginal lesion is considered a recurrent cancer unless proven otherwise by discriminating pathology or greater than 5 years have intervally passed since prior diagnosis.

D. Risk factors for vaginal cancer include HPV infection, chronic vaginal irritation, prior treatment for cervical cancer, prior CIN, and a history of in-utero exposure to DES.

E. DES was used from 1940 to 1971. Vaginal adenosis and vaginal adenocarcinoma are characteristics of exposure. Other physical representations are a cockscomb cervix. The risk of clear cell carcinoma is 1:1000 with a history of DES. The peak age at diagnosis was 19 years. Surveillance for women who were exposed includes Pap smears and colposcopy with indicated biopsies every 6 months to 1 year starting at the age of 16 years old, continuing indefinitely.

F. The route of spread is direct, lymphatic, or hematogenous. The route of lymphatic spread depends on the location of the lesion. If the lesion is in the upper two-thirds of the vagina, metastasis is often directly to the pelvic lymph nodes. If the lesion is in the lower one-third of the vagina, metastasis can often be to the inguinal-femoral lymph nodes, and/or to pelvic lymph nodes. Hematogenous spread often occurs late in the disease process.

G. The most important prognostic factor is stage of disease. Age is also an important factor. Melanomas and sarcomas have the worst prognosis. Lesions of the distal vagina tend to have a worse prognosis than proximal lesions. Size less than 3 cm has a better prognosis than if larger than 5 cm. LN status also confers prognosis, with a 5 YS of 33% for positive lymph nodes compared to 56% for negative LNs.

II. Pretreatment Workup

The pretreatment workup is colposcopy of the entire genital tract and physical examination. Diagnosis is via biopsy often guided with colposcopy. It may be necessary to perform an examination under anesthesia with cystoscopy and proctoscopy. These procedures may also help with initial staging. Chest x-ray, IVP, cystoscopy, proctoscopy, and barium enema are FIGO-approved diagnostic studies. CT, MRI, and PET imaging may assist in evaluation and for extent of disease.

III. Histology

A. 80% of vaginal cancers are of squamous cell histology.

B. 5% to 9% are adenocarcinomas.

C. Malignant melanoma represents 2.8% to 5% of vaginal neoplasms. Vaginal melanomas are more often found in the lower one-third of the vagina.

D. Rhabdomyosarcoma is usually found as the botryoid variant of embryonal rhabdomyosarcoma and is the most common malignant tumor of the vagina in infants and children; 90% of patients are younger than 5 years of age. On clinical examination, grape-like edematous masses may protrude from the vagina. The histologic pearl is the presence of a cambium layer beneath an intact vaginal epithelium.

E. Leiomyosarcoma can also be found, and this can occur in women with a prior history of radiotherapy.

IV. Staging: Staging continues to be clinical, closely following cervical cancer parameters.

A. FIGO Staging

Stage I: Limited to the vaginal wall

Stage II: Involves subvaginal tissue, does not extend to the pelvic wall.

Some practitioners consider:

- Stage IIA: without parametrial involvement
- Stage IIB: with parametrial involvement

Stage III: Extension to the pelvic wall

Stage IV: Invading adjacent pelvic organs or distant metastasis

- IVA: Involves the bladder or rectal mucosa
- IVB: Disease is beyond the true pelvis, metastasis to distant organs

B. AJCC Staging

Primary tumor (T):

- TX: Primary tumor cannot be assessed
- T0: No evidence of primary tumor
- T1: I Tumor confined to vagina
- T2: II Tumor invades paravaginal tissues but not to pelvic wall
- T3: III Tumor extends to pelvic wall*
- T4: IVA Tumor invades mucosa of the bladder or rectum and/or extends beyond the true pelvis (bullous edema is not sufficient evidence to classify a tumor as T4)

  *Pelvic wall is defined as muscle, fascia, neurovascular structures, or skeletal portions of the bony pelvis.

Regional LN (N):

Pelvic or inguinal lymph node metastasis

- NX: Regional lymph nodes cannot be assessed
- N0: No regional lymph node metastasis
- N1: Regional lymph node metastasis (pelvic or inguinal)

Distant metastasis (M)

- M0: No distant metastasis (no pathologic M0; use clinical M to complete stage group)
- M1: IVB Distant metastasis

TNM Stage Grouping

- Stage I: T1 N0 M0
- Stage II: T2 N0 M0
- Stage III: T1–T3 N1 M0
- T3 N0 M0
- Stage IV:
  - IVA: T4 any N M0
  - IVB: Any T any N M1

V. Treatment: Treatment depends on the location and depth of the lesion, the stage of the cancer, and medical comorbidities.

A. Treatment for Stage I squamous cell or adenocarcinomas that involve the upper two-thirds of the vagina can include a radical hysterectomy with upper vaginectomy and LN dissection, or an upper vaginectomy and parametrectomy with LN dissection if the uterus has previously been removed. Radiation without surgery has equivalent outcomes. Concurrent platinum-based chemotherapy has been adopted to follow cervical cancer guidelines. If the lower one-third of the vagina is involved, external beam radiotherapy fields should include the groins. Dosing is 50.4 Gy to a total of 80 to 85 Gy with interstitial or Fletcher-Suit brachytherapy.

B. Treatment for Stages II, III, and IV is definitive radiotherapy with concurrent platinum-based chemotherapy. If the lesion size is 2 cm or greater, surgical resection can be considered to potentially optimize radiotherapy. Radiotherapy usually includes external beam radiation and intracavitary or interstitial therapy to a total dose of 85–90 Gy. If the lower one-third of the vagina is involved, the groins should also be irradiated.

C. Treatment for melanoma is radical surgical resection if possible. Exenterative surgery has not been found to provide additional survival benefit. Chemotherapy with biologic therapy may provide adjuvant benefits.

D. The treatment of rhabdomyosarcoma is usually multimodal with therapy consisting of surgical resection, radiation, and systemic chemotherapy. Commonly used agents are vincristine, actinomycin, and cyclophosphamide. Another regimen is cyclophosphamide, doxorubicin, and DTIC.

E. Leiomyosarcoma is treated with radical surgical resection and the consideration of adjuvant radiation and/or chemotherapy.

VI. Recurrent Disease: If recurrent disease is identified, a full metastatic workup should be employed. If only local disease is confirmed, a wide local excision or a partial (radical) vaginectomy can be performed. If central disease is identified, a pelvic exenteration can be considered. If there is distant metastasis, chemotherapy with or without radiation can be considered.

VII. Survival

    A. 5-year survival

        Stage I: 80%

        Stage II: 45%

        Stage III: 35%

        Stage IV: 10%

VIII. Follow-up

    A. Physical and pelvic examinations are recommended: A Pap smear may help with detection of recurrence.

    Every 3 months for the first 2 years

    Every 6 months for the next 3 years

    Annual examinations thereafter

Gestational Trophoblastic Disease

I. Characteristics

A. Gestational trophoblastic disease (GTD) describes a group of tumors that arise from trophoblastic cells. This is usually the result of an abnormal fertilization event and includes molar pregnancy, choriocarcinoma, and placental site trophoblastic tumor.

B. Hydatidiform molar pregnancy occurs in approximately 1 out of 1,000 pregnancies in North America. Clinical features of a mole are vaginal bleeding in the first trimester or early second trimester; uterine size large for dates; ovarian theca-lutein cysts (seen in 46% of patients, 2% of which may torse); early preeclampsia < 20 weeks (12%–17%); hyperthyroidism due to the similarity between the alpha subunit of both hCG and TSH hormones; hyperemesis gravidarum (20%); passage of vesicles per vagina; and respiratory complaints due to tumor emboli or increased progesterone (27%).

C. Risk factors for a molar pregnancy include age (< 20 years or > 40 years of age), history of a prior mole, and Asian ethnicity.

D. The WHO has classified GTD into two states: premalignant and malignant. The premalignant tumors are the complete and the partial moles. The malignant tumors are the invasive mole, gestational choriocarcinoma, and placental site trophoblastic tumor (PSTT). Within the malignant tumors are the categories of nonmetastatic and metastatic. Within the metastatic category are low-risk metastatic and high-risk metastatic disease.

E. There is an increased risk for a second mole after a first molar pregnancy. This is usually paternally related. The risk of another molar pregnancy increases from 1 out of 1,000 to 1 out of 100. There is a familial molar syndrome which is not paternally related.

F. Twin pregnancies with a mole and fetus have been diagnosed at a rate of 1 out of 100,000 pregnancies. There is data to suggest a 40% chance of a live birth. Persistent GTD is diagnosed in 55% of these patients, and 22.7% are found to have metastatic disease. There is an increased risk for hemorrhage, preeclampsia, and metastatic disease. The pregnancy should be terminated if these life-threatening complications occur.

II. Histology

A. Complete and partial moles are usually diagnosed at the time of uterine evacuation. Histopathology is the main diagnostic method. Other abnormal pregnancies/fetuses can be mistaken for a partial mole. These include Turner's, Beckwith-Wiedemann, and Edward's syndromes.

B. A complete mole has no fetal components. Furthermore, the placental villi are hydropic (or edematous) with no identifiable vasculature. The origin of this mole is considered to arise from fertilization of an anuclear oocyte with either two sperm or one sperm that duplicates itself, thus all nuclear DNA is paternal, while the mitochondrial DNA is maternal. Fluorescence in situ hybridization (FISH) can confirm the diagnosis. The rate of persistent GTD after a complete mole is 15% to 20%.

C. The partial mole's origin is thought to arise from the dual fertilization of an egg by two sperm, or duplication of a paternal chromosome. Fetal components can be seen, along with fetal vasculature and hydropic villi. FISH can aid with the diagnosis if necessary, and immunohistochemistry can add information with positive staining for p57. The rate of persistent GTD after partial mole is 0.5% to 5%.

Characteristic	Complete Mole	Partial Mole
Hydatidiform edematous villi	Diffuse	Focal
Trophoblastic hyperplasia	Cyto and syncytial	Syncytial
Embryo	Absent	Present
Villous capillary	No fetal RBC	Many fetal
Gestational age at diagnosis	8–16 weeks	10–22 weeks
Beta hCG titer mIU/mL	> 50,000 mIU/mL in 75%	< 50,000

Malignant potential	15%–25%	0.5–5%
Karyotype	46XX 95%, 46XY 5%	Triploid (69XXY) 80%
Size for dates:		
Small	33%	65%
Large	33%	10%

D. Choriocarcinoma occurs in 1 of 20,000 pregnancies and is inherently a high-risk disease at diagnosis, regardless of metastasis. It should be treated aggressively. 50% of tumors follow a term gestation, 20% occur after molar gestations (both partial and complete), and 25% occur after a spontaneous or elective abortion. These tumors have diverse, nonspecific ploidies and are highly malignant. Both cytotrophoblasts and syncytiotrophoblasts are present, with syncytiotrophoblasts predominating, but there are no chorionic villi. Metastasis occurs frequently to the lung (80% with symptoms such as hemoptysis or dyspnea), vagina (30% with bleeding), brain (10% with focal neurologic deficits, headache, mass effect), and liver (10% pain, hemoperitoneum).

E. Placental-site trophoblastic tumors (PSTT) may follow a term gestation, a nonmolar abortion, a complete mole, and, in theory, a partial mole. These tumors are mostly diploid and produce very low amounts of beta hCG as well as serum human placental lactogen (HPL). This is due to the presence of intermediate cytotrophoblast cells. There is an increased proportion of free beta hCG. These tumors stain for HPL, B1-glycoprotein, and Ki-67. PSTTs grow slowly and can be seen years after any type of pregnancy. It can produce a nephrotic syndrome or hematuria. The prognosis depends on the time until diagnosis; if it presents less than 4 years since a pregnancy, the prognosis is better than if later.

F. Quiescent gestational trophoblastic disease is the state of elevated beta hCG without documented hyperglycosylated hCG. There has never been a documented case of quiescent GTD with a beta hCG level that is higher than 230 mIU/mL. In this disease state, the residual mole lacks a cytotrophoblastic cell population. Therefore, there is no hyperglycosylated hCG production, and as a result, no invasion. Usually the residual mass of tissue dies after 6 months. In 10.4% of cases, however, quiescent GTD can activate and lead to persistent trophoblastic disease. Therefore, when a hyperglycosylated hCG is detected, the patient should be treated with chemotherapy. This is similar to a low malignant potential tumor. There is some data to suggest waiting to treat until a threshold beta hCG level of 3,000 mIU/mL is detected (1,2).

III. Diagnosis

A. Diagnosis of a mole is by ultrasound and serum beta hCG level. Invasive hydatidiform moles/GTD occur usually after evacuation of a complete mole or partial mole.

B. The diagnosis of an invasive mole/GTD is made if there is: persistent beta hCG for 6 months after evacuation of a molar pregnancy, an elevating beta hCG (a 10% rise over 3 values in 2 weeks), a plateauing beta hCG (a plateau of plus or minus 10% over 4 values in 3 weeks), evidence of metastatic disease (mainly lung). In addition, some may consider the presence of an hCG value > 20,000 IU 4 weeks after evacuation diagnostic for an invasive mole. It is imperative to perform dual serum and urine hCG testing to rule out phantom hCG, which is due to heterophilic/cross-reacting antibodies in the serum hCG test.

IV. Workup

A. The pretreatment workup of GTD is a pelvic ultrasound (which can document the primary tumor as a uterine mass and give its dimensions) and a chest x-ray. If the chest x-ray is negative, a CT of the chest should be obtained. If the lungs show metastatic disease, it is then necessary to obtain an MRI of the abdomen and the brain. Alternatively, some practitioners routinely obtain a CT of the chest, abdomen, and pelvis for initial evaluation. A urine beta Hcg and serum beta Hcg both need to be performed to confirm beta Hcg presence. Serum laboratories include a quantitative beta Hcg, CBC, renal function tests, liver function tests, thyroid function tests, a physical examination, and consideration of a lumbar puncture if central neurologic symptoms are present and the brain MRI is negative. The plasma to CSF ratio of hCG can be < 60 in cases with cerebral metastasis, but this ratio is not always reliable.

B. Repeated D&Cs are contraindicated. With a second D&C, the risk of needing chemotherapy is 21%; with a third D&C, the risk of needing chemotherapy more than doubles to 47% (3).

V. Serum beta hCG is a very representative tumor marker. The half-life of beta hCG is 24 to 36 hours. It is a very sensitive and specific marker for trophoblastic tissue. The amount of hCG correlates to

the amount of viable tissue: 5 IU is approximately equal to 10,000 to 100,000 viable cells. However, it is also produced by many other carcinomas, including lung, and ovarian cancers.

VI. Staging

A. FIGO Staging

Stage I: Confined to uterus

Stage II: Metastasis to vagina or pelvis

Stage III: Metastasis to lung

Stage IV: Metastasis to liver, brain, kidney, GI tract

B. AJCC TNM Staging

Clinical TNM Grouping

I: T1 M0 Unknown

IA: T1 M0 Low risk

IB: T1 M0 High risk

II: T2 M0 Unknown

IIA: T2 M0 Low risk

IIB: T2 M0 High risk

III: Any T M1a Unknown

IIIA: Any T M1a Low risk

IIIB: Any T M1a High risk

IV: Any T M1b Unknown

IVA: Any T M1b Low risk

IVB: Any T M1b High risk

Pathological TMN Grouping

I: T1 Unknown

IA: T1 M0 Low risk

IB: T1 M0 High risk

II: T2 M0 Unknown

IIA: T2 M0 Low risk

IIB: T2 M0 High risk

III: Any T M1a Unknown

  IIIA: Any T M1a Low risk

  IIIB: Any T M1a High risk

IV: Any T M1b Unknown

  IVA: Any T M1b Low risk

  IVB: Any T M1b High risk

C. Prognostic factors required for staging

Patients are classified into low-risk or high-risk metastatic disease based on the WHO score below. If the score is less than 7, they are considered low risk. If the score is 7 or greater, they are considered high risk.

WHO Prognostic Scoring System as Modified by FIGO (2002)				
Score	0	1	2	4
Age	≤ 39	≥ 40		
Antecedent pregnancy	mole	abortion	term	
Interval months from index pregnancy	< 4	4–7	7–12	> 12
Pretreatment serum hCG level (IU/L)	< 10^3	10^3–10^4	10^4–10^5	≥ 10^5
Largest tumor size including uterus		3–4 cm	> 5	
Site of metastasis	Lung	Spleen, kidney	GI	Brain, liver
Number of metastases	–	1–4	5–8	> 8
Prior failed chemotherapy drugs	–	–	1	≥ 2

VII. GTD Metastatic Sites

GTD Metastatic Sites	Percent
Lungs	80%
Vagina	30%
Pelvis	20%
Brain	10%
Liver	10%
Bowel, kidney, spleen	5%

VIII. Treatment

A. Molar pregnancy:

1. Evacuation via suction D&C is the primary treatment. Some clinicians avoid sharp curettage due to the increased risk of uterine perforation and possible metastasis. If fertility is not desired, a hysterectomy with ovarian preservation can be the primary treatment of a molar pregnancy.

2. Medications such as Prostin have been shown to increase the need for chemotherapy due to hematogenous spread via contraction of the uterine arteries. Pitocin administered after cervical dilation can assist in uterine involution in addition to expression of uterine contents extracorporeally and not into the vascular system. RhoGAM should be given if the patient is Rh negative.

3. Some patients with molar pregnancies are considered high risk for developing persistent or metastatic disease. Chemoprophylaxis with a one-time dose of single-agent chemotherapy can be considered. In these patients, data has shown the rates of persistent disease have gone from about 50% to 15%. Chemoprophylaxis in lower-risk patients can also be considered if they are seen as potentially noncompliant.

4. Clinical features predictive of high-risk persistent/metastatic disease:

Clinical Feature	Percent Risk of GTD
Delayed postmolar evacuation hemorrhage	75%
Theca lutein cysts > 5 cm	60%
Acute pulmonary insufficiency following molar evacuation	58%
Uterus large for dates (16-week size)	45%
Serum hCG > 100,000 mIU/mL	45%
Second molar gestation	40%
Maternal age > 40	25%

B. Invasive disease/GTD

1. Stage I disease can be managed surgically or with chemotherapy. A hysterectomy with ovarian preservation can be performed if fertility is not desired. A single dose of either methotrexate or dactinomycin immediately prior to the surgical procedure can be considered for prophylaxis against embolism of tumor cells from surgical manipulation. Single-agent chemotherapy is administered if hysterectomy is not performed. Chemotherapy is either with methotrexate or dactinomycin.

2. Stage II disease follows the same chemotherapy principles as those of Stage I disease.

3. Stage III disease is categorized as either low risk or high risk based on WHO risk scoring.

   a. If the patient is considered low risk, initial single-agent chemotherapy is administered.

   b. If the patient is high risk, combination chemotherapy with EMA-CO should be initiated.

4. Stage IV disease is high risk, by definition, and is initially managed with combination chemotherapy. Treatment is usually with EMA-CO, but the methotrexate dose is increased to 1 g/m². If there are cerebral metastases, craniotomy to prevent herniation from mass or hemorrhage may be indicated. Consideration of intrathecal methotrexate or whole brain irradiation to 30 Gy is important. Intrathecal methotrexate is dosed at 12.5 mg, followed in 24 hours with 15 mg of oral folinic acid. This is given once with each course of CO during EMA-CO therapy.

C. Chemotherapy is continued for 2 courses beyond normalization of the beta hCG for Stages I to III. For Stage IV disease or a WHO score > 12, 4 additional courses are recommended after normalization of the beta hCG level. This is due to data suggesting that 100,000 viable cancer cells remain when the beta hCG becomes undetectable.

D. Optimal therapy for placental-site trophoblastic tumors is a hysterectomy with pelvic and para-aortic LN dissection. Ovarian preservation has not been found to be detrimental. This is a relatively chemoresistant tumor, so if the disease is found to be advanced, surgery with adjuvant chemotherapy is likely the best option. Chemotherapy can consist of EMA-EP or EMA-CO. The only prognostic factor identified regarding survival is time from the last pregnancy. If this time is < 4 years, patients usually do well; if it is > 4 years, this is usually universally fatal.

   E. Choriocarcinoma by definition is high-risk disease and should be treated with combination EMA-CO therapy.

IX. Management of Acute Disease-Induced Complications Can Be Lifesaving

   A. If there is uterine hemorrhage, vaginal packing, blood transfusion, and emergent uterine artery embolization can be performed. Laparotomy may be necessary for hysterectomy.

   B. Respiratory failure either from tumor embolization, pulmonary embolization, tumor burden, or hemorrhage may occur. Mechanical ventilation is contraindicated due to a high risk of trauma and iatrogenic hemorrhage, but CPAP is a good alternative. Risk factors for respiratory failure are as follows: 50% opacification of lung fields on chest x-ray, dyspnea, anemia, cyanosis, and pulmonary hypertension.

   C. If cerebral metastases are identified, vigilance for cerebral hemorrhage, edema, and herniation should be maintained. If a solitary lesion is found, site directed vs. whole brain radiation can be considered. If multiple lesions are identified, whole brain radiation is recommended. Premedication with 24 mg of dexamethasone twice daily during treatment with whole brain radiotherapy is important.

X. Chemotherapy Regimens

   A. Single agent

   1. 5-day regimen:

   MTX: 0.4 mg/kg IV or IM daily $\times$ 5 days

   Repeat every 2 weeks

   2. Weekly regimen:

   MTX 30 to 50 mg/m^2 IM

   Leucovorin rescue 15 mg PO 30 hours after each MTX injection

    3. Biweekly regimen:

        a. MTX: 1 mg/m^2 days 1/3/5/7

          Folinic acid: 1 mg/kg daily days 2/4/6/8

          Repeat every 2 weeks

        b. Actinomycin D:

          10 to 12 mcg/kg IV daily × 5 days

          Repeat every 2 weeks

              or

          0.5 mg IV daily × 5 days repeated every 2 weeks

              or

          1.25 mg/m^2 IV every 2 weeks

B. MAC regimen:

    Daily for 5 days repeated every 2 to 3 weeks

    MTX 0.3 mg/kg IM

    Actinomycin D 8 to 10 mcg/kg IV

    Cyclophosphamide 250 mg IV

C. EMACO regimen

    Week 1: EMA

    Day 1: Etoposide 100 mg/m^2 IV

      Actinomycin D 0.5 mg IV

      MTX 100 mg/m^2 IV push with subsequent

      12-hour infusion of 200 mg/m^2

    Day 2: Etoposide 100 mg/m^2

      Actinomycin D 0.5 mg IV

      Leucovorin TID for 24 hours

    Week 2: CO

    Day 8: Vincristine 1 mg/m^2 IV

      Cyclophosphamide 600 mg/m^2 IV

    70% of patients require G-CSF for support

XI. Resistant Disease

A. Stage I resistant disease is seen with an elevating beta hCG. If this occurs, a switch to the other single-agent chemotherapy drug is indicated. If resistance continues, it is important to start combination chemotherapy with MAC (to avoid potential myeloid cancers) or EMA-CO. A hysterectomy or local uterine resection may be considered in addition to chemotherapy if there is persistent disease.

B. Stage II resistant disease is treated in a similar fashion as that for Stage I resistant disease. Hysterectomy with ovarian preservation may be offered if this is the sole site of resistant disease.

C. Stage III resistant disease:

  1. For Stage III low-risk resistant disease, treatment with MAC or EMA-CO should follow single-agent chemotherapy.

  2. For high-risk Stage III resistant disease, treatment with other regimens is indicated. These include MAC, CHAMOCA, VPB, VIP, or ICE.

D. Stage IV resistant disease: Second-line combination chemotherapy with MAC, CHAMOCA, VPB, VIP, or ICE is indicated. Hysterectomy with ovarian preservation may be indicated if this appears to be the sole site of resistant disease.

XII. Recurrent Disease

A. At diagnosis, re-imaging with a CT of the chest, abdomen, and pelvis and MRI of the brain should be obtained. If all are negative, it may be helpful to then perform a lumbar puncture.

B. Experimental imaging techniques can be employed to include anti-hCG radioisotope scanning and PET.

C. If there are lung metastases and this appears to be the only site of resistant disease on comprehensive workup, a thoracotomy with lobectomy may be considered. If there are isolated liver metastases, a wedge resection may also be considered.

XIII. Follow-Up

A. For Stages I–III, weekly quantitative beta hCG levels are drawn until they normalize for 3 weeks. Monthly quantitative beta hCG then continue until they are normal for 12 consecutive months.

B. For Stage IV disease it is important to follow beta hCG levels monthly for 2 years after the weekly beta hCG levels have normalized.

C. Contraception with OCPs (preferably) or Depo-Provera is important. Pregnancy may be attempted after 12 to 24 months of normal beta hCGs.

IMPORTANT GESTATIONAL TROPHOBLASTIC DISEASE TRIALS

A. GOG 55 (4): 266 patients were randomly assigned to either oral contraceptive pills (OCP) vs. barrier method contraception after molar evacuation. The median time to spontaneous regression in the oral contraceptives group was 9 weeks, whereas the median time to regression in the barrier group was 10 weeks. Twice as many patients in the barrier group became pregnant in the immediate follow-up period; 23% of patients receiving OCPs had postmolar trophoblastic disease, and 33% of patients using barrier methods had postmolar trophoblastic disease. OCPs are the preferred method of contraception after evacuation of a hydatidiform mole.

B. GOG 79 (5): Patients with nonmetastatic gestational trophoblastic disease were initially treated with 30 mg/m^2 of weekly IM methotrexate. If no major toxicity was encountered, the weekly dose was escalated by 5 mg/m^2 at 3-week intervals until a maximum dose of 50 mg/m^2 each week was achieved. 81% had a complete response to weekly IM methotrexate. Duration of therapy ranged from 3 to 19 weeks, with a median of 7 weeks. No major toxicity occurred.

C. GOG 79 follow-up study (6): This study evaluated 62 patients with nonmetastatic gestational trophoblastic disease who were initially treated with 40 mg/m^2 weekly of IM methotrexate. If no major toxicity was encountered, the weekly dose was escalated by 5 mg/m^2 at 2-week intervals until a maximum dose of 50 mg/m^2 per week was achieved; 74% had a complete response. Duration of therapy ranged from 3 weeks to 16 weeks with a median of 7 weeks. No major toxicity occurred. The 40 mg/m^2 dose of weekly IM methotrexate therapy is no more effective and of similar toxicity to the 30 mg/m^2 regimen.

D. GOG 174 (7): This trial evaluated 216 eligible patients with a WHO score of 0 to 6 and metastatic disease limited to lung lesions < 2 cm, adnexa, or vagina, and/or histologically proven nonmetastatic choriocarcinoma. Patients were randomized to either biweekly IV actinomycin D 1.25 mg/m² vs. weekly IM methotrexate 30 mg/m². Biweekly actinomycin D was superior to weekly methotrexate (CR 70% vs. 53%; $P = 0.03$). If the risk score was 5 to 6, or the diagnosis was choriocarcinoma, the CR to MTX was 9% and the CR was 42% with actinomycin D. Primary chemotherapy should then consist of EMA-CO in these intermediate and high-risk patients.

REFERENCES

1. Cole LA, Muller CY. Hyperglycosylated hCG in the management of quiescent and chemorefractory gestational trophoblastic diseases. *Gynecol Oncol*. 2010;116(1):3–9.
2. Cole LA, Laidler LL, Muller CY. USA hCG reference service, 10-year report. *Clin Biochem*. 2010;43(12):1013–1022.
3. Pezeshki M, Hancock BW, Silcocks P, et al. The role of repeat uterine evacuation in the management of persistent gestational trophoblastic disease. *Gynecol Oncol*. 2004;95(3):423–429.
4. Curry SL, Schlaerth JB, Kohorn EI, et al. Hormonal contraception and trophoblastic sequelae after hydatidiform mole (a Gynecologic Oncology Group study). *Am J Obstet Gynecol*. 1989;160(4):805–809; discussion 809–811.
5. Homesley HD, Blessing JA, Rettenmaier M, et al. Weekly intramuscular methotrexate for nonmetastatic gestational trophoblastic disease. *Obstet Gynecol*. 1988;72(3 Pt. 1):413–418.
6. Homesley HD, Blessing JA, Schlaerth J, Rettenmaier M, Major FJ. Rapid escalation of weekly intramuscular methotrexate for nonmetastatic gestational trophoblastic disease: a Gynecologic Oncology Group study. *Gynecol Oncol*. 1990;39(3):305–308.
7. Osborne RJ, Filiaci V, Schink JC, et al. Phase III trial of weekly methotrexate or pulsed dactinomycin for low-risk gestational trophoblastic neoplasia: a Gynecologic Oncology Group study. *J Clin Oncol*. 2011 1;29(7):825–831.

Hereditary Cancer Syndromes

I. Hereditary Breast and Ovarian Cancer (HBOC)

A. HBOC is usually attributed to the *BRCA* mutations 1 and 2. The genetic mutation is found on chromosomes 17q21 and 13q12–13 for *BRCA1* and *BRCA2*, respectively, and 80% of patients have a frame shift mutation. The mutation causes a defect in DS DNA repair and E3 ubiquitination. *BRCA1* is known to co-localize with *Rad51*. Inheritance is autosomal dominant and *BRCA* is known to be a tumor suppressor gene. Up to 30% of ovarian cancers have a genetic mutation. Many are found in the Fanconi anemia pathway. These mutated genes include: Rad50/51/51C, BRIP1, BARD1, CHEK2, MRE11A, MSH6, NBN, PALB2, TP53 (1).

B. The lifetime risk of ovarian cancer for *BRCA1* is 25% to 40% and for *BRCA2* is 18% to 27%. For patients who are found to harbor *BRCA1* or 2 mutations, bilateral salpingo-oophorectomy is indicated after the age of 35 years, or when childbearing is completed. PFTC is seen in 2% to 17% of patients at the time of risk, reducing salpingo-oophorectomy.

C. The risk reduction for ovarian cancer is over 80%, but there is still an inherent risk of primary peritoneal cancer, which is 2% to 4.3%. OCPs for at least 6 years can provide a 60% risk reduction for ovarian cancer for *BRCA*-positive patients (2).

D. The presence of a *BRCA* mutation has been found to alter disease prognosis: The disease-free interval after chemotherapy was 14 months for mutation carriers vs. 7 months in sporadic cancer patients. The CR was found to be 3.2 times higher if the patient was *BRCA* positive. The OS was found to be 101 months in *BRCA* carriers vs. 51 months in sporadic cancer patients. The age of onset for patients who are *BRCA1* positive was 52 years old.

E. Oophorectomy may decrease the incidence of breast cancer for both *BRCA1* and *2* carriers. *BRCA*-positive women are recommended to undergo a BSO before age 40 or after childbearing is completed. BRCA1 breast cancers are often ER negative and commonly are triple negative (ER, PR, Her-2-neu negative). The risk of breast cancer was decreased 56% in BRCA1 patients who underwent a BSO, and was decreased 46% in BRCA2 patients. There was an increase in risk reduction from breast cancer the earlier the BSO was performed (3).

F. Patients who have BRCA mutations are categorized as "high risk." If these patients do not opt for surgical management, chemoprophylaxis with OCPs or bilateral salpingectomy and delayed oophorectomy can be considered. Screening with every-6-to-12-month pelvic examinations, transvaginal ultrasound, and serum CA-125 levels has not proven beneficial.

II. Hereditary Nonpolyposis Colon Cancer (HNPCC)

A. HNPCC can contribute to about 10% of hereditary ovarian cancers. HNPCC is also called **Lynch II syndrome**. There is an increase in colon, endometrial, ovarian, pancreatic, CNS, and urothelial cancers. The mutations responsible for these cancers are: *MLH1, MSH 2, MSH6, PMS1,* and *PMS2*. These mutations cause defects in DNA mismatch repair mechanisms. 60% of the cancers present as colon cancer, and 60% present as endometrial cancer.

B. Screening tests usually start around age 25 years old.

1. Colonoscopy should start between ages 20 to 25 years old or 2 to 5 years prior to the earliest diagnosed proband. Screening should occur every 1 to 2 years.

2. Prophylactic hysterectomy with BSO is a risk-reducing option in women. Annual EMB is an option for those not having completed childbearing.

3. There is no data to support annual ovarian ultrasound and serum CA-125.

4. EGD with extended duodenoscopy should be considered every 2 to 3 years beginning at age 30 to 35 years.

5. Urinalysis should start at age 25 to 30 years and continue annually.

6. A CNS annual physical examination should also start at age 25 to 30 years, but no imaging recommendations have been made.

REFERENCES

1. Walsh T, Casadei S, Lee MK, et al. Mutations in 12 genes for inherited ovarian, fallopian tube, and peritoneal carcinoma identified by massively parallel sequencing. *Proc Natl Acad Sci USA*. 2011;108(44):18032–18037. doi:10.1073/pnas.1115052108.
2. Narod SA, Risch H, Moslehi R, et al. Oral contraceptives and the risk of hereditary ovarian cancer. Hereditary Ovarian Cancer Clinical Study Group. *N Engl J Med*. 1998;339(7):424–428.
3. Eisen A, Lubinski J, Klijn J, et al. Breast cancer risk following bilateral oophorectomy in BRCA1 and BRCA2 mutation carriers: an international case-control study. *J Clin Oncol*. 2005;23(30):7491–7496.

Ovarian Cancer Screening

I. An **ideal screening test** has a sensitivity of 100% and a specificity of 95%. A PPV of 10% or greater is the goal of any screening test. This means that 1 diagnosis per 10 interventions is needed for the test to be considered worthwhile.

II. **HE4** alone has a sensitivity of 78%; specificity of 95%; PPV of 80%; and NPV of 99%. It has no sensitivity for borderline tumors.

III. **CA-125** alone has a sensitivity of 83%; specificity of 59%; PPV of 16%; and NPV of 97%.

IV. **Risk of Malignancy Index (ROMI)**

A. The ROMI incorporates ultrasound findings with menopausal status (M) and the CA-125 level. It is written as: ROMI = U × M × CA-125. A score of either 1 or 3 is given to the U. U = 1 for an ultrasound score of 1. U = 3 for an ultrasound score of 2 to 5. A score of either 1 or 3 is given for menopausal status. M = 1 for premenopausal women or M = 3 for postmenopausal women.

B. On ultrasound, 1 point is given for each of the following morphologies: multiloculation, solid components, bilaterality, ascites, or intra-abdominal metastasis. The stated sensitivity is 81%, specificity is 85%, PPV is 48%, and NPV is 96%. If the calculated level is greater than 200, referral to a gynecologic oncologist is recommended.

1. The Ueland Morphology Index (MI) (1) provides the morphology component to the ROMI. When the MI is < 5, most adnexal masses are found to be benign with a NPV of 99%. If the MI is > 5, the PPV has been stated at 40%.

2. The Kentucky University Algorithm has identified women at higher risk for ovarian cancer. A baseline ultrasound is obtained. If it is abnormal, it is repeated in 6 weeks. If the repeat ultrasound is found to still be abnormal, a CA-125 is drawn and the MI is calculated. The stated sensitivity is 85%, the specificity is 98%, the PPV is 14%, and the NPV is 99%. Disease was found at an earlier stage (i.e., stage migration) if there was strict adherence to the above guidelines. 64% of cancers were found at Stage I (2).

V. ROMA (Risk of Ovarian Malignancy Algorithm)

A. The combination test of HE4 and CA-125 is called the **predictive probability algorithm** or **ROMA**. This predictive algorithm is calculated for premenopausal and postmenopausal women separately, using the equations below. To calculate the algorithm the assay values obtained from the HE4 EIA and CA-125 II assays are inserted into the applicable equation.

1. Premenopausal woman

$$\text{Predictive Index (PI)} = -12.0 + 2.38 \times LN\ (HE4) + 0.0626 \times LN\ (CA\text{-}125)$$

2. Postmenopausal woman

$$\text{Predictive Index (PI)} = -8.09 + 1.04 \times LN\ (HE4) + 0.732 \times LN\ (CA\text{-}125)$$

B. To calculate the ROMA value (the predictive probability), insert the calculated value for the predictive index into the following equation:

$$\text{ROMA value \%} = \exp\ (PI)/(1 + \exp\ (PI)) \times 100$$

The following cutoff points were used in order to provide a specificity level of 75%:

1. Premenopausal women

ROMA value $\geq$ 13.1% = High risk of finding epithelial ovarian cancer

2. ROMA value $<$ 13.1% = Low risk of finding epithelial ovarian cancer

Postmenopausal women

ROMA value $\geq$ 27.7% = High risk of finding epithelial ovarian cancer

ROMA value < 27.7% = Low risk of finding epithelial ovarian cancer

This test is stated to have a sensitivity of 94%; specificity of 75%; PPV of 58%; and NPV of 97%.

VI. The **ROCA** is the risk of ovarian cancer algorithm. This test represents the slope of serial CA-125 levels drawn over a period of time and correlated with patient age time. If there is greater than 1% change in the slope of the line, a TVUS is recommended. The UK ROCA study showed a PPV of 19% and a specificity of 99.8%.

VII. The **OVA-1 test** utilizes 5 well-established biomarkers: prealbumin, apolipoprotein A-1, beta$_2$-microglobulin, transferrin, and CA-125. A proprietary algorithm is used to determine the likelihood of malignancy in women with a pelvic mass for whom surgery is planned. The sensitivity is stated to be 92.5%; with a specificity of 42.8%; PPV of 42.3%; and NPV of 92.7%. It is important to remember not to perform this test if the patient has a rheumatoid factor greater than or equal to 250 IU/L or has a triglyceride level greater than 450 mg/dL.

VIII. The **ovarian cancer symptom index (SI)** associates specific symptoms with ovarian cancer. These symptoms are: pelvic/abdominal pain, urinary urgency/frequency, increased abdominal size/bloating, and difficulty eating/feeling full. These symptoms become significant when present for < 1 year and when they occur >12 days per month. The overall sensitivity was 64% and specificity of 88%. For women who are found to have early-stage disease, the sensitivity is stated to be 56.7%, and for women with advanced-stage disease is 79.5%. When age stratified, the specificity is stated at 90% for women age > 50 years and 86.7% for women age < 50 years (3).

A. The symptom index in combination with a CA-125 has also been used to risk stratify adnexal masses. The combination of CA-125 and the symptom index has been shown to identify 89.3% of women with cancer, 80.6% of early-stage cancers, and 95.1% of late-stage cancers. The false-positive rate was 11.8% (4).

B. The symptom index in combination with both CA-125 and HE4 has been found to have a sensitivity of 95% and specificity of

80%. If any 2 of the 3 tests were positive, a sensitivity of 84% and specificity of 98.5% were found. When all 3 tests were used, the specificity was 98.5% and the sensitivity was 58% (5).

IX. **The UK Collaborative Trial of Ovarian Cancer Screening (UKCTOCS)** (6) combined the ROCA and transvaginal ultrasound. 202,638 women aged 50–74 years were randomized to no treatment, annual screening with transvaginal ultrasound, or annual CA-125 (interpreted as a ROCA) with transvaginal ultrasound as a second-line test (designated multimodal screening, MMS). The sensitivity, specificity, and positive predictive values for all primary ovarian cancers were 89.4%, 99.8%, and 43.3% for MMS, and 84.9%, 98.2%, and 5.3% for transvaginal ultrasound screening. 2.9 surgeries were needed per cancer detected in the MMS arm, compared to 35.2 in the ultrasound group.

X. **The Prostate, Lung, Colon, and Ovarian Cancer Trial (PLCO)** This study compared CA-125 levels and ultrasound imaging vs. observation in 78,216 women aged 55–74 with annual transvaginal ultrasound for 4 years and CA-125 for 6 years. 42 of 61 ovarian cancers were found, but 28 (67%) of these were advanced stage. The PPV was 1.1%; the number needed to treat was 20:1. 15% of patients had serious complications related to surgery. There was no evidence of stage migration. Additional data discovered in this trial revealed that 14% of postmenopausal women had simple ovarian cysts, at an 8% incidence; and 32% of these cysts spontaneously regressed (7).

REFERENCES

1. Ueland FR, DePriest PD, Pavlik EJ, et al. Preoperative differentiation of malignant from benign ovarian tumors: the efficacy of morphology indexing and Doppler flow sonography. *Gynecol Oncol.* 2003;91(1): 46–50.
2. van Nagell JR Jr, Miller RW, DeSimone CP, et al. Long-term survival of women with epithelial ovarian cancer detected by ultrasonographic screening. *Obstet Gynecol.* 2011;118(6):1212–1221.
3. Goff BA, Mandel LS, Drescher CW, et al. Development of an ovarian cancer symptom index: possibilities for earlier detection. *Cancer.* 2007;109(2):221–227.
4. Andersen MR, Goff BA, Lowe KA, et al. Combining a symptoms index with CA125 to improve detection of ovarian cancer. *Cancer.* 2008;113(3):484–489.

5. Andersen MR, Goff BA, Lowe KA, et al. Use of a symptom index, CA125, and HE4 to predict ovarian cancer. *Gynecol Oncol.* 2010;116(3): 378–383.

6. Menon U, Gentry-Maharaj A, Hallett R, et al. Sensitivity and specificity of multimodal and ultrasound screening for ovarian cancer, and stage distribution of detected cancers: results of the prevalence screen of the UK Collaborative Trial of Ovarian Cancer Screening (UKCTOCS). *Lancet Oncol.* 2009;10(4):327–340.

7. Buys SS, Partridge E, Black A, et al. Effect of screening on ovarian cancer mortality: the Prostate, Lung, Colorectal and Ovarian (PLCO) Cancer Screening Randomized Controlled Trial. *JAMA.* 2011;305(22): 2295–2303.

Cervical Cancer Screening

I. **The HPV (human papilloma virus)** has been found to cause over 90% of cervical cancers. The virus is organized into 3 regions: the upstream regulatory regions, the early region containing genes E1–E7, and the late region containing genes L1–L2.

    A. The Early, or E, region proteins have the following activities:

        E1: ATP-dependent helicase for replication

        E2: Transcriptional regulatory activities, regulates E6/7

        E3: Uncertain activity

        E4: Structural proteins, expressed in late stages. These proteins disrupt the intermediate filaments and cornified cell envelopes. They facilitate the release of assembled virions. Produces koilocytosis.

        E5: Stimulates cell growth, complexes with EGFR. It is lost during cancer development.

        E6: Binds to p53 and gets ubiquitinized, thus decreases the amount of this regulatory protein

        E7: Transforming and immortalizing capacities; cooperates with activated Ras and binds Rb, it activates cyclins E and A

    B. The Late, or L, proteins are necessary for the virion capsid production:

        L1: major capsid

        L2: minor capsid

    C. HPV infects the host by binding to alpha 6 integrin on basal epithelial cells in the lower reproductive tract. The host cell replicative machinery is activated by HPV when normally it would go dormant, and the basal cells divide with the potential for malignant transformation.

D. Detection of HPV is either by PCR or ELISA. PCR is the gold standard. Type-specific primers or consensus primers can be used to amplify highly conserved regions. The hybrid capture 2 HPV DNA assay uses a pooled set of probes. The sensitivity for this assay is lower than PCR, and it cannot identify specific high-risk HPV types.

E. Transmission is mainly via sexual contact. HPV has been detected in 3% of sexually naïve persons, in 7% of women with only one male partner, and in 53% of women with 5 or more male partners. The use of condoms has consistently reduced the rate of infections by 50%. Fomite transmission is debatable.

F. Most exposures produce a transient productive viral infection. One-third of women develop low-grade cytological changes. Most changes clear spontaneously within 2 years. Less than 20% of women are still HPV+ at 2 years. Long-term or persistent infections occur in fewer than 10% of women at 2 years. Rates of HPV infection differ by age: if older than 29 years old, there is a 31% infection rate; if younger than 29, there is a 65% rate of infection.

G. The ATHENA study has documented the prevalence of cervical cytologic abnormalities in 7.1% of all screened women. The prevalence of HR HPV, HPV 16, and HPV 18 was 12.6%, 2.8%, and 1.0% respectively. HR HPV was detected in 31% of women aged 21 to 24 years old, 7.5% of women aged 40 to 44 years old, and 5% of women older than 70 years old. Currently, virus typing in CIN 2/3 patients has revealed that HPV 16 is present in 45.3%, HPV 18 is present in 6.9%, and HPV 31 is present in 8.6%.

II. Screening with Pap smears has caused significant decreases in the rates of cervical cancer. The incidence of cancer declined 43% between 1972 and 1994, along with a decline in mortality by 45%.

A. The false-negative rate of Pap smears is between 6% and 25%. The conventional Pap smear has a sensitivity of 58% and a specificity of 69%. Liquid-based cytology (LBC) screening has been widely adopted. Liquid based cytology has the same sensitivity and specificity as conventional Pap smears. The Thin Prep and Mono Prep Pap tests both use a filter for cell separation. SurePath uses density centrifugation for cell separation. There is no evidence that LBC is better than conventional cytology but there are advantages to LBC: Reflex HPV testing can be done in ASC-US Pap tests and postmenopausal women with LSIL. Testing for other pathogens and STDs can also be performed.

B. Screening can be discontinued for women with an intact cervix who are aged 65 years and older and who have had 3 or more normal Pap tests within a 10-year period or 2 negative co-tests in a 10-year period. For women with a hysterectomy performed for benign indications, screening can be discontinued. Women with a supracervical hysterectomy should continue screening until age 65 years and can discontinue screening when 3 or more negative consecutive Pap tests occur in a 10-year period or there are 2 negative co-tests in a 10-year period.

C. Annual screening indefinitely is recommended for women with a history of intrauterine DES exposure or who are HIV positive.

D. Women with a history of an abnormal Pap should continue screening until there are 3 negative consecutive Pap tests in a 10-year period or 2 negative co-tests (Pap and HPV testing) in a 10-year period. Women with a history of CIN should continue screening for 20 years after diagnosis and/or treatment—screening interval guidelines may be followed if normal Pap smears are obtained. Women with a history of hysterectomy due to CIN should continue vaginal Pap smear screening for 20 years after surgery—screening interval guidelines may also be followed if a normal Pap smear is obtained. Women with a history of cervical cancer should continue annual screening indefinitely.

E. Screening should be initiated no earlier than age 21 years. The interval should be every 3 years between ages 21 and 29 years with a Pap smear. The Pap smear screening interval can continue every 3 years for women ages 30 to 65 years, or can change to every 5 years if co-testing with HPV is done. There is no evidence that screening victims of sexual abuse provides an earlier diagnosis of dysplastic lesions.

III. Pap smear reports should include terminology that reports an estimate of adequacy. General categorization should follow: negative, whether there is an abnormality, or other. A descriptive diagnosis should then follow and include the level of Pap smear abnormality, organisms/reactive, radiation changes, or atrophy.

A. Squamous cell abnormalities are reported as LSIL, HSIL, squamous cell carcinoma, or atypical squamous cells (ASC). ASC is divided into ASC-US (the risk of CIN 2/3 is 7%–17%) or ASC-H (the risk of CIN 2/3 is 40% and the risk of invasive cancer is 1 of 1,000).

B. Glandular cell abnormalities include atypical glandular cells (AGC), adenocarcinoma in situ (AIS), and adenocarcinoma. AGC is divided into AGC–not further classified or AGC–favor neoplasia.

C. The median rate of ASC is 5%. In the ASCUS/LSIL Triage Study for Cervical Cancer Study (ALTS study), rates of CIN 1 were 20%, and rates of CIN 2/3 were 15%. HPV DNA testing identified more cases of CIN 2/3 than a single repeat Pap and referred equivalent numbers of women for colposcopy. Cost-effective modeling revealed that HPV DNA testing was cheaper than colposcopy. Thus, all 3 methods (immediate colposcopy, re-Pap, or HPV testing) were found to be safe and effective, but HPV testing was the preferred approach for triage.

D. ASC-H is relatively proportional to HSIL. Immediate colposcopy and ECC are recommended. If no CIN is found, a repeat Pap smear at 6 and 12 months, or HPV testing at 12 months, is recommended.

E. LSIL is found at a median rate of 2.6%. In the ALTS study, 83% of LSIL Pap tests were found to harbor HR HPV. CIN 2/3 was identified in 15% to 30% of these patients. Therefore, all LSIL Pap smear tests should be dispositioned to colposcopy and ECC. The only caveat to this is if the patient is postmenopausal. Reflex HPV testing can be done for this subgroup of women. If negative for HPV, a repeat Pap in 12 months can follow; if positive for HPV, then colposcopy is indicated.

F. HSIL is found at a median rate of 0.7%. CIN 2/3 is found in 53% to 66% of women with HSIL. Therefore, all patients with HSIL should receive colposcopy with ECC or be dispositioned to an immediate conization. If no CIN is found on biopsy, and the exam was satisfactory with a negative ECC, a LEEP should be considered. Colposcopy and cytology every 6 months for 1 year should be done if LEEP is declined or the patient is nulliparous. If repeat HSIL is found at Pap smear, LEEP should definitively be performed.

G. AGUS Pap smears should be managed with a colposcopy, directed biopsy, ECC, HPV testing, and EMB based on risk factors (obesity, PCOS, age over 35 years).

H. A meta-analysis of Pap smear results was performed to review progression and regression rates at 24 months after the first abnormal Pap. Progression to HSIL from ASCUS was 7.1%, and LSIL 20.8%. Progression to invasive cancer was 0.2% for ASCUS, 0.15% for LSIL, and 1.44% for HSIL. Regression to normal was 68.2% for ASCUS, 47.4% for LSIL, and 35% for HSIL (2).

IV. **Cytologic guidelines** can be found at the following:
www.asccp.org (Cytology Algorithms)
www.nccn.org (NCCN Guidelines for Detection, Prevention, and Risk Reduction; Cervical Cancer Screening)

REFERENCES

1. Wright TC Jr, Stoler MH, Behrens CM, et al. The ATHENA human papillomavirus study: design, methods, and baseline results. *Am J Obstet Gynecol*. 2012;206:46.e1–46.e11.
2. Melnikow J, Nuovo J, Willan AR, et al. Natural history of cervical squamous intraepithelial lesions: a meta-analysis. *Obstet Gynecol*. 1998;92(4, Pt. 2):727–735.

Anatomy

I. **Layers of the abdomen** (from superficial to deep): Skin, Camper's fascia, Scarpa's fascia, deep fascia (composed of the aponeuroses of the external oblique, internal oblique, and transversus muscles). The transversalis fascia lies below the transversus muscle. Superior to the arcuate line, the internal oblique aponeurosis splits to envelop the rectus abdominis muscle. Inferior to the arcuate line, the internal oblique and transversus abdominis aponeuroses merge and pass superficial (i.e., anteriorly) to the rectus muscle.

II. **Ligaments**

   A. Infundibulopelvic: Contains ovarian vessels and nerves

   B. Round: Originates from the uterine cornua, passes through the inguinal ring, the inguinal canal, and inserts into the labia majora. The male counterpart to this ligament is the gubernaculum testis. A small evagination of peritoneum (canal of Nuck) accompanies the round ligament through the inguinal ring.

   C. Utero-ovarian: These contain the utero-ovarian vessels between the ovary and the uterus. They represent the proximal portion of the gubernaculum testis.

   D. Cardinal (Mackenrodt's ligaments): Located laterally to the cervix, they originate from thickening of the endopelvic fascia. They are the main support for pelvic organs.

   E. Uterosacral: Located posterior to the cervix, they originate from thickening of the endopelvic fascia. They insert on the anterior surface of S2 to S4.

III. **Vasculature**

   A. Ovarian vessels: Travel through the infundibulopelvic ligaments. The ovarian arteries arise from the abdominal aorta, below the renal arteries. The left ovarian vein drains to the left renal vein. The right ovarian vein drains to the inferior vena cava.

B. Artery of Sampson: Travels through the round ligament

C. External iliac artery and vein: Become the femoral vessels after they pass under the inguinal ligament. There are two branches of the external iliac artery and vein: the deep circumflex iliacs and the inferior epigastrics.

D. The internal iliac artery and vein are also known as the hypogastrics. Branches of the internal iliac artery:

    1. Posterior division: iliolumbar, lateral sacral (superior and inferior), superior gluteal

    2. Anterior division: inferior gluteal, internal pudendal, obturator, middle rectal, uterine, vaginal, inferior vesicle, superior vesicle, obliterated umbilical

E. Branches of the celiac trunk: left gastric, common hepatic (branches: right gastric, gastroduodenal), splenic

F. Omental blood supply: right and left gastroepiploics, from the gastro-duodenal and splenic vessels respectively

G. Short gastric arteries originate from the splenic artery.

H. Marginal artery of Drummond: collateral blood supply for the large bowel

I. Blood supply to bowel is from two main arteries, the superior and inferior mesenteric arteries.

    1. Superior mesenteric artery supplies (SMA) the:

        a. Small bowel is supplied by the SMA

        b. Right colon is supplied by right colic and ileocolic arteries which are branches of the SMA

        c. Appendix: Ileocolic branch of the SMA

        d. Transverse colon: Middle colic branch of the SMA

    2. Inferior mesenteric artery supplies the:

        a. Descending colon: Left colic branch of the inferior mesenteric artery (IMA)

        b. Sigmoid colon and rectum: Sigmoid arteries, superior hemorrhoidal artery branches of the IMA

IV. Nerves: The following nerves are composed of contributing spinal nerve roots:

A. Brachial Plexus: C5, C6, C7, C8, and T1

Injury can cause paresthesias of the radial, ulnar, or median nerves. Etiology of injury is from traction on the extended arm or neck.

B. Genitofemoral Nerve: L1 and L2

It arises on the medial border of the psoas muscle. It is a sensory nerve to the medial thigh, and motor innervation to the cremaster muscle.

Injury can cause paresthesia or anesthesia of the labia or skin of the superior thigh.

Etiology of injury is transection or traction of the nerve along the psoas muscle.

C. Ilioinguinal Nerve: L1

It arises on the anterior abdominal wall between the internal oblique and transversus abdominis muscles. It supplies the skin over the pubic symphysis.

Injury can cause paresthesia or anesthesia of the lower abdomen. Etiology of injury is commonly from scar fibrosis.

D. Lateral Femoral Cutaneous Nerve: L2 and L3

Injury can cause parasthesia or anesthesia to the anterior and lateral thigh.

E. Femoral Nerve: L2, L3, L4

Injury can cause paresthesia or anesthesia to the anterior and medial thigh, groin pain, weakness of knee extension and thigh flexion. Etiology of injury is often from retractor placement, stirrup positioning, tumor invasion.

F. Obturator Nerve: L2, L3, L4

It emerges from the medial border of the psoas muscle, traverses the obturator space.

Injury can cause sensory loss to the upper and medial thigh, and weakness in hip abductors.

Etiology of injury is commonly transection during lymph node dissection.

G. Accessory Obturator Nerve: L3 and L4

It is present in 5% to 30% of patients.

H. Internal Pudendal Nerve: S1, S2, and S3

Injury can cause sensory loss to the labia.

I. Sciatic Nerve: L5 and S1

Injury can cause paresthesias of the posterior leg skin and hamstring areas and difficulty with knee flexion.

Etiology of injury is from stretch injury from poor stirrup positioning.

J. Common Peroneal Nerve: L4, L5, S1, S2

Symptoms are foot drop

Etiology of injury is usually from poor stirrup positioning.

K. Autonomic nerves

Symptoms are large bowel dysfunction and urinary retention.

Etiology of injury is from radical pelvic surgery or tumor invasion of the autonomic plexus.

V. Vulvar and Groin Anatomy

A. The anatomical boundaries of the groin form the femoral triangle. This is bounded superiorly by the inguinal ligament, the sartorius muscle laterally to medially, and the adductor longus muscle medially to laterally. The base of the triangle consists of the iliacus, iliopsoas, and pectineus muscles, laterally to medially.

B. Through the triangle run the femoral nerve and 3 other smaller nerves. The femoral nerve consists of the anterior femoral cutaneous branch and the medial femoral cutaneous branches from the L1, L2, and L3 nerve roots. The lateral femoral cutaneous nerve runs on top of the iliopsoas muscle and originates from L1. The genital-femoral nerve runs medial to the psoas muscle in the abdomen and originates from the L1 and L2 nerve roots. The ilioinguinal nerve also runs through the triangle and originates in the L1 root.

C. Innervation to the vulva is from branches of the genito-femoral nerve and the perineal branch of the posterior femoral cutaneous nerve (a branch of the femoral nerve). The internal pudendal nerve also provides innervation to the vulva.

D. The femoral artery gives off branches to form the superficial circumflex, the external pudendal, and the superficial epigastric arteries. The femoral vein receives branches from the superficial circumflex, external pudendal, and superficial epigastric veins. These enter the femoral vein near the saphenous vein, or sometimes drain into the saphenous prior to entry into the femoral vein.

E. The lymphatics drain first into the superficial inguinal LNs. Around the clitoris and prepuce, the lymph nodes may drain directly into the deep inguinal LNs or the pelvic LN, but this has little clinical relevance. The superficial inguinal LNs lie around the branches of the femoral vein. The deep inguinal LNs lie medial to the femoral vein beneath the cribriform fascia. The most superior deep inguinal node is Cloquet's node, which is medial to the femoral vein. Jackson's node is the most distal of the external iliac nodes; thus, Jackson's node is first exiting the pelvic LNs and last entering from the groin route.

F. The blood supply to the vulva is not anomalous. The internal pudendal artery (a branch of the posterior division of the internal iliac) divides to form the perineal, clitoral, and inferior rectal arteries. The superficial external pudendal (a branch of the common femoral) supplies the lower abdominal wall, pubis, and labia majora. The deep external pudendal (a branch of the common femoral) supplies the labial fat pad. The veins commonly follow arteries except that the superficial epigastric and superficial and deep external pudendal drain into or near the saphenous and may not drain directly into the femoral vein.

Surgical Devices

I. Suture

The smallest gauge suture needed to obtain hemostasis is used to decrease the degree of foreign body reaction.

	Name	Composition	Indication	Filament	Tensile Strength (lb)	Absorption	Number of Knots Needed	Gauge	Method of Degradation
Natural Absorbable									
	Plain catgut	Collagen from animal submucosa	Tubal ligation	Monofilament	4.4–8.4	70% at 7 days; Full digestion at 70 days	3	0, 1-0	Enzyme digestion
	Chromic catgut	Collagen and chromic salts from animal submucosa	Serosal, visceral, vaginal tissues	Monofilament	4.4–8.4	50% at 10 days	3	0, 1-0	Enzyme digestion
Synthetic Absorbable									
	Dexon	Glycolic acid	Serosal, visceral, vaginal tissues, fascia in low-risk patients	Braided	6.2–11.6	50% at 14 days; 30% at 21 days	4	0, 1-0, 2-0	Hydrolysis
	Vicryl	Polyglactin 910	Serosal, visceral, vaginal tissues, fascia in low-risk patients	Braided	6.2–11.6	50% at 14 days; 30% at 21 days	4	0, 1-0, 2-0	Hydrolysis
	Maxon	Polyglyconate	Fascia	Monofilament	6.2–11.6	90% at 7 days; 25% at 6 weeks	8–9	0, 1-0	Hydrolysis
	PDS	Polydioxanone	Fascia	Monofilament	6.2–11.6	90% at 7 days; 25% at 6 weeks	8–9	0, 1-0	Hydrolysis
	Monocryl	Poliglecaprone 25	Serosal, visceral, vaginal tissues under no tension	Monofilament	6.2–11.6	50% at 7 days; 30% at 21 days	8–9	0, 1-0	Hydrolysis

Category	Generic	Brand	Tissue/Use	Construction	Size range	Degradation		Sizes	Mechanism
Nonabsorbable Natural	Silk	Silk	Serosal, visceral tissues, inappropriate in infected tissue	Braided	3.2–6.0	50% at 1 year; Full degradation at 2 years	3–4	0, 1-0, 2-0	Hydrolysis
Synthetic Nonabsorbable	Nylon	Neurolon	Suture drains and catheters to skin	Braided	2.3–4.0	Degrades 15% per year	4	0, 1-0, 2-0	Hydrolysis
	Nylon	Dermalon	Suture drains and catheters to skin	Monofilament	2.3–4.0	Degrades 15% per year	8–9	0, 1-0, 2-0	Hydrolysis
	Polyester	Mersilene, Dacron	Visceral tissues	Uncoated, braided	2.3–4.0	Degrades 15% per year	4	0, 1-0, 2-0	Hydrolysis
	Polyester	Ethibond	Visceral tissues, hernia repair	Polybutilate coated, braided	2.3–4.0	Degrades 15% per year	8–9	0, 1-0, 2-0	Hydrolysis
	Polyester	Polydek	Visceral tissues	Teflon coated, braided	2.3–4.0	Degrades 15% per year	8–9	0, 1-0, 2-0	Hydrolysis
	Polypropylene	Prolene	Fascia, vascular procedures, ureteral anastomosis, sacrospinous fixation	Monofilament	4.0–10.5	Degrades 15% per year	8–9	0, 1-0	Hydrolysis

II. Drains

A. **Gastric tube (G-tube):** Indicated for decompression of the stomach to avoid long-term use of a nasogastric tube. It can also be used for feeding patients with swallow difficulties. When placed to gravity, it can be used as an outlet for bowel contents to decrease nausea and vomiting in patients with bowel obstruction.

B. **Chest tube:** Indicated for pleural effusions, hemothorax, or pneumothorax (if greater than 15%). When used with pleurovac, negative pressure is set at 20 cm of H_2O. A pursestring stitch is placed subcutaneously to secure it to the skin. Petrolatum-impregnated gauze should be placed over the incision to make it airtight. Obtain chest x-ray daily.

   1. Pneumothorax: Place to suction for 2 days, then to water seal for the third day. CXR should be obtained daily to evaluate size of pneumothorax. Leave water sealed until the output is <100 mL in 24 hours; and check for the presence of an air leak daily. Pull when output is <100 mL in 24 hours and there is no air leak.

   2. Hemothorax or pleural effusion: Place to suction for 1 day and then to water seal for the second day. Pull when output is <100 mL in 24 hours.

   3. Resolution normally occurs at 10% to 20% per day.

   4. When it is ready to be pulled, the patient should take a deep breath and then Valsalva and the tube pulled as the pursestring stitch then pulled tight around the prior incision. Another petrolatum gauze should be placed on top.

C. **Jackson Pratt:** Indicated for subcutaneous or intraperitoneal wound drainage. Used to decrease the incidence of seroma and infection. It is a closed drain; placed to bulb suction.

   1. Subcutaneous: Removal is recommended when output is less than 30 mL per day. Subcutaneous drainage decreases the incidence of seromas and infections if not used in conjunction with a subcutaneous stitch.

   2. **Peritoneal/intra-abdominal placement:** Removal is recommended when the peritoneal output is less than 50 mL per day. If there was significant preoperative ascites, discontinuation of the drain is when the fluid turns mainly serous.

D. **Penrose drain and T-tubes:** Indicated for drainage of pelvic or subcutaneous infections. It is a passive drain.

E. **Nasogastric tube:** Indicated for postoperative ileus or for bowel obstruction. It is placed to low intermittent suction or Gomco suction.

III. **Central Venous Catheters**

Used to administer systemic cytotoxic agents, blood products, antibiotics, or in patients with poor peripheral access.

A. The Mediport is a subcutaneous port and catheter used for central venous access. It is accessed using a Huber needle. It needs a monthly flush with heparin. A chest x-ray is needed after placement unless it is placed under fluoroscopic guidance.

B. A PICC line is a central venous line placed through a peripheral vein. Indications are for systemic cytotoxic agents, antibiotic therapy, or in patients with poor peripheral access. A daily flush is needed but it can be left in place for 6 months. A chest x-ray after placement is needed.

C. A Hickman catheter is a subclavian catheter used for central venous access. It has no subcutaneous pocket reservoir, so the rate of infection is higher. Indications are similar to the above. It necessitates a daily flush. A chest x-ray after placement is needed.

D. A Groshong catheter has similar indications for central venous access. It is a semi-permanent central venous catheter. It needs a weekly flush. A chest x-ray after placement is needed.

IV. **Peritoneal Catheters**

A. The Tenckhoff catheter is a type of intraperitoneal port-a-cath. It can be irrigated with 500 units of heparin in 15 mL normal saline flush qid × 3 days after placement. It needs a weekly maintenance flush.

B. The Bardport or Mediport 8–9.6F nonfenestrated port can also be used for intraperitoneal placement. It does not need a flush.

V. **Catheter Troubleshooting**

A. If a blood clot obstructs the use of any vascular catheter, attempts at salvage with a thrombolytic agent are indicated. Patency can be checked by injection of hypaque contrast or visualization under fluoroscopy. An example of a thrombolytic protocol is a urokinase flush with 5,000 units/mL solution. A 1-mL injection into the port is performed followed by a 3-mL normal saline flush. This is allowed to remain for 1 hour, then fluid withdrawal is attempted.

B. Fibrin sheath: Difficulty withdrawing is encountered but the flush is smooth or has only moderate resistance. Treatment is placement of a new port if difficulty continues.

Surgical Procedures

I. Laparotomy Incisions

A. The most common vertical incision used for an exploratory laparotomy in oncology is a vertical midline incision. A less commonly used vertical incision is the paramedian incision.

B. There are 3 common transverse skin incisions, with differences in fascial entry:

1. Pfannenstiel: Dissects fascia from rectus muscles

2. Cherney: Dissects the tendons of the rectus abdominis muscles from the pubic bone. A major complication with this incision is the development of osteomyelitis due to suturing of muscles back to bone.

3. Maylard: Muscle cutting. Involves ligating the inferior epigastrics prior to transection of the muscle bodies. This incision does not separate the transversalis fascia from the rectus muscles.

II. Incision Closure

A. Abdominal wall closure:

1. Mass closure: Made with one continuous length of suture material; includes all body wall layers, and incorporates the peritoneum, fascia, and muscles.

2. Smead-Jones (far-near, near-far): A double loop, interrupted matress suture technique that incorporates all the body layers in the outside suture ("far") and fascia and peritoneum in the inner suture ("near")

3. Fascial incision strength after surgery: Week 1: 10%, Week 2: 25%, Week 3: 30%, Week 4: 40%, 6 months: 80%

B. Subcutaneous tissue: If the wound is greater than 2-cm deep, subcutaneous suture or placement of a JP drain is indicated.

C. Skin closure:

1. Staples

2. Subcuticular suture with mononcryl or vicryl with or without a dermabond overlay

3. Vertical mattress skin closure: Useful in delayed primary closure of abdominal incisions and in perineal wound closure (place the knot lateral to the line of incision)

III. Lymph Node Dissection

A. The boundaries for the pelvic LN dissection are the following: superiorly the distal half of the common iliac vessels; laterally the anterior and medial aspect of the external and internal iliac vessels, the ureter medially, the circumflex iliac vein inferiorly, and the obturator nerve posteriorly.

B. The boundaries for the para-aortic LN dissection are the following: the fat pads over and lateral to the inferior vena cava and aorta, the inferior mesenteric artery superiorly, and the proximal half of the common iliac vessels inferiorly.

C. For a high para-aortic LN dissection, the LNs up to the renal vessels are removed lateral and anterior to the great vessels.

IV. Bowel Diversion

A. When an ostomy is considered preoperatively, an ostomy consult should be obtained. The consult is for patient education in addition to identification of best placement; this includes evaluation of her waistline, her common pant line, and any other individual body nuances.

B. A mucous fistula is the distal segment of bowel remaining at the time of end ostomy. It is brought through a separate ostomy site when an end ostomy is placed. The mucous fistula is performed when the remaining distal bowel is more than 10 cm from the anus. These mucous fistulas have minimal drainage. It is important to ensure that both ends are distant enough from each other so that cross fecal contamination and infection cannot occur.

C. Complications:

1. Stricture: there is a 3% stricture rate for all ostomies. Dilation or surgical correction can be performed for strictures.

2. Prolapse: the descending colon has the least risk of prolapse

3. Hernia

D. There are two common types of ostomy:

1. An end ostomy is performed when a take-down is not planned. A mucous fistula needs to be constructed in most cases. The distal end of resected bowel needs management because it still produces mucous and sloughed cells, and could become dilated and perforate. Permanent colostomies prolapse in 1% to 3%. If the resection of the colon occurs at the rectosigmoid and 5 to 10 cm remains, this remaining rectum is then called a Hartmann's pouch and functions as a mucous fistula with output through the anus.

2. A loop ostomy should be performed when there are plans to take the ostomy down. The bowel is brought through the abdominal wall and opened on its antimesenteric side. Both sides of the opened bowel are sutured to the skin. A Hollister bridge or glass rod is placed under the bowel loop for support. The proximal end functions as the colostomy and the distal opening functions as the mucous fistula. It is easier to take down because it is not mandatory to know which end is proximal and which is distal.

E. Ileostomy: Indications include diversion when no distal bowel is available, when small bowel is too dilated to perform an anastomosis, for protection of a distal anastomosis when an anastomotic leak is likely, or in the presence of a bowel perforation with peritonitis. These are high-output ostomies, so as distal an ostomy as possible is preferred. A Turnbull loop is recommended.

F. Gastrostomy tube (G-tube): G-tubes are indicated for decompression of the stomach and intestine to avoid long-term use of a nasogastric tube. They are also used for intractable small bowel obstructions associated with carcinomatosis and fistulas. The body or antrum of the stomach is chosen. A size 18 to 20 Malecot or Foley catheter can be used. The greater curve of the stomach is incised with a scalpel 0.5 cm in length. Two pursestring sutures of 2-0 gauge silk are placed to secured the tube to the stomach. The gastrostomy site is brought to the peritoneal surface and secured with interrupted vicryl sutures. The catheter is then exteriorized through a skin incision and secured to the skin with 2-0 gauge prolene sutures. The G-tube needs to be changed every 2 months.

V. Bowel Resection

A. Bowel anastomosis can be performed using either hand-sewn or stapled technique.

1. Types:

   a. End to end: The bowel is aligned with cut ends together and hand-sewn together using a two-layer technique (the inner layer using 3-0 gauge vicryl and the outer imbricating layer using 3-0 gauge vicryl or silk). Alternatively, using a stapler, the bowel ends are aligned on their antimesenteric borders. An enterotomy is made on the antimesenteric corner of the 2 bowel sections. One prong of the GIA stapler is then advanced through each enterotomy and fired. The TA stapler is then used to close the connected bowel segments to create a functional end-to-end anastomosis. The mesentery should be closed and silk stay sutures are placed along the antimesenteric borders to reduce tension.

   b. Side to side: 5-mm enterotomies are made with the Bovie on each segment of the resected bowel 5–10 cm back from the primary transection site. One prong of the GIA stapler is then advanced through each enterotomy and the stapler is then fired. The TA stapler is then applied to close the defect transversely or longitudinally, whichever narrows the lumen least.

   c. Low rectal anastomosis is often performed after a rectosigmoid resection. It is important to consider placing a diverting loop colostomy or loop ileostomy to protect the anastomosis and allow for healing. The anastomosis should preferably be performed out of the irradiated field. The largest staple cartridge available and accommodated by the patient should be used. If a very low anastomosis is performed, consider construction of a J pouch to increase reservoir capacity and to decrease tenesmus.

2. Anastomotic leaks complicate bowel surgery in 0% to 30%. Rectal anastomosis have a higher complication rate of about 6%.

3. Requirements for a good anastomosis include: an adequate lumen of at least 2–3 cm, the anastomosis be tension free, there be adequate vascular supply from the mesentery with evidence of bleeding (viability) of the cut edges, and the presence of peristalsis.

4. Watershed areas of the bowel include the ileocecal junction/terminal ileum, the splenic flexure of colon (Griffith's point), and the rectosigmoid flexure (Sudeck's point).

B. Meckel's diverticulum represents persistence of the vitelline yolk sac. It is present in 2% of people. It is twice as common in men as women. It is usually located within 2 feet of the ileocecal valve. It should be removed when found, due to the presence of ectopic gastric tissue in 2% of patients, i.e., Zollinger-Ellison syndrome.

VI. Urinary Diversion: Stents, Conduits, and Bladder Reconstructions

A. Ureteral stents should be placed in most ureteral injury cases. They can be placed via retrograde cystoscopy, retrograde cystotomy, via ureterotomy, or antegrade through a percutaneous nephrostomy. A 6 French double pigtail stent or a pediatric feeding tube can be placed. These should be changed every 3 to 6 months. They can often be removed 2 to 6 weeks after surgery via cystoscopy.

B. Urinary conduits/neobladders are often placed in the settings of pelvic exenteration, intractable hemorrhagic cystitis, a neurogenic bladder, or decreased bladder capacitance from surgery or radiation therapy. Decreased capacity is defined as an intravesical pressure greater than 30 cm of H_2O with minimum volume.

C. Bladder reconstruction can be performed when there has been surgical resection with the urethra safely preserved.

D. Principles of urinary conduits are: a low-pressure system (less than 20-cm water), high-volume, anti-refluxing system to prevent ascending infection, and low water and solute reabsorption.

    1. Universal techniques are needed. There has to be a wide uretero-bowel anastomosis, the intestinal segment should be isoperistaltic, the stoma should be protruding, the conduit should be stabilized within the abdominal cavity, and there should be an adequate diameter of the efferent loop with a straight path through the abdominal wall for urine outlet.

    2. There are two types of conduits, incontinent and continent.

        a. Incontinent types include:

            i. Percutaneous nephrostomy tube

            ii. Cutaneous ureterostomy. The ureters should be brought out 2 cm past the skin, and the skin incision should be an inverted V pointing down.

            iii. The right colon pouch is another incontinent conduit. It does not use nipple valves. It is made from nonirradiated, detubularized colon. It has an increased risk of ureteral obstruction, angulation of the distal ureters, fibrosis of the submucosal ureteral tunnels, devascularization, and distension of the pouch. The left ureter requires more mobilization to reach the colon.

iv. The ileal conduit uses a longer intestinal segment. The Bricker type incorporates a horizontal internal orientation for the body of the reservoir. The ureters are anastomosed laterally. The Leadbetter modification orients the body of the conduit vertically. The ureters are brought to the midline for the anastomosis. The ureteroileal anastomoses are end to end. A Turnbull stoma is used to overcome the complications of nipple ischemia. A short ileal segment of 15 to 18 cm is used. The conduit is sutured at its proximal end to the sacral prominence. The Daniels modification is used for obese patients, and the Wallace modification is used for double ureters (where both ureters are split and sewn together).

v. A jejunal conduit has a higher incidence of electrolyte imbalances: hyperchloremic acidosis occurs in 25% to 65% of patients. There is reabsorption of potassium (K) and urea and a concomitant increase in aldosterone. It is more often outside the fields of radiation.

vi. The sigmoid conduit has the advantages of avoiding small bowel anastomosis and fewer stomal complications. Disadvantages are that it cannot be used with inflammatory bowel syndromes or diverticulosis. There is an increased risk of secondary cancers inside the conduit. The ureters should be tunneled submucosally if no prior radiation was given.

vii. The transverse colon conduit has advantages in that it is good for the obese patient, in those with a history of pelvic radiation as it is outside the field of radiation, and in those with short ureters.

b. Continent diversions are contraindicated in persons with short life expectancies, in those with physical problems accessing/maintaining the conduit (dementia/arthritis), those with right colon diseases (prior bowel cancer, IBD, cecal radiation), those with morbid obesity (making this a short system), and in those with compromised renal function.

i. The ureterosigmoidostomy maintains continence through the anal sphincter. The ureters directly into the sigmoid colon and efflux is through the rectum. There are high rates of pyelonephritis, obstruction, hyperchloremic acidosis, nocturnal incontinence, and frequent bowel evacuation. Secondary carcinomas of the colon can occur.

ii. The ileocolic continent diversion (Indiana Pouch) uses 10 to 15 cm of terminal ileum, the cecum, and 30 cm of ascending colon. The right colonic segment is detubularized. The terminal ileum is plicated over a red robin catheter to the level of the ileocolic valve—this provides the continence mechanism. The plicated ileum is brought to the abdominal wall. Intestinal integrity is re-established after resection. Drains are placed to follow: stents for each ureter; a Malecot catheter placed into the right colon pouch and exists superior to the ileal stoma; a red robin/Foley catheter placed in the plicated ileum maintaining patency from the right colonic pouch through the abdominal wall, and a JP placed in the abdomen.

iii. The Miami Pouch uses the same principles as above, but extends the intestinal resection to the level of the transverse colon. Postoperative maintenance includes irrigation of the Malecot every 4 to 6 hours with 40 mL normal saline, and irrigation of the ureteral stents only if plugged. Both drains are removed at 14 days after an IVP and pouchogram are normal. If the patient had prior radiation, 21 days of stenting and drainage is recommended. The JP should be removed at the same time as the ureteral stents. Active catherization every 2 hours the first week, every 3 hours the second week, every 4 hours the third week, every 5 hours the fourth week, and every 6 hours the fifth week are recommended. The pouch should be irrigated daily to weekly with 50 mL of normal saline. An IVP, pouchogram, and CMP should be obtained at 3 months.

iv. The Kock ileal pouch is specifically contraindicated for chronic inflammatory or neoplastic disease of the colon, as well as in patients with short ureters. A portion of ileum is isolated and marked into segments measuring

17 cm, 22 cm, 22 cm, and 17 cm. 15 cm of distal ileum remains at the ilealcecal junction to protect the watershed area. The 22-cm (central portion) lengths are sutured together, then opened along their antimesenteric borders to make the reservoir. The pouch is then folded over. The 17-cm lengths are then each intussuscepted and secured with a GIA or TA stapler. The ureters are brought in to the proximal end. Mesh is attached to each intussusception to secure the intussuscepted nipples. A Marlex strut is attached from the distal mesh to the rectus muscle. The 2 ends of the ileal segment become the nipples: the afferent end prevents reflux into the kidneys and the efferent end is the continence mechanism. Complications include stone formation around staples, prolapse, extussusception, and stenosis from ischemia.

C. Bladder reconstruction can be performed with:

1. Right colon augmentation (enterocystoplasty)

2. A hemi-Kock ileal bladder can also be constructed. With this technique no efferent nipple is constructed.

3. The psoas hitch provides bladder reconstruction by mobilizing the bladder to reach a shortened ureter on the ipsilateral side. The bladder is distended with water, then opened along the dome. A suture is placed through the lateral side of the bladder to the psoas muscle on the affected side, at the level of the proximal external iliac artery. The ureter is anastomosed to the bladder and the cystotomy is closed in 2 layers.

4. The Boari bladder flap is used in combination with the psoas hitch for a more extensively shortened ureter. The bladder is again distended, and opened in the dome with a U-shaped incision. The base of the created flap is then oriented toward the psoas muscle and the flap is rotated upward. The flap is tubularized around the ureter, and the bladder is then sutured to the psoas muscle. The bladder defect is then closed in 2 layers. This technique provides 3 to 5 cm of additional length for a shortened ureter.

D. There are three methods for ureteral reanastomosis after transection:

1. The ureteroureterostomy (UU), which is a primary reanastomosis

2. The transureteroureterostomy, which is an anastomosis to the contralateral ureter

3. The ureteroneocystostomy (UNC), which reimplants the ureter directly into the bladder, with or without psoas hitch or Boari flap

4. All ureteral injuries and diversions should be stented unless minimal crush injury is seen and immediately released.

VII. Reconstructive surgery: Reconstructive surgery is useful in gynecologic oncology for coverage of perineal defects and for neovaginal construction. There are different methods of reconstruction.

A. Split thickness skin grafts (STSG) are often used to cover epidermal/dermal defects encountered with simple vulvectomy. The Zimmer dermatome can produce an optimal graft thickness of 0.020 inches.

B. Tissue expansion can be produced with inflatable balloons and the area harvested after an appropriate time.

C. Skin flaps are used to reconstruct deeper resections. There are 3 types of flaps: rotational, advancement, and transpositional (pass over).

1. Common rotational flaps include the rhomboid and perineal thigh flaps. The rotational flap most often used is the rhomboid flap/Limberg flap. This flap can cover anterior, lateral, or posterior vulvar defects in addition to defects of the perianal region. The donor sites are the buttocks and posterior thigh. The blood supply is the inferior gluteal artery. The perineal thigh flap is used to cover a defect to the labial crural fold. The donor site is the medial thigh. This blood supply is unreliable. The length of the flap should be a ratio of 2:1 to the vulvar defect.

2. Advancement flaps are used to provide defect coverage when there is enough adjacent skin mobility. This is usually called a V-Y advancement flap.

3. Transpositional axial flaps move the flap on an axis (its vascular pedicle) to another site.

    a. The Martius/bulbocavernosus flap is used for repair of vaginal fistulas, for vaginal reconstruction, and for repair of 4th-degree lacerations. The donor site is the labial fat pad and the blood supply is the superficial external pudendal artery and the perineal branch of the internal pudendal artery.

    b. The SEPA (superficial external pudendal artery) flap is often used for vulvar reconstruction and repair of urethral defects.

The donor site is the area directly above the mons pubis. This type of flap should not be performed if a groin node dissection is planned. The blood supply is related to the flap's name and originates from the common femoral artery. This is a sensate flap.

c. The SCIA (superficial circumflex iliac artery) flap is indicated for anterior perineal and vaginal defects. The donor site is the skin around the anterior superior iliac spine to 2.5 cm below the inguinal ligament. The blood supply again relates to its name.

d. The posterior labial artery flap is also known as the pudendal thigh flap and the Singapore flap. It too covers perineal defects and is good for vaginal reconstruction. The donor site is the labial crural fold and the inguinal crease. The blood supply is related to its name and originates from the deep external pudendal artery. This flap is sensate and innervation is from branches of the pudendal nerve and the posterior cutaneous nerves.

e. The inferior gluteal fasciocutaneous flap can cover vulvar, vaginal, and rectal defects. The donor site is the buttocks. The blood supply is the axial artery of the inferior gluteal artery, originating from the internal iliac artery. This flap can be up to 35 cm long. It too is a sensate flap and the nerve supply is from the posterior cutaneous nerve of the thigh.

D. Myocutaneous flaps are distinguished by the number of vascular pedicles that supply the flap. There are 5 types. Type I flaps consist of a single vascular pedicle. Type II flaps have one dominant vascular pedicle and one or more minor vascular pedicles. Type III flaps obtain their blood supply from 2 dominant pedicles. Type IV flaps obtain their blood supply from 3 dominant pedicles. Type V flaps obtain their blood supply from 4 dominant vascular pedicles. To test flap viability, IV fluorescein (10 mL of 10% solution, or a dose of 15 mg/kg administered over 5 minutes) can be given and a Wood's light can be placed over the flap site. Twice the dose should be used in African American patients.

1. The rectus abdominis myocutaneous flap (RAM) is often used for vaginal/pelvic reconstruction. The blood supply is the superior and inferior epigastrics and it is a type III flap.

2. The gracilis myocutaneous flap (GMC) is used for vaginal, groin, or perineal reconstruction. It can be used as an island flap, or directly rotated into the defect. The blood supply is the medial femoral circumflex artery from the deep femoral artery. It is a type II flap.

3. The tensor fasciae latae flap is indicated for vulvar and groin defects, as well as for ischial and deep abdominal wall defects. The donor sites are the gluteus medius and sartorius muscles. The blood supply is the terminal branch of the lateral circumflex femoral artery. It is a type I flap. Side effects can be lateral instability of the knee, a long scar on the medial thigh, thigh pain, and vascular spasm from torsion. It is not a suitable flap for vaginal reconstruction after a supralevator exenteration. The latissimus dorsi flap is a good flap for breast reconstruction. It is a type V flap.

E. Neovaginal techniques are also varied. These include the following:

1. McIndoe Split thickness skin graft (STSG): The McIndoe neovagina is constructed using a STSG formed around a mold. It is placed in the perineal defect and the patient should then be immobilized to allow the STSG to anneal. Daily dilation should follow indefinitely.

2. The RAM flap is a more reliable neovaginal flap and is less likely to prolapse than other neovaginal flaps.

3. Two gracilis myocutaneous flaps are needed for neovaginal reconstruction if this procedure is performed. There can be vascular pedicle spasm with this type of flap. It does have a tendency to prolapse.

4. The Martius flap is a durable and pliable flap to use for neovaginal reconstruction.

5. The posterior labial artery thigh flap is a sensate flap but has a less reliable blood supply.

6. The perineal thigh skin flap tends to prolapse and can stenose.

7. Intestinal segments, including the cecum, small bowel, sigmoid colon, and rectum, can also be used for neovaginal reconstruction. The sigmoid colon is used the most often. It is important to detubularize it. The benefits of this type of neovagina are its large caliber, and low-volume mucous output. Risks include secondary malignancies, including HPV related.

VIII. Splenectomy is often indicated with splenic trauma, or when tumor has involved this organ and optimal debulking is feasible if the spleen is removed.

    A. Anatomy: The splenic artery originates at the celiac trunk. The splenic vein combines with the hepatic veins to join the IVC.

    B. Technique: When performing a splenectomy, it is necessary to take down the splenogastric, splenocolic, and splenophrenic ligaments. The artery and vein should be clamped and ligated separately to decrease the risk of arteriovenous fistula.

    C. Complications: There is a risk of thrombocytosis post splenectomy, as well as an increased risk of DVT.

    D. Necessary vaccines after splenectomy include immunization against *Meningococcus, Haemophilus influenzae,* and *Pneumococcus.* Ideally, these vaccines should be given 14 days prior to the anticipated splenectomy. If not done prior, they should be done as soon as possible after surgery.

IX. Diaphragmatic stripping is performed when optimal debulking can be achieved. The peritoneum is removed with varied techniques.

    A. The liver usually needs to be mobilized inferiorly with release of the falciform and triangular ligaments.

    B. Complications include pneumothorax when the diaphragm is perforated. To rectify this, a Foley or red rubber catheter is placed through the defect and connected to suction. A pursestring suture is placed around the Foley catheter and the patient is placed in Trendelenberg. The anesthesiologist is asked to perform an expiratory Valsalva for the patient with the ventilator, and the catheter is removed with the suture tied. A chest tube is usually placed and a CXR is checked postoperatively.

X. Minimally Invasive Surgery: Minimally invasive surgery (MIS) has emerged as a growing area in procedural medicine and has specifically found to be useful in gynecologic surgery.

    A. Three laparoscopic approaches are typically used: traditional laparoscopy; robotic-assisted laparoscopy; and laparoendoscopic single-site surgery.

    B. Advantages of minimally invasive surgery include a shorter hospitalization; a more rapid recovery; smaller incisions; and a trend for fewer analgesics.

    C. Limitations of minimally invasive surgery are a longer learning curve and the costs of instrumentation.

Intraoperative Complications

I. Vascular Injury

A. Venous lacerations should be repaired using 6-0 gauge prolene sutures, in an interrupted or running fashion. Irrigation with heparinized saline can be used to visualize the repair. If the vein is large caliber, distal and proximal control should be obtained using pressure or Judd-Allis clamps. If there is a large hole, a lesser vein can be harvested and opened using Potts scissors to create a patch and sewn in place with interrupted sutures. Omentum can be placed on top to help vascularize. If sutures start to tear through the vein, pledgets (small pieces of cellulose) can be used to avoid suture tension.

B. Arterial damage should be approximated in a similar fashion. If the edges are ragged, consider complete resection and approximation. If there is a large hole, a vein graft can be used to patch the artery; 100 to 150 units/kg of IV heparin can be given before cross clamping the vessel. This dosing can continue every 50 minutes until circulation is reestablished.

II. Nerve Injury:
The nerve should be repaired using 7-0 gauge prolene sutures to align the fascicle bundles. Only the perineurium should be approximated. Nerve growth is estimated at 1 mm per day, or 1 inch per month.

III. Gastrointestinal Injury

A. Small bowel injuries:

1. Serosal injuries can be observed if they are small, but should be primarily oversewn with 3-0 gauge silk or vicryl sutures if large. If radiation therapy has been administered, serosal injuries should always be oversewn.

2. A seromuscular injury is evident if bulging of the bowel wall is seen. Repair should be double layered with 3-0 gauge silk or vicryl.

3. If there is luminal injury, a double-layered closure is indicated. Double-layered repair can be with 3-0 gauge vicryl for the mucosal layer and either vicryl or silk for the serosal layer.

B. Large bowel injury should be evaluated for a transmural defect. If no transmural defect is identified, a primary single-layered repair can be performed using 3-0 gauge silk or vicryl. If there is a transmural defect and no evidence of fecal contamination, a primary double-layer closure can be attempted. If there is an extensive defect, consideration should be given to resection with reanastomosis. If no bowel preparation was given, consideration should be given to a diverting loop or end colostomy with mucous fistula.

IV. Urinary Tract Injury

A. Urinary tract injury occurs in 1% to 2.5% of gynecologic surgeries. Intraoperative cystoscopy with IV indigo carmine should follow most hysterectomy procedures to detect and provide early repair of these injuries (1).

B. Bladder injury should be identified with direct visualization or IV indigo carmine. The bladder should be closed in 2 layers using absorbable suture. This is usually with an inverting stitch of 2-0 gauge vicryl or chromic for the first layer, and vicryl for the second. If there is trigone injury, cystoscopy should be performed to ensure the ureters are intact. The bladder should be drained with a Foley catheter for 5 to 14 days.

C. Ureteral injury is recognized at the time of surgery in 20% to 30% of cases. Injury can be via transection, ligation, crush injury, angulation, or ischemia. Injury is commonly at the level of the uterine artery, at the infundibulopelvic ligament, or at the level of the pelvic brim. Ureteral stenting should occur for most ureteral injuries. This is done via cystoscopy, cystotomy, or ureterotomy. A JP drain should be placed in all cases. If there is concern for further ureteral leakage, the JP fluid can be checked for a creatinine level and compared to a serum creatinine. Stenting is maintained for 6 to 12 weeks followed by IVP after stent removal.

1. If there is a crush injury identified, the clamp should be released, and the ureter observed and mobilized. An ampule of IV indigo carmine should be given. If no extravasion is seen, consideration should be given to stenting the ureter.

2. A partial transection can be treated with stenting and primary closure using 4-0 gauge to 6-0 gauge delayed absorbable suture (PDS).

3. If there is complete transection, the ends should be dissected out, mobilized, and trimmed. The location of transection dictates repair.

   a. A distal transection (below the pelvic brim) can be managed with ureterneocystostomy/reimplantation. There is debate as to the benefit of tunneling the ureter into the bladder. Reimplantation can also be via a Boari flap, a psoas hitch, the Demel technique, or use of intestinal interposition with an ileal segment.

   b. If there is middle pelvic transection, ureteroureterostomy or ureteroileoneocystostomy can be performed.

   c. If the transection is above the pelvic brim, a transureteroureterostomy or ileal intestinal interposition can be performed. Care should be taken with a TUU as this procedure can compromise the opposite kidney.

V. **Intraoperative Hemorrhage**

When there is life-threatening, severe intraoperative hemorrhage, the use of a "massive transfusion protocol" may be indicated. This transfusion protocol decreases the use of blood components, as well as turnaround times, costs, and mortality (2).

A. Initiate massive transfusion protocol.

   1. Issue 4 units PRBC and 4 units FFP in cooler.

   2. Once first package is issued, prepare second package as a "Stay Ahead" order.

3. Once second package is issued (RBC, FFP, and platelets), begin preparing cryoprecipitate dose and set up next "Stay Ahead" package (RBC, FFP, platelets).

4. Repeat as necessary.

Blood Component Prepared			
1st package	4 units PRBC	4 units FFP	
2nd package	4 units PRBC	4 units FFP	1 dose platelets
	Prepare cryo after 2nd package issued		1 dose cryoprecipitate
3rd package	4 units PRBC	4 units FFP	1 dose platelets
	Prepare cryo after 3rd package issued		1 dose cryoprecipitate

REFERENCES

1. Ibeanu OA, Chesson RR, Echols KT, et al. Urinary tract injury during hysterectomy based on universal cystoscopy. *Obstet Gynecol.* 2009; 113:6–10.
2. O'Keeffe T, Refaai M, Tchorz K, et al. A massive transfusion protocol to decrease blood component use and costs. *Arch Surg.* 2008;143(7): 686–690.

Postoperative Care Protocols

I. Radical Vulvar Surgery

   A. Drains:

      1. Groin JP drains should be discontinued when output is less than 30 mL per day.

      2. Foley catheter: Depending on site of resection and reconstruction, the Foley can be left in for 7 days with prophylactic antibiotics, or removed postoperative day 1.

   B. Antibiotics: Oral prophylactic antibiotics can be given starting on postoperative day 1 and until groin and vulvar wounds are well healed. The antibiotics decrease the incidence of lymphedema due to beta-hemolytic streptococcus.

   C. Wound Care: this is mainly peri-care with soap and water squirt bottle to the perineum TID and after each bowel movement. The area can be blown dry with a hairdryer on cool setting after each cleaning.

   D. DVT Prophylaxis: Combination injectable anticoagulant and SCDs should be employed until the patient is fully ambulatory. Ambulation should occur as soon as pain is controlled, strength permits, and wound integrity is documented.

   E. Nutrition: Low-residue diet as tolerated

   F. Complications: Lymphocysts: Percutaneous drainage can be performed if symptomatic. If they are recurrent, they can be sclerosed with talc, tetracyclines, or alcohol.

   G. Follow-up: 6 weeks

II. Radical Hysterectomy

A. Drains:

1. JP Drains: Discontinue when less than 30 mL/day output.

2. Foley Catheter: Should be discontinued POD 3 to 4. A post-void residual should be checked immediately after the first self-void. The Foley should be replaced if the residual volume is greater than 75 mL, and the Foley then continued for 1 week. If at recheck, the PVR is still elevated, the patient should be educated on self-catheterization. Bladder dysfunction can occur in up to 10% of patients due to denervation from cardinal and uterosacral ligament resection.

B. Antibiotics: Consider daily PO antibiotics for suppression when a Foley catheter is in place.

C. Wound Care: Keep clean and dry. Staples: Remove staples postoperative day 3 for transverse or Maylard incisions. Remove staples postoperative day 10 for midline incisions.

D. DVT Prophylaxis: Combination injectable anticoagulant and SCDs should be used until the patient is fully ambulatory. Four weeks of postoperative anticoagulation should be considered. Ambulation should occur as soon as pain is controlled and strength permits.

E. Nutrition: Regular diet as tolerated

F. Complications: Lymphocysts: Can occur in up to 25% of patients but are symptomatic in about 5% of patients. If infected or symptomatic, broad-spectrum antibiotics should be employed. Percutaneous drainage can be attempted if spontaneous resolution does not occur or if vessel or organ obstruction/compression occurs. They can also be sclerosed with talc, alcohol, or tetracyclines.

G. Follow-up: 6 weeks

III. Urinary Conduits and Pelvic Exenteration

A. Drains:

1. If a nasogastric tube was inserted during surgery, it should be removed at the end of the operation.

2. Malecot (for continent conduits): Should be placed to dependent drainage for 7 to 10 days. Irrigation every 4 to 6 hours with 40 cc of normal saline should be performed to prevent the accumulation of mucus.

      3. Red rubber catheter: In continent conduits: It should be left sewn in place until ready to self-catheterize at 7 to 10 days.

      4. JP drains: should be left in place for 7 to 10 days or until output is less than 30 mL/day.

      5. Gracilis flap JP leg drains: Leave for 7 days or until output is less than 30 mL/day.

B. Antibiotics: If the patient has a conduit, consider sending her home on PO prophylaxis.

C. Wound and Flap Care: Keep clean and dry. Peri-care should be performed TID. The area can be blown dry with a hairdryer on cool setting after each cleaning. Staples should be left in place for 10 days, including those on the legs for gracilis flaps.

D. DVT Prophylaxis: Combination injectable anticoagulant and SCDs should be employed until the patient is fully ambulatory. Consider 4 weeks of postoperative injectable anticoagulation. Ambulation should occur as soon as pain is controlled, strength permits, and wound integrity is documented.

E. Nutrition: TPN should be started postoperatively if the patient is suspected to be NPO for greater than 7 days or if the patient was malnourished prior to surgery. Begin PO feedings with bowel sounds.

F. Complications: Evaluation of the urinary tract by IVP or ultrasound should be part of a postoperative fever workup. Stomas should be checked daily; if they are dusky, endoscopy should be performed.

G. Other:

      1. Ureteral stents: Should be sewn in with chromic suture, which will spontaneously dissolve and separate between days 10 and 14.

      2. CXR on admission to the recovery room should be obtained if a central line was inserted.

H. Follow-up: Should occur at 2 weeks and 6 weeks. Lab tests: BUN and creatinine should be obtained at each visit. Radiologic studies: An IVP should be obtained at discharge, 6 weeks, 6 months, 18 months, 3 years, and 5 years. A CT of abdomen and pelvis can be considered every 6 months to 1 year.

IV. Bowel Resection

A. Drains:

1. NGT can be removed immediately after surgery. If there was obstruction preoperatively, it can remain until bowel function returns.

2. JP peritoneal drains can be placed if multiple enterotomies occurred to check for bowel leak or fistula. Leave drains in until fluid output is serosanguinous.

3. Subcutaneous JP drains: These can be discontinued when the output is less than 30 mL/day.

4. Foley: This can be discontinued on postoperative day 1.

B. Antibiotics: These should only be used postoperatively if gross peritoneal contamination occurs with bowel contents. They can be discontinued on POD 2 to 3 if the patient is afebrile.

C. Wound Care: Vertical midline staples should remain for 10 days. Patients with transverse incisions can have their staples removed between days 3 and 5.

D. DVT Prophylaxis: Combination injectable anticoagulant and SCDs should be employed until the patient is fully ambulatory. Consider 4 weeks of injectable postoperative anticoagulation. Ambulation should occur as soon as pain is controlled and strength permits.

E. Nutrition: Consider TPN if there is prolonged ileus for more than 7 days; postoperative obstruction occurs; or the patient was malnourished preoperatively.

V. Ovarian Cancer Debulking

A. Drains:

1. If a nasogastric tube was placed due to obstruction, remove when bowel function returns.

2. JP Peritoneal drain: These will always have output, especially if there was a large amount of ascites.

3. Subcutaneous drains: Discontinue when output is less than 30 mL/day.

4. Foley: Discontinue on postoperative day 1 if adequate urine output.

B. Antibiotics: These should only be used postoperatively if gross peritoneal contamination occurs with bowel contents. They can be discontinued on POD 2 to 3 if the patient is afebrile.

C. Wound Care: Vertical midline staples should remain for 10 days. Patients with transverse incisions can have their staples removed between days 3 and 5.

D. DVT Prophylaxis: Combination injectable anticoagulant and SCDs should be employed until the patient is fully ambulatory. Consider 4 weeks of postoperative injectable anticoagulation. Ambulation should occur as soon as pain is controlled and strength permits.

E. Nutrition: Consider TPN if there is prolonged ileus for more than 7 days; postoperative obstruction occurs; or the patient was malnourished preoperatively.

VI. Bowel Obstruction

A. Partial obstructions can resolve in 50% of cases. Complete obstructions usually need surgical intervention.

B. Large bowel obstruction

1. To manage conservatively:

   a. CT scan of abdomen and pelvis with Gastrografin should be obtained. This can document the site of obstruction and may occasionally be therapeutic.

   b. Barium enema: Can occasionally be therapeutic. This study should be performed before a CT scan or small bowel follow-through.

   c. The patient should be made NPO; a NGT should be placed to LIWS; IV fluids and pain control should be instituted; antiemetics should be given.

2. To manage surgically:

   a. IV second-generation cephalosporins should be given prior to surgical correction.

   b. Resection with end-to-end anastomosis, loop, or end ostomy with mucous fistula can be performed.

   c. Stenting may occasionally be useful if the patient is a poor surgical candidate.

    d. Enemas in partial large bowel obstruction can either be therapeutic or can convert the obstruction to a complete obstruction by inducing colonic spasm.

C. Small bowel obstruction

  1. To manage conservatively:

    a. CT scan of abdomen and pelvis with Gastrografin should be obtained. This can document a transition point and may occasionally be therapeutic.

    b. The patient should be made NPO; a NGT should be placed to LIWS; IV fluids and pain control should be instituted; and antiemetics should be given.

  2. To manage surgically:

    a. IV second-generation cephalosporins should be given prior to surgery.

    b. Resection with end-to-end, side-to-side, or end-to-side anastomosis can be performed. An ileostomy or jejunostomy can also be considered with mucous fistula.

  3. If the patient chooses to forego extensive surgery, consider endoscopy with stent placement or diversion via end ostomy.

  4. When considering whether to perform surgical reduction of an obstruction in a cancer patient, it is important to take into account the patient's social factors; the expected outcome; the patient's life expectancy; and the etiology and the extent of obstruction (e.g., recurrent cancer, radiation stenosis).

Postoperative Complications

I. Gastrointestinal Complications

A. Ileus

1. The etiology is often intraoperative manipulation, electrolyte abnormalities, narcotics, peritonitis, abscess, hematoma, or fistula.

2. Signs are nausea and vomiting, hypoactive or absent bowel sounds, and abdominal distension.

3. Workup is with laboratories and physical examination.

4. Treatment: The patient can be made NPO, IVF initiated, and consideration given to a NGT. If the ileus does not resolve, imaging can be obtained with a CT scan of the abdomen and pelvis with PO Gastrograffin contrast to rule out an obstruction. An abdominal x-ray will provide no difference in clinical treatment between obstruction and ileus as they will both be managed with NPO/NGT/electrolyte replacement. If abscess is seen, a percutaneous drain can be placed with antibiotics as indicated.

B. Small bowel obstructions (SBO)

1. The etiology can be adhesions or herniation from surgery, bowel kinking, tumor, radiation-induced ischemia and stricture.

2. Signs are nausea and vomiting. Bowel sounds are present and can be high-pitched and hyperactive. Abdominal distension is present, and absence of flatus is common.

3. Workup is with lab tests, a physical examination, and CT scan of the abdomen and pelvis with PO Gastrografin contrast.

4. The patient should be made NPO, a NGT placed to LIWS, and IVF should be initiated. Correction of electrolyte abnormalities is important in addition to antiemetics and pain management.

Occasionally, high-dose steroids can reduce peri-luminal inflammation and have antiemetic properties. Partial obstructions can resolve with conservative management, but fewer than 50% of complete obstructions resolve similarly.

C. Large bowel obstructions (LBO) present in a similar fashion.

1. The etiology can be a mass causing obstruction intrinsically (bowel tumor) or extrinsically (pelvic tumor).

2. Signs: They can have a delayed time to presentation with a lower amount of emesis.

3. Workup: Imaging is indicated. A barium enema should be ordered first, followed by CT scan of the abdomen and pelvis with PO Gastrografin contrast or a small bowel follow-through.

4. Treatment: If resolution does not occur with conservative management as outlined for SBOs, surgical intervention is indicated. If the patient is not a surgical candidate, stent placement via endoscopy can be considered.

D. Bowel perforation

1. Etiology: Perforation can occur from an unrecognized enterotomy, intestinal devascularization, tumor infiltration of the bowel wall, bowel infarction (from thrombus, atrial fibrillation), or even certain chemotherapy agents (bevacuzimab up to 11%, paclitaxel 2%).

2. Signs are peritonitis, pain, abdominal distension, and fever.

3. Workup: Imaging with abdominal x-ray or CT demonstrating free air under the diaphragm. Treatment is with emergent surgical exploration and antibiotics. Cecal perforation tends to occur if the cecum is dilated to, or greater than, 10 cm as seen on imaging.

4. Treatment is with loop or end ostomy with mucous fistula, or ileostomy.

E. Pneumoperitoneum after laparotomy should be considered when ruling out a bowel perforation. The following table demonstrates the time from surgery and percent of patients with residual abdominal air present:

Time	Radiograph Percent Positive	CT Scan Percent Positive
Postoperative day 3	53% positive	87% positive
Postoperative day 6	8% positive	50% positive

F. Anastomotic bowel leak after a bowel resection can occur in up to 15% of patients. Prevention is avoidance of the bowel watershed areas. When performing an anastomosis, universal principles should be followed ensuring adequate vascularization of both ends of the bowel, absence of tumor at the anastomotic site, a tension-free anastomosis, and an adequate bowel lumen. Bowel viability is ascertained with IV fluroscene dye and a Wood's lamp at the time of resection and reanastomosis, or with Doppler ultrasound.

1. Signs: Leaks tend to present with nausea, ileus, abdominal pain, fever, and occasionally leakage of feculent material through the wound.

2. Workup: Includes physical exam, lab tests, and a CT of the abdomen and pelvis with PO Gastrografin.

3. Treatment: A drain needs to be placed, the patient made NPO, broad-spectrum antibiotics given, and consideration for surgical intervention with intestinal diversion. The diversion can usually be taken down in about 2 months, after imaging with PO contrast shows no evidence of continued leakage.

G. Bowel fistula

1. Signs: Fistulae can present as feculent discharge from a surgical wound or the vagina.

2. Workup: Diagnosis is with a CT of the abdomen and pelvis with PO Gastrografin contrast or a fistulagram.

3. Treatment: A NGT should be placed, the patient made NPO, and TPN initiated. Wound care should be performed, and consideration given to administration of somatostatin. If there is no resolution of the fistula with these conservative measures, surgical resection of the fistulous tract with bowel resection and reanastomosis should be performed. Staged repair with a diverting loop colostomy, primary fistula repair, and ostomy take down approximately 2 months later is another option.

H. Stoma complications usually involve stomal retraction or devitalization.

1. Etiology: This occurs from tension or decreased blood flow to the distal bowel edges.

2. Signs include a dusky appearance, necrosis, or retraction.

3. Workup: Evaluation of viability includes placement of a test tube or blood vial inside the stoma to assess the depth/extent of damage.

4. Treatment is based on location of devitalization. If it is limited to the distal segment above the fascia, observation and wound care are indicated. If there is necrosis beneath the fascia, surgical revision is necessary.

I. Ostomy herniation or prolapse usually occurs in patients whose ostomy was placed lateral to the rectus muscles.

1. Prolapse occurs in 1% to 3% of patients with an ostomy.

a. Etiology: It is often due to a stoma that is too long or wide, increased intra-abdominal pressure, extensive weight loss, or a redundant sigmoid colon.

b. Treatment: Conservative measures are placement of a rigid appliance with a tight belt. Treatment is resection of the protruding segment of colon with nipple reconstruction. Care should be taken to rule out those with a hernia so there is no loop transection risk.

2. Parastomal hernia: One half of patients with a prolapse also have a parastomal hernia.

a. Etiology: Parastomal hernias occur more often with loop ostomies than with end stomas. 2% to 3% of all end colostomy patients require hernia repair. Predisposing factors are often too large of an opening in the abdominal wall, placement lateral to the rectus muscle, placement in the laparotomy incision itself, or increased intra-abdominal pressure due to COPD, coughing, heavy lifting, obesity.

b. Repair is indicated if the hernia does not reduce easily, there is evidence of incarceration, or if the hernia interferes with appliance security. If the hernia is small, primary fascial repair without relocation can often be accomplished. If it is large, the ostomy can be placed at a different site (to a higher midrectus position, to the opposite side, or to the umbilicus) with repair of the primary ventral hernia. Mesh can otherwise be placed over part of the fascial defect to reduce the defect size (Sugarbaker) and the stoma can be brought out in-between an aperture between the mesh and the skin. To initiate the repair, the repair skin should be elliptically excised, and a finger swept circumferentially around the bowel between it and the fascia.

J. Short bowel syndrome is defined as malnutrition due to the lack of absorptive bowel length.

    1. Etiology: This can occur from significant bowel resection or from radiation injury. A length of 6.6 feet of bowel is necessary for nutrient absorption.

    2. Signs: Symptoms include diarrhea, steatorrhea, fluid depletion, fatigue, and occasionally abdominal pain.

    3. Diagnosis is made by malnutrition indices and weight loss.

    4. Treatment is with caloric, vitamin, and mineral supplementation. Hyperalimentation with TPN or continuous gastrostomy tube (G-tube) nutrition should be considered if there is significant weight loss. Additionally, antacids, antidiarrheals, and lactase supplements should be given.

K. Blind loop syndrome

    1. Etiology: Occurs after bowel resection and bypass producing a nonfunctional but retained loop of bowel.

    2. Signs: Increased flatulence, steatorrhea, weight loss, fatigue, and malabsorption.

    3. Diagnosis: A hydrogen breath test using glucose or lactulose can assist in the diagnosis. Bacterial overgrowth causes the majority of symptoms.

    4. Treatment: Antibiotics can reduce the bacterial load and decrease symptoms. Vitamin B_{12} supplementation is also often indicated.

II. Hemorrhage

A. Blood loss from the gastrointestinal system can occur from a stomach ulcer, esophageal varices, a Mallory-Weiss tear, a Boerhaave tear, NGT/catheter erosion, or radiation enteritis.

B. Inadequate hemostasis from a slipped suture, coagulopathy, or over-anticoagulation.

C. Tumor can spontaneously bleed from neovascularization.

D. Symptoms can include tachycardia, ectopy, pain, abdominal distension, decreased perfusion with mental status changes from hypoxia, low urine output from renal compromise, or extremity cyanosis due to centralization of the blood supply. Diagnosis is geared to identification of the source.

E. Workup: Laboratories include CBC and electrolytes. Imaging studies include CT, MRI, ultrasound, or angiography.

F. Treatment is focused on the "ABCs." Resuscitation is with IVF (in a 3:1 replacement ratio to loss), blood products, and oxygen. Treatment is surgical re-exploration or angiographic embolization.

G. If hemorrhage is due to a large cervical tumor, vaginal packing with Monsel's solution is indicated. The packing should be changed every 24 to 48 hours. Embolization can be considered but this will decrease oxygenation needed for radiotherapy to the primary tumor. Emergent radiotherapy can also be given.

III. Postoperative Fever: Postoperative fever is the most common postoperative complication. The definition of a fever is a temperature elevation taken 2 times, 6 hours apart. If the fever occurs within the first 24 hours of surgery, the temperature must be above 101.5°F (38.6°C). If the fever occurs greater than 24 hours after surgery, the temperature must be greater than or equal to 100.4°F (38.1°C).

A. The source of the fever usually follows the "five Ws."

Wind: This can represent atelectasis or pneumonia. Obtain a CXR.

Water: This can represent a UTI or pyelonephritis. Obtain a urine analysis.

Wound: This can represent a superficial infection, a seroma, cellulitis, or abscess. Evaluation involves examination and occasionally opening of the incision.

Walk: This can represent a DVT, septic pelvic thrombophlebitis, or a PE. Diagnosis is via examination, measurement of calf diameter, Doppler ultrasound, and occasionally CT angiogram.

Wonder Drugs: This can result from drug fevers. This is a diagnosis of exclusion. After ruling out other causes, consideration of discontinuing all drugs and observing the patient may be beneficial. Evaluation of the WBC differential may be helpful by assessment for the degree of eosinophilia.

IV. Wound Infection

A. Surgical site infections account for 40% of nosocomial infections. Risk factors for infection include: surgery lasting longer than 2 hours, higher blood loss, preoperative anemia, hypothermia, poor nutrition, cancer, prior pelvic radiation, diabetes, obesity, peripheral vascular disease, and a history of prior surgical infections.

1. Whole body scrubs including chlorhexidine can reduce bacterial skin counts, but they do not reduce the rate of wound infection. Patients may shower normally before surgery.

2. Hair clipping, not shaving, reduces the rate of wound infections.

3. Antibiotics given 1 hour before the skin incision are recommended, except for vancomycin and the fluoroquines, which should be given 2 hours prior. Cefazolin has a longer half-life and a broad spectrum of coverage. Cefotetan is preferred in longer, radical gynecologic operations and in colorectal surgery. An alternative is cefazolin plus metronidazole or Unasyn. If the patient's weight is greater than 70 kg, it is important to double the dose or weight-base dose the antibiotics.

4. Repeat dosing is recommended if surgery lasts longer than 3 to 4 hours, or if there is greater than 1,000 mL blood loss. Antibiotics should be stopped within 24 hours of surgery to decrease bacterial resistance and complications.

5. Obese patients have a higher risk for postoperative complications due to their body habitus and medical comorbidities. Some providers suggest these patients have baseline PFTs, assisted intubation, and delayed extubation until they are fully awake. Higher weight capacity hospital beds and operating room (OR) tables, specialized retractors, and extra-long instruments for surgery are important. A panniculectomy can be performed to improve surgical exposure.

B. Classification of operative wound infections is standardized.

1. A clean operative wound has a 1% to 2% risk of a surgical wound infection. This means that the GI and respiratory tracts were not entered, no drains were placed, and there was no break in aseptic technique. Examples of these surgeries are elective hernia repair.

2. A clean contaminated wound has a 4–10% risk of a surgical wound infection in uninfected patients. The GI or respiratory tracts were entered but minimal contamination occurred.

This includes hysterectomy, appendectomy, and most elective bowel surgery.

3. A contaminated operative wound has a 20% risk of surgical wound infection. This means there may have been a major break in sterile technique, the wound was made through nonpurulent inflammation, there was gross spill from the GI tract, or the wound was in or near contaminated skin. An example of this is a laparotomy in a patient with a colostomy.

4. An infected/dirty surgical wound has a 50% risk of wound infection. This occurs in a wound in which purulent infection or a perforated viscus was encountered. An example is a localized bowel perforation.

V. Urinary Tract Injury

A. Unrecognized injury occurs in 70% of patients.

1. Signs of injury include flank pain, fever, ileus from urine, hematuria, an elevated creatinine, or serous wound drainage (vaginal or abdominal).

2. Diagnosis is with renal ultrasound, IVP, CT with IV contrast, or cystoscopy with an attempt to pass ureteral stents.

3. Treatment is with antibiotics and ureteral stenting or percutaneous nephrostomy (PCN) to decompress the kidney and preserve renal function. Delay of definitive repair until 4 to 6 weeks should occur if the patient is unstable from other comorbidities. Recent data supports repair at the time of diagnosis if the patient is stable.

B. Postoperative fistulae can be either ureteral-vaginal or vesico-vaginal. Symptoms are leakage of clear fluid vaginally. Diagnosis is with a tampon test: This is performed with retrograde filling of the bladder using indigo carmine and placement of a vaginal tampon. If the tampon turns blue, the fistula originates in the bladder. If the tampon does not turn blue, pyrimidine can be given PO. If the tampon then turns orange, the fistula is most likely of ureteral origin.

1. Uretero-vaginal fistula tend to become apparent 5 to 14 postoperatively. Attempts at retrograde stenting should be made first. Percutaneous nephrostomy with antegrade stenting is the next best step. If stenting is not possible, percutaneous nephrostomy with drainage should be performed.

2. Vesicle-vaginal fistulas should first be treated with prolonged bladder drainage, in an attempt to allow spontaneous healing. If this does not work, repair is vaginal or abdominal. Vaginal repairs are with a modified Latzko technique, or a bulbocavernosus flap. If prior radiation therapy was given, a flap is needed to provide vascularized tissue.

3. Fistula that occur from a neobladder should be managed conservatively. An abdominal drain and percutaneous nephrostomy should be placed. If surgical intervention is attempted, there is a 9% mortality rate and 53% rate of complications.

VI. Lymphatic Complications

A. Lymphedema mainly occurs from surgical lymph node dissection. It can less commonly be due to radiation or tumor infiltration. Woody edema is the main symptom. Treatment is with elevation of the leg, support hose, or pneumatic compression devices.

B. Lymphangitis can present as acute erythema of the extremity, fever, and pain. It usually occurs after surgical lymph node dissection with superimposed infection. Treatment is with elevation of the leg, antibiotics, and NSAIDs.

C. Lymphocysts occur after lymph node dissection. Signs are a palpable cystic mass and pain. Diagnosis is via ultrasound, CT, or MRI. Treatment depends on symptoms. If the patient is asymptomatic, observation is enough. If there are symptoms, from pressure or mass effect, the cyst can be aspirated or sclerosed. If there are symptoms from infection, drainage with broad-spectrum antibiotics and NSAIDs are indicated.

VII. Nerve Injury

A. Neuropathy can complicate any surgical procedure. This stems from positioning, retractors, or direct nerve injury from dissection. Symptoms are sharp or burning pain, paresthesias, and weakness in the affected muscle groups. Treatment is often supportive care with physical therapy. If there is extensive deficit, a neurology consult can be obtained and electromyograms can assist in assessment.

B. Nerve transection: *See* Chapter 5D.

Preoperative Risk Assessment

I. Recommended laboratories include: CBC, PTT, PT, CMP. Other recommended studies include an EKG, a CXR, and pelvic imaging as appropriate. Further workup depends on patient medical history and physical findings.

II. ASA Score: The American Society of Anesthesiologists Score (ASA Score) provides risk information regarding surgical patients. There are 5 score classifications. Gynecologic oncology patients usually fall into classes 2 or 3. Class 1 is usually healthy and young persons. Class 2 patients have mild to moderate systemic disease. Class 3 patients have severe systemic disease. Class 4 patients have severe life-threatening systemic disease, and Class 5 patients are usually moribund.

III. Cardiac Risk Score: Cardiac risk evaluation is important because 1 of 12 patients over the age of 65 will have coronary artery disease. 30% of those undergoing major elective surgery have at least 1 cardiac risk factor. The Goldman multifactorial index helps to stratify patients based on their history and studies ordered. The index of cardiac risk factors includes:

Sign/Symptom	Points
S3 gallop or increased JVP	11
Myocardial infarction in last 6 months	10
More than 5 PVCs/min	7
Any rhythm other than sinus or PAC	7
Age greater than 70 years	5
Emergenct noncardiac operative procedure	4
Aortic stenosis	3
Poor general health	3
Abdominal or thoracic surgery	3

Patients then fall into risk factor classes:

Class	Points	Morbidity	Mortality
Class I	0–5 points	0.7%	0.2%
Class II	6–12 points	5%	1.6%
Class III	13–25 points	11%	2.3%
Class IV	≥ 26 points	22%	55.6%

IV. Functional status is commonly determined by METS. The ability to climb one flight of stairs is equal to 4 METS, and considered a decent functional status.

V. Subacute Bacterial Endocarditis: Prophylaxis for subacute bacterial endocarditis (SBE) should still be remembered. There are three categories of risk that require different levels of antibiotic protection.

A. The low-risk category includes isolated secundum atrial septal defect; prior surgical repair of an ASD, VSD, or PDA more than 6 months from surgery; a prior CABG, MVP without valve regurgitation; physiologic heart murmurs; prior Kawasaki disease without valve dysfunction; pacemakers and defibrillators; and prior rheumatic fever without valve dysfunction.

B. The moderate-risk category includes acquired valve dysfunctions, hypertropic cardiomyopathy, mitral valve prolapse with valve regurgitation or thickened leaflets, and other congenital cardiac malformations.

C. The high-risk category includes patients with prosthetic cardiac valves, prior BSE, complex cyanotic congenital heart disease, tetralogy of Fallot, transposition of the great arteries, patients with a single ventricle, or surgically constructed systemic pulmonary shunts or conduits.

D. Treatment is directed at the moderate and high-risk patients: Those who are moderate risk should get ampicillin 2 g IV within 30 minutes of the procedure. If they are allergic to ampicillin, they should receive vancomycin 1 g IV over 1 hour within 2 hours of starting the procedure. High-risk patients should receive ampicillin 2 g and gentamicin 1.5 mg/kg IV 30 minutes prior to surgery and again 8 hours after the surgery. If the patient is allergic to ampicillin, the patient should then receive vancomycin 1 g and gentamicin 1.5 mg/kg IV2 hours prior to surgery and 8 hours after surgery.

Perioperative Management in Gynecologic Oncology

I. Bowel Preparation

A. The administration of a preoperative bowel preparation is debatable. The pros include easy palpation of the entire colon, improved exposure, a decrease in operative time due to easier handling, and the removal of solid material from the GI tract. The cons include more anastomotic leaks from liquid stool, more sepsis due to trauma from the prep, and nonsignificant differences in operative times or facilitated exposure.

B. There are a number of different preparations: PEG can be given in 4 liters, magnesium citrate can be given in 300-mL bottles × 2 with or without a Dulcolax suppository, and antibiotic preparations. Antibiotic preparations include erythromycin base 1 g and neomycin 1 g; each given by mouth at 1, 2, and 10 p.m. the day before surgery. The erythromycin is given for both its antibiotic and its stimulant mechanisms of action. Another option is metronidazole 1 g and neomycin 1 g by mouth given at 1, 2, and 10 p.m. the day before surgery.

C. It is important to rehydrate with electrolytes (Gatorade) after the preparation, and care should be taken in patients with renal, heart, or liver failure.

II. Vascular Thromboembolism

A. DVT/VTE prophylaxis should be given to most hospitalized patients. The gynecologic oncology patient population is an especially high-risk group. Pneumatic sequential compression devices (SCDs) should be used. Use should start preoperatively, continue intraoperatively, and continue postoperatively.

B. A low-dose injectable anticoagulant should be considered prior to surgery. The normal dose of heparin is 5,000 units SC before surgery. Dalteparin dosed at 5,000 units SC can be given before surgery. Enoxaparin can also be used at 40 mg SC before surgery.

C. The combination of SCDs and injectable anticoagulants is especially helpful for the prevention of VTE complications. The use of SCDs has taken the incidence of VTE from 25% to 8%. The use of combination therapy then took the VTE occurrence from 8% to 2%. The risk of DVT with laparoscopic surgery in high-risk cancer patients with appropriate prophylaxis is 1.2% (1). Care should be taken and SCDs not used if an active DVT is present because of potential embolization.

D. Risk factors for VTE include known malignancy, surgery, surgical time greater than 2 to 3 hours, postoperative immobility, a past history of VTE, BMI > 30, hereditary coagulopathy, age 60 years or older, hypertension, renal disease, pulmonary disease, estrogen use, inflammatory bowel disease, and hereditary coagulopathies (MTHFR deficiency, protein C protein S deficiencies, prothrombin gene mutation, antithrombin III, and factor V Leiden gene mutations, antinuclear antibodies, antiphospholipid antibodies).

E. Symptoms of a DVT are leg edema, erythema, size discrepancy between the legs, and pain. Positive physical signs are the Pratt's, Homan's, and Moses's tests. Diagnosis is with Doppler ultrasound.

F. Pulmonary embolism can occur following a DVT. If untreated, 15% to 25% of DVTs progress to PE. If treated, 1.6% to 4.5% can still progress to PE, with 0.9% being fatal. Symptoms include tachypnea (90%), tachycardia (45%), hemoptysis (30%), cyanosis (20%), and a sense of impending doom (50%–65%).

1. Workup includes: CT angiogram of the chest, identification of the original thrombus with lower extremity Doppler's, a CXR, an ELISA D-dimer (which has a NPV 99.5%), an ABG (the PO_2 is often < 80 in 85% of patients) with calculation of the A-a gradient.

a. A normal A-a gradient is: age +4 years.

b. A CXR has a sensitivity of 33%, a specificity of 59%. Signs on CXR are an elevated hemidiaphragm (50%), the Hampton's hump due to a pleural-based infiltrate pointed toward the hilum, Westmark's sign (dilated proximal vessels with a distal cutoff), a pleural effusion, and atelectasis.

    c. An EKG showing RBBB or a right axis shift can be helpful. If spiral CT is contraindicated, a V/Q scan can be obtained with probabilities of PE represented as low, intermediate, or high. If the probabilities are intermediate or high, it is important to confirm with ECHO to evaluate right heart strain.

G. Treatment of DVT is with heparin, dalteparin, enoxaparin, or fondaparinux. It is important to not use SCDs when a DVT is diagnosed due to the risk of clot embolization.

    1. Dosing:

        a. Heparin is given IV and dosed at 80 units/kg bolus, then 18 units per hour.

        b. Dalteparin is dosed at 200 units/kg SC every 24 hours or 100 units/kg SC every 12 hours.

        c. Enoxaparin is dosed at 1 mg/kg SC every 12 hours. It is possible to convert to a daily dosing schedule of 1.5 mg/kg after 3 days of every-12-hour dosing.

        d. Fondaparinux is dosed at 5 mg if < 50 kg; 7.5 mg if 50 to 100 kg, or 10 mg if > 100 kg body weight SC daily.

H. Treatment of PE is with supportive care and anticoagulation. O_2 is titrated to keep saturations > 92%. Echocardiogram can evaluate for pulmonary hypertension and right heart failure. Cardiac support can be given with IV or PO medications. Occasionally, embolectomy can be performed. Anticoagulants are dosed the same as for DVT.

I. Conversion to PO anticoagulation is usually with warfarin. This is to start after 3 days of IV heparin or SC therapeutic anticoagulatoin with overlap due to rebound coagulopathy. It is important to follow the INR to keep it 2 to 3 × normal. Duration of treatment is 3 to 6 months for DVT diagnosis, and 6 to 12 months for a diagnosis of PE. Consider lifetime anticoagulation if there is a diagnosis of cancer, hereditary coagulopathy, or arterial thrombosis.

J. Drug interactions with Coumadin can affect the INR. These include erythromycin, sulfas, INH, fluconazole, amiodarone, corticosteroids, cimetidine, omeprazole, lovastatin, phenytoin, and propranolol. If the patient is malnourished, is vegetarian, or has liver disease, a lower dose may be needed. If the patient eats high amounts of green leafy vegetables, the patient may have increased levels of vitamin K and be more difficult to anticoagulate.

K. There is data to suggest that continued injectable anticoagulation is better in patients with malignancy than warfarin (CANTHANOX and LITE studies). There is also data to suggest better PFS and OS in patients receiving injectable anticoagulation (FAMOUS and CLOT studies).

L. Complications from anticoagulation do occur:

   1. Hemorrhage from over anti-coagulation;

   2. Heparin-induced thrombocytopenia (HIT)

      a. Type I: There is a decrease in platelet count to around 20,000. This is not life threatening but the patient should be removed from heparin treatment.

      b. Type II: There is a significant decrease in the platelet count, and an increased risk of both arterial and venous thrombi. There is also an increased risk of bleeding. The patient should be removed from heparin treatment.

      c. To diagnose HIT, heparin antibody testing should be ordered. Probability scoring should be calculated according to NCCN guidelines. If the score is 4 or more, unfractionated and LMW heparins as well as warfarin should be discontinued. The INR should be reversed with vitamin K. A direct thrombin inhibitor (DTI) or fonadparinux should be administered. If the HIT antibody is positive, serotonin release assay (SRA) testing should be ordered and DTIs continued for 6 weeks if no VTE is identified, or 6 months if a VTE is found.

M. Mechanisms of action:

   1. Heparin binds to antithrombin III. It enhances the inhibition of thrombin, and factors Xa and IXa. It increases the PTT and the level of anticoagulation can be monitored in this fashion. Heparin does not cross the placenta. Reversal is with protamine sulfate dosed at 1 mg/100 units of heparin. FFP can also be used if there is acute bleeding.

   2. Enoxaparin binds to and accelerates the action of antithrombin III. It preferentially potentiates the inhibition of factors Xa and IIa. Enoxaparin also has bleeding complications, but there is a lower incidence of induced thrombocytopenia. Monitoring is through anti-factor Xa.

3. Warfarin inhibits the synthesis of vitamin K-dependent clotting factors II, VII, IX, and X. It also inhibits proteins C and S. It is usually effective in 48 hours. It does cross the placenta. It increases the PT and INR and the level of anticoagulation can be monitored in this way. Reversal is with PO or IV vitamin K given at 1 to 10 mg depending on the INR.

N. Anticoagulation

1. Preoperative discontinuation: Anticoagulants such as warfarin should be stopped 4 to 5 days prior to surgery if the desired PT is 1 to 1.5 and the patients were maintained at an INR of 2 to 3. Aspirin should be stopped 7 days prior to surgery due to the irreversible binding to platelets. Clopidogrel should be stopped 10 days prior to surgery.

2. The patient needs an anticoagulant bridge if the patient has a mechanical valve, there is a history of thromboembolism, or there is atrial fibrillation with a history of stroke.

3. Some patients may not be responsive to medical prophylaxis or therapeutic management of DVT. An IVC filter can be placed to prevent embolization. Indications for an IVC filter are: VTE/PE in patients with a contraindication to anticoagulation, a PE despite anticoagulation, significant heparin-induced thrombocytopenia, chronic PE with associated pulmonary hypertension, or the patient is status post a pulmonary embolectomy. Another indication is the need for urgent surgery in a patient with a recent history of DVT, on anticoagulation, but needing temporary discontinuation for a procedure.

4. Naturopathic supplements are commonly used and it is important to discontinue the following prior to surgery as they can alter clotting time: vitamin E, garlic, gingko, and ginseng.

O. Arterial Embolic Events

1. Arterial occlusion usually occurs from direct injury or trauma to a vessel or extremity. It may also represent a thrombotic insult from the left heart or a patent foramen ovale.

2. Symptoms are related to the arterial occlusion and the extremity usually has pallor, pulselessness, paresthesia, pain, and is cold. The diagnostic workup includes a Doppler and an angiogram.

3. Treatment is via vascular surgery with a thrombectomy, followed by anticoagulation as soon as the diagnosis is made.

4. Acute mesenteric ischemia is a medical emergency. Characteristics are abdominal pain out of proportion to the examination, and a history of atrial fibrillation. Diagnosis is via EKG and CT. Treatment is emergency laparotomy with bowel resection if indicated and surgical revascularization followed by anticoagulation.

III. Nutrition

A. 50% of gynecologic oncology patients are malnourished when admitted. A weight loss of over 10% from the patient's normal weight usually means he or she is malnourished. There are a few ways to measure the level of malnutrition.

1. The prognostic nutritional index includes: measurement of the triceps skin fold, the serum albumin level, the serum transferrin level, and assessment of the delayed hypersensitivity response to mumps, TB, and *Candida* Ag.

2. Laboratory measurements of malnutrition can include the total lymphocyte count, or the serum albumin level (which has a half-life of 20 days). The serum albumin test is the single test with the most predictive value: levels less than 2.1 mg/dL are associated with morbidity from 10% to 65%.

B. A rapid postoperative feeding schedule has proven benefits and is usually encouraged in gynecologic surgeries. Clear liquids orally are started as soon as the patient is alert and without nausea, vomiting, or significant abdominal distension. Advancement to a regular diet after proven tolerance to liquids follows. Rapid postoperative feeding has been shown to decrease hospital length of stay with no additional adverse events.

C. The Harris-Benedict equation calculates the daily basal caloric need: BEE = 655 + (9.6 × kg) + (1.8 × cm height) − (4.7 × age in years). Stress factors should be added to this caloric need as indicated: 1.2× for a minor insult, 1.3× for an elective surgical patient or with moderate stress (SIRS, sepsis), and 1.5× for severe stress (burn patients).

D. TPN composition includes: glucose at 3.4 kcal/g to yield 70% of the calculated calories. The remaining 30% is from lipids (at 9 kcal/kg). Protein is added at 1 to 1.5 g nitrogen/kg. TPN should be considered if the patient has a nonfunctioning GI tract due to ileus or obstruction, is unable to tolerate PO for 7 days or more after surgery, has short bowel syndrome, or is severely malnourished.

IV. Endocrine Management

A. Diabetes

    1. Diabetes mellitus can increase perioperative complications. It is important to get a preoperative ECHO for baseline cardiac function, renal labs, an HgA1c, and a urine analysis to check for protein.

    2. Postoperative infections cause 20% of deaths in diabetics. To optimize glycemic control, the serum glucose should be maintained between 80 and 110 mg/dL using a weight based sliding scale regimen. This yields a 46% reduction in septicemia and 34% reduction in hospital mortality. It is recommended to stop metformin and sulfonylurea medications 24 to 48 hours before surgery and restarted when the patient tolerates a regular ADA diet.

B. Steroid therapy: Steroid therapy is indicated for patients who have medical comorbidities that need additional adrenal support.

    1. Indications for stress dosing of steroids would be more than 3 weeks of, or an equivalent to, 20 mg of prednisone daily within 1 year of surgery.

    2. Stress dosing is administered preoperatively with IV hydrocortisone or methylprednisolone 100 mg. Postoperative treatment is 100 mg IV every 8 hours for 3 doses. When the patient can tolerate PO, it is okay to resume scheduled dosing or to start a steroid taper. If the patient is clinically Cushingoid, he or she also then requires stress dosing.

Steroid Taper	Hydrocortisone (IV)	Prednisone (PO)
POD 0	100 mg IV q 8 hours	—
POD 1	100 mg IV q 8 hours	37.5 mg PO q 12 hours
POD 2	80 mg IV q 8 hours	30 mg PO q 12 hours

Steroid Taper	Hydrocortisone (IV)	Prednisone (PO)
POD 3	60 mg IV q 8 hours	22.5 mg PO q 12 hours
POD 4	40 mg IV q 8 hours	15 mg PO q 12 hours
POD 5	20 mg IV q 8 hours	7.5 mg PO q 12 hours
POD 6	May discontinue	

    3. It is important to perform Accu-Chek measures and place the patient on a sliding scale of insulin due to the risk of diabetic insult and systemic hyperglycemia.

  C. Thyroid disease: Thyroid disease can complicate surgery. It is important to check a TSH and a T4 prior to surgery in patients with a known thyroid disorder, in diabetic patients, or in undiagnosed patients who are symptomatic.

    1. Patients who are hypothyroid have more ileus, delirium, and infection without fever.

    2. If the patient is severely hypothyroid, it is important to give IV thyroxine, and stress dose steroids. The half-life of thyroxine is 5 to 9 days.

    3. Patients who are hyperthyroid can have major complications as well. These can be cardiac related to both inotropic and chronotropic factors. Atrial fibrillation can occur in 10% to 20% of patients.

    4. Thyroid storm should be suspected if there is fever, tachycardia, confusion, CV collapse, or death. Preoperative treatment is with a beta blocker, continuation of PTU or methimazole, and administration of stress dose steroids.

V. Hepatic Disease: Hepatitis is divided into acute and chronic diseases. It is important to check for coagulopathies in liver disease. It is also important to reduce narcotic dosing by 50% in these patients.

  A. Surgery should be delayed if there is acute hepatitis. The mortality ranges up to 58% if surgery is pursued in the acute phases.

  B. If the hepatitis is chronic, there is no change in mortality and surgery does not need to be delayed.

  C. The Child-Turcotte classification system predicts mortality in patients with liver disease. Class A has a 10% postoperative mortality, Class B has 30% mortality, and Class C has 80% mortality.

VI. Neurologic Disease

A. There are a number of different etiologies that may explain altered mental status. Common causes include metabolic abnormalities, sepsis, meningitis, brain metastasis, or stroke. The initial treatment for a patient with acute-onset altered mental status is to maintain an airway, establish IV access, and provide oxygen, if necessary; laboratories and imaging follow.

1. Workup for metabolic causes includes: CBC, CMP, urine analysis, urine drug screen, cardiac enzymes and pulse oximetry and blood cultures.

2. Workup for sepsis or meningitis includes: CBC, CMP, blood, and urine cultures. Lumbar puncture is appropriate for cell count, culture, and cytology, but should only be performed after a CT of the head demonstrates no brain lesions causing mass effect.

3. Workup for metastatic disease or stroke: CT of the head is usually ordered without contrast to evaluate for evidence of an acute hemorrhagic stroke. If negative, a study with contrast is better for evaluation of metastatic lesions. MRI is the most sensitive and specific study to evaluate for evidence of brain metastasis or stroke.

B. Treatment for specific clinical situations:

1. Narcotic drug overdose: Naloxone: 1 ampule (0.01 mg/kg IV)

2. Seizure: Dilantin 1,000 mg load then 200 to 300 mg QD, valium 5 mg IV

3. Brainstem herniation: Hyperventilate PCO_2 to 25 to 30 mm Hg, dexamethasone 10 mg IV then 4 mg IV q 6 hours, mannitol 12 g/kg IV then 50 to 300 mg/kg IV q 6 hours. Surgical intervention may be necessary.

VII. Alcohol Withdrawal: Alcohol withdrawal can cause significant morbidity. Patients with a history of alcohol abuse should be assessed for withdrawal. A well-lit room, social support, and reassurance are first steps. Seizures can occur 12 to 48 hours after alcohol cessation. Delirium tremens complicates 5% to 10% of alcohol withdrawal cases, and mortality can approach 15%. Beer can be ordered while a patient is hospitalized.

A. CIWA Scoring is a cumulative score that provides the basis of a treatment plan for patients undergoing alcohol withdrawal.

Nausea and Vomiting		Tremor	
Score		Score	
0	No nausea and no vomiting	0	No tremor
1	Mild nausea with no vomiting	1	Not visible, but can be felt fingertip to fingertip
4	Intermittent nausea with dry heaves	4	Moderate, with patient's arms extended
7	Constant nausea, frequent dry heaves and vomiting	7	Severe, even with arms not extended

Paroxysmal Sweats		Anxiety	
Score		Score	
0	No sweat visible	0	No anxiety, at ease
1	Barely perceptible sweating, palms moist	1	Mildly anxious
4	Beads of sweat obvious on forehead	4	Moderately anxious, or guarded, so anxiety is inferred
7	Drenching sweats	7	Equivalent to acute panic states as seen in severe delirium or acute schizophrenic reactions

Agitation		Tactile Disturbances	
Score		Score	
0	Normal activity	0	None
1	Somewhat more than normal activity	1	Very mild itching, pins and needles, burning or numbness
4	Moderately fidgety and restless	2	Mild itching, pins and needles, burning or numbness
7	Paces during most of the interview, or constantly thrashes about	3	Moderate itching, pins and needles, burning or numbness
		4	Moderately severe hallucinations
		5	Severe hallucinations
		6	Extremely severe hallucinations
		7	Continuous hallucinations

Auditory Disturbances		Visual Disturbances	
Score		Score	
0	Not present	0	Not present
1	Very mild harshness or ability to frighten	1	Very mild sensitivity
		2	Mild sensitivity
2	Mild harshness or ability to frighten	3	Moderate sensitivity
		4	Moderately severe hallucinations
3	Moderate harshness or ability to frighten	5	Severe hallucinations
4	Moderately severe hallucinations	6	Extremely severe hallucinations
		7	Continuous hallucinations
5	Severe hallucinations		
6	Extremely severe hallucinations		
7	Continuous hallucinations		

Headache, Fullness in Head		Orientation and Clouding of Sensorium	
Score		Score	
0	Not present	0	Oriented and can do serial additions
1	Very mild		
2	Mild	1	Cannot do serial additions or is uncertain about date
3	Moderate		
4	Moderately severe	2	Disoriented for date by no more than 2 calendar days
5	Severe		
6	Very severe	3	Disoriented for date by more than 2 calendar days
7	Extremely severe		
		4	Disoriented for place and/or person

Cumulative	
Score	
0–8	No medication is necessary
9–14	Medication is optional for patients with a score of 8–14
15–20	A score of 15 or over requires treatment with medication
>20	A score of over 20 poses a strong risk of delirium tremens
67	Maximum possible cumulative score

B. Basic orders include seizure precautions, aspiration precautions, and restraints if the patient has safety risks. Admission lab tests include: CBC, CMP, LFTs, PTT, INR, and a urine analysis. Blood alcohol levels should also be drawn. A urine toxicology screen is usually indicated. A CXR to evaluate for pneumonia should be considered. A daily CMP is important.

C. IV fluids should be initiated with normal saline. D5 should be added if the patient is NPO but thiamine should be given first. When the patient becomes euvolemic, the IVF should be switched to one-half normal saline (or D5 one-half normal saline) at 125 mL/hour.

D. Medications should include vitamins, benzodiazepines, and antipsychotics as indicated.

    1. Vitamins include: thiamine dosed at 100 mg IV for 3 days, then daily by mouth; folate 1 mg daily by mouth; and a multivitamin daily.

    2. Benzodiazepines include chlordiazepoxide and lorazepam. Chlordiazepoxide (Librium) is dosed at 25 to 100 mg PO q 4 to 6 hours. Lorazepam (Ativan) is dosed at 1 to 4 mg PO/SL/IM/IV. It may be given every 4 to 6 hours or every 15 to 30 min in cases of severe withdrawal. Lorazepam should be first choice in patients with liver compromise (AST > 200, INR > 1.5); in patients who need IV dosing and cannot take PO well; and in patients who exceed the maximum chlordiazepoxide dose of 600 mg in 24 hours.

E. Treatment per CIWA score.

    1. For a CIWA score of < 8, scheduled doses of benzodiazepine should be considered. Patients should be assessed and assigned a CIWA score every 6 hours. Total benzodiazepine dose should be tapered by 25% per day after an initial 72-hour period. Initially, this can be achieved by decreasing the q 6 hour dose. Once the dose is at the smallest unit interval (0.5 to 1 mg lorazepam, or 25 mg chlordiazepoxide), the dosing interval should be lengthened.

    2. For patients in active withdrawal with a CIWA score of 8 to 25, symptom-triggered treatment should be initiated. These patients are categorized according to the severity of their current symptoms: mild = CIWA 8 to 13; moderate = CIWA 14 to 20; marked = CIWA 21 to 25. Patients should be assessed every 4 hours, in addition to 1 hour after medication administration.

    3. For patients with severe withdrawal who are assigned a CIWA score greater than 25, ICU admission is required. Nursing staff assessment is every 2 hours. Treatment is with lorazepam and these patients may require a continuous infusion of lorazepam. The initial rate may be estimated by averaging the hourly dose of benzodiazepine delivered over the first

6 hours. The infusion rate should then be titrated with the goal of sedation scale of 3 to 4.

4. Treatment of disorientation or hallucinations without autonomic signs of alcohol withdrawal (such as tremor and diaphoresis) may benefit from the addition of haloperidol instead of additional benzodiazepine use.

VIII. Blood Transfusion

A. Transfusion is recommended in an asymptomatic patient for a Hg level below 6 g/dL. If a perioperative patient has an Hg of 7 g/dL and surgery is expected to have significant blood loss, or if the risks associated with anesthesia are high, the patient may be transfused before the procedure. If the patient has medical comorbidities such as cardiovascular, pulmonary, or cerebrovascular disease, an optimal Hg is around 10 g/dL and the patient can be transfused to reach that parameter. If the patient is expected to receive adjuvant therapies, an optimal Hg is 10 g/dL. If the patient is symptomatic with orthostatic hypotension, dizziness, or has new physical symptoms such as cardiac murmur, transfusion should be entertained.

B. The current risk of viral infection from transfusion is 1:2.3 million for HIV, 1:350,000 for hepatitis B, and 1:2 milion for hepatitis C.

C. Allogeneic blood transfusions are an alternative to standard transfusions, but need to be obtained 6 weeks prior to surgery and are screened in the same fashion as all other blood donations. Normovolemic hemodilution is an alternative to blood transfusion.

D. Immunomodulation from blood transfusion may lead to postoperative infections as well as increased morbidity and mortality. Multiorgan failure is now an important concept such as transfusion-related acute lung injury (TRALI) and transfusion associated circulatory overload (TACO) are now major causes of complications.

REFERENCE

1. Nick AM, Schmeler KM, Frumovitz MM, et al. Risk of thromboembolic disease in patients undergoing laparoscopic gynecologic surgery. *Obstet Gynecol.* 2010;116(4):956–961.

Critical Care

I. Pulmonary

A. Complications related to pulmonary factors occur in 20% to 30% of postoperative patients. The functional residual capacity (FRC) is reduced when patients are supine, or have had a laparotomy. Vital capacity is decreased 45% and FRC is reduced 20%.

B. Risk factors are obesity, surgery longer than 2 hours, COPD, CHF, renal failure, poor mental status, immunosuppression, NGT use, narcotics, smoking, sleep apnea, and asthma. COPD patients can benefit from a preoperative ABG and PFTs.

C. Atelectasis usually occurs postintubation, and is due to surgical pain with its associated decreased inspiratory effort. Dyspnea, tachypnea, and fever can be present. Examination reveals crackles at the lung bases. Diagnosis is with CXR. Treatment is incentive spirometry.

D. Pneumonia can present with dyspnea, tachypnea, fever, and decreased O_2 saturation. Examination reveals decreased breath sounds segmentally. Diagnosis is via CXR and documentation of infiltrate or consolidation. Treatment is with antibiotics, incentive spirometry, chest physiotherapy, and pulmonary toilet.

E. Respiratory failure is defined as altered pulmonary function that yields hypercarbia, acidemia, or hypoxemia.

1. The etiology can be a decreased respiratory drive, airway obstruction, decreased pulmonary function, COPD, asthma, anaphylaxis, pulmonary edema from CHF, ARDS, pneumonia, abscess, tuberculosis, pneumothorax, pleural effusion, hemothorax, cancer, anemia, or pulmonary embolus.

2. Diagnosis is via physical examination, imaging, and laboratories. It is important to obtain a CXR, oxygen saturation monitor, an ABG, a CBC, electrolytes, a CT angiogram if

suspicion for a PE is present, and potentially an ECHO to rule out cardiogenic etiology.

F. Oxygen is not as good as we think. 100% O_2 for greater than 6 hours has been shown to decrease macrophage activity, mucous velocity, cardiac output, and can cause irreversible pulmonary damage if given for greater than 60 hours. Oxygen can be delivered via nasal prongs, a rebreathing face mask, a nonrebreathing face mask, CPAP, BiPAP, and intubation with mechanical ventilation. Delivery via nasal prongs has been shown to be as good as a rebreathing face mask.

G. Parameters

PaO_2: Arterial oxygen tension

Normal: 70 to 100 mm Hg

PAO_2: Alveolar oxygen tension $(FiO_2 \times 713) - (PaCO_2/0.8)$

Normal: 100 mm Hg

$PaCO_2$: Arterial CO_2 tension

Normal: 35 to 44 mm Hg

AA Gradient: Alveolar − arterial O_2 tension or $[(FiO_2) \times$ (Atmospheric pressure − H_2O Pressure) − $(PaCO_2/0.8)] - PaO_2$

Normal is 3 to 16 mm Hg or (Age/4) +4

Vital Capacity: Volume of expired air after maximal inspiration

Normal: 3 to 5 L

Tidal Volume: Volume of inspired air for each peak breath

Normal: 6 to 7 mL/kg

FEV_1: Maximum volume forcefully expired in 1 second

Normal: > 83% of vital capacity

PEF: Peak expiratory flow rate

Normal: > 400 L/minute

NIF: Negative inspiratory force

Normal: 60 to 100 cm H_2O

H. Parameters for intubation in respiratory failure: Indications for mechanical ventilation include hypoxemia, hypercarbia, respiratory acidosis, the inability to maintain or protect the airway including changes in mental status, and respiratory fatigue. The largest endotracheal tube possible should be chosen: This is usually a 7.5 to 8 for women. This is to decrease airway resistance. Vitals and laboratory benchmarks are listed below:

Mechanics	Results
FiO_2	> 60 mm Hg
$PaCO_2$	> 55–60 mm Hg
Respiratory rate	> 30–35 bpm
Arterial pH	< 7.25
Negative inspiratory force	More positive than –20 cm H_2O
Vital capacity	< 10 mL/kg
PO_2	< 80 mm Hg

I. The A-a gradient is calculated to determine shunt and help rule out a pulmonary embolus. The A-a gradient = $[(FiO_2) \times$ (Atmospheric pressure $- H_2O$ Pressure) $- (PaCO_2/0.8)] - PaO_2$. A normal gradient estimate = $(Age/4) + 4$.

J. Ventilation by machine can be run by volume or by pressure. The volume cycled setting has a preset tidal volume. The pressure cycled setting stops the cycle at a preset pressure; this setting is useful in hypoxic patients.

1. Continuous mandatory ventilation (CMV) delivers a preset minute ventilation determined by a set respiratory rate and tidal volume. It is useful in heavily sedated patients, those given paralytic agents, and those who do not tolerate assisted ventilation.

2. Assist-control (A/C or volume controlled) ventilation presets the tidal volume, and this tidal volume is delivered when a breath is initiated by the patient. This is the most common mode of mechanical ventilation used in the ICU. A control back up rate is set to prevent hypoventilation.

3. Intermittent mandatory ventilation (IMV) has a set rate and tidal volume, but allows unassisted spontaneous breaths and provides a full breath in relation to the amount of patient effort.

4. Synchronized IMV (SIMV) delivers breaths at regular intervals that are based on a preset tidal volume and rate which are synchronized with the patient's respiratory efforts.

5. Pressure supported (PS) ventilation provides constant airway pressure, which is delivered during inspiration. It is the most frequently used mode during "weaning". In this mode, each time the patient inhales, the ventilator delivers a pressure-limited breath. The patient controls the rate, volume and duration of the breaths.

K. To initially set the ventilator, IMV or A/C cycles are usually chosen. The FiO_2 is started at 60% (maximum), and weaned down to a patient O_2 saturation of 90% to 95% and a FiO_2 of 21% (room air). The rate is usually initiated at 8 to 12 breaths per minute. The tidal volume is chosen at 8 to 12 mL/kg, but should be lower at 6 mL/kg if the patient is suspected or diagnosed with ARDS. A PEEP of 5 cm H_2O is also chosen. It is important to check an ABG and adjust the settings further based on those results.

L. Extubation should be a rapid goal. A spontaneous breathing trial or t-tube trial should be performed daily to assess patient status. Weaning settings on the ventilator are with SIMV or PS ventilation. To be extubated, the patient must be conscious and can protect the airway, the FiO_2 must be less than 50% (optimally at 21% room air [RA]), the PEEP should be less than 5 cm H_2O, the negative inspiratory force should be greater than 20 cm H_2O.

Weaning Parameters	Acceptable for Extubation
Respiratory rate	< 30–35 (> 8) bpm with FiO_2 < 0.5
PaO_2	> 60 mm Hg with FiO_2 < 0.5
$PaCO_2$	< 50 with respiratory rate < 25 bpm
Negative inspiratory force	More negative than –20–25 cm H_2O
Vital capacity	> 10–15 mL/kg
Tidal volume	> 3 mL/kg
The patient is awake and can protect the airway	

M. Ventilator acquired pneumonia (VAP) occurs in 30% of patients after 72 hours of intubation. The mortality of VAP is 25% to 50%.

N. Monitoring of pulmonary and cardiac status can be with a central line. The central venous pressure (CVP) is an assessment of volume status and crude cardiac function. It consists of multiple measurements, and is not a single number. A normal CVP is 8 to 10 cm H_2O, or 2 to 6 mm Hg.

O. A pulmonary artery (PA or Swan) catheter can be helpful when it is important to know critical cardiac output or fluid status. Complications of a Swan include pneumonthorax, arrhythmia, line sepsis (2%), or pulmonary artery rupture. Cardiac output is calculated thermodynamically. An estimation of preload is obtained by wedging the end of the catheter into an afferent pulmonary capillary. This is called the PAOP or PCWP. A normal PCWP is 6 to 12 mm Hg. The PCWP is a crude reflection of the left arterial pressure. If the PCWP is elevated, then the preload is adequate or excessive; if it is low, then the patient is likely volume depleted. The mixed venous blood sample is blood obtained from the tip of the PA catheter and reflects the most desaturated blood in the body.

P. Acute respiratory distress syndrome (ARDS) occurs after a defined insult to the lungs. This can include hemorrhage, sepsis, shock, or pneumonia. An ABG should be drawn.

    1. Symptoms are tachypnea, dyspnea, and respiratory failure.

    2. There are several criteria for the diagnosis of ARDS:

        a. Bilateral diffuse infiltrates are seen on CXR

        b. CHF and iatrogenic volume overload are ruled out by ECHO (showing an EF > 35%)

        c. There is impaired oxygenation with documented oxygen saturation less than 92%

        d. The calculated PAO_2/FiO_2 is < 200 for the diagnosis of ARDS

        e. If the PAO2/FiO2 < 300, the diagnosis is acute lung injury (ALI)

    3. The mortality of ARDS is 30% to 40%.

    4. Treatment is with intubation, mechanical ventilation, antibiotics, and treatment of the underlying cause. Steroids have not been proven beneficial. Better survival has been seen with ventilatory support maintaining low tidal volumes to prevent barotrauma (6 mL/kg), and elevated PCO_2—permissive hypercapnia.

II. Cardiac

A. Reinfarction can occur after a recent myocardial infarction. Rates have decreased from 37% to now 5–10%; due to better medications used for reperfusion. The rate further decreases the longer the time from the initial insult. The rate is 2% to 3% after 4 to 6 months, and 1% to 2% if greater than 6 months have elapsed after a recent MI.

B. Perioperative beta blockers have been studied. Laughton, in 2005, showed there were fewer infarctions and lower mortality when used after surgery. The rates of infarction with use were 24% vs. 39% without. The 2-year mortality was 16% with use vs. 32% without. A more recent study, the POISE study in 2008, refutes the benefit of beta blocker use postoperatively. There were fewer MIs in the beta blocker group (4.2% vs. 5.7%, $P < .05$), but there were more deaths (3.1% vs. 2.3%, $P < .05$) and more CVAs (1% vs. 0.5%, $P < .05$) with beta blocker use (1).

C. The role of a pulmonary artery catheter (Swan-Ganz) for surgery remains controversial and has been decreasing in indications. There are no definitive studies that provide evidence of benefit in the surgical setting. The current indications are active CHF, severely depressed LV function, and critical aortic stenosis.

D. Parameters

Cardiac output: Heart rate × Stroke volume

Normal: 4 to 8 L/min

Cardiac index: Cardiac output/BSA m²

Normal: 2.5 to 4 L/min

MAP: Mean arterial pressure = 1/3 × (SBP – DBP) + DBP

Normal: 70 to 105 mm Hg

PAP Systolic: Systolic pulmonary arterial pressure

Normal: 15 to 30 mm Hg

PAP Diastolic: Diastolic pulmonary arterial pressure

Normal: 5 to 12 mm Hg

PAP mean: Mean pulmonary arterial pressure

Normal: 5 to 10 mm Hg

PAWP: Pulmonary artery wedge pressure = LA and LV filling pressure

Normal: 5 to 12 mm Hg

SVR: Systemic vascular resistance (MAP – MRAP)(80)/CO

Normal 900 to 1400 dynes/sec/cm^{-5}

PVR: Pulmonary vascular resistance (mean PAP – PAWP)/CO

Normal 100 to 240 dynes/sec/cm^{-5}

VO_2: O_2 consumption

Normal 115 to 1165 mL/min/m^2

DO_2: O_2 delivery

Normal 640 to 1000 mL O_2/min

E. Ischemic heart disease

1. Ischemic heart disease (myocardial infarction) can oftentimes be identified by its symptoms. Angina, nausea, vomiting, dyspnea, sweating, diaphoresis, SOB, weakness, anxiety, elevated BP, tachycardia, bradycardia, JVD, or tachyarrhythmias are often present.

2. Workup includes: an EKG, cardiac enzymes × 3 q 6 to 8 hours (CK, CKMB, troponin I), BNP, CXR, and consideration of angiography, especially if a ST elevation myocardial infarction (STEMI) is diagnosed.

3. Medical treatment is with transfer to the critical care unit (CCU) for telemetry.

Myocardial infarctions are classified as: STEMI, NSTEMI, and unstable angina.

Pulse oximetry should be obtained, aspirin administered, and oxygen placed to keep saturations greater than 90%. A CXR should be obtained in addition to an EKG and laboratories.

Initial stabilization should include administration of sublingual NTG at 5 minute intervals for 3 doses if there is chest pain. IV morphine dosed at 4–8 mg repeated every 5–15 minutes is recommended for chest pain and to decrease the myocardial workload. Atropine can be given to increase blood pressure if hypotension is present and reflects bradycardia. Beta blockers should be administered in the absence of contraindications. Contraindications include: SBP < 90, bradycardia, findings suggesting right ventricle infarction.

a. Treatment of patients with STEMI include: IV thrombolysis within 30 minutes or cardiac catheterization for PCTA within 90 minutes of arrival or occurrence.

b. Treatment of patients with NSTEMI include: Observation and monitoring in a CCU with administration of stool softeners, stress ulcer prophylaxis, antipyretics, and bedrest. Beta blockers should be administered in the absence of contraindications. ACE inhibitors may be additionally beneficial in limiting infarct size. If chest pain continues, angiography and revascularization via PCTA, stenting, or surgery is indicated. IV NTG titrated to 10–200 mg/min to prevent hypotension can be given to alleviate coronary artery spasm and decrease infarct size. Thrombolytic therapy is not indicated in NSTEMI MI's.

c. Treatment of patients with unstable angina is angiography with PCTA, stenting, or surgery.

An EKG should be obtained with each set of enzymes. An ECHO is usually ordered as well for ejection fraction and ventricular assessment. PCTA should be administered within 90 minutes. Angiography should be considered.

For severe LV dysfunction and cardiogenic shock, angioplasty, thrombolysis, and revascularization with multivessel stenting may be indicated.

4. Interventional treatment:

a. Angioplasty is used to dilate a stenosed artery mechanically with a balloon catheter.

b. A stent can also be placed simultaneously. The stent can be mechanical alone or medicated (impregnated with paclitaxel). The medicated stents keep occluded arteries open and decrease local plaque. Surgery can be performed 6 weeks after a medicated stent as antithrombotics are needed for this duration. A nonmedicated/bare metal stent is indicated if surgery is urgent. Surgery can be performed 2 weeks after bare metal stent placement.

c. Thrombolysis is another option for removing coronary artery occlusion. This occurs after localization with angiography and if the diagnosis occurs within 6 hours of the onset of pain. The clot is lysed with antithrombotics.

F. Heart failure is defined as an EF less than 35%. The etiology is most commonly a MI, but can be viral, or hereditary.

1. Symptoms are SOB, lower extremity edema, or JVD. There can be ascites if there is significant right heart failure, progressing to anasarca if not managed.

2. Workup includes a CXR, which will show bilateral infiltrates, an EKG, an ECHO, cardiac enzymes × 3 every 6 to 8 hours, BNP, electrolytes, and a CBC. A spiral CT can help rule out a PE.

3. Treatment is with O_2 supplementation, water restriction to 2 liters per day, morphine, and diuretics (furosemide to start at 20 mg IV, doubling of the dose is indicated if minimal response is seen). If there is a need to increase the cardiac output (CO), inotropes such as dopamine or dobutamine can be considered. Digoxin can be administered to improve contractility (1 mg load 0.5 mg IV, then 0.25 mg q 6 hours × 2, maintenance 0.125 mg per day, checking the level the first day then every 5 days). A daily weight and strict salt management (<2 g per day) are important.

G. Pulmonary edema is characterized by SOB.

1. Diagnosis is with a physical examination demonstrating bilateral rales and low oxygen saturation. Confirmation is with CXR showing bilateral infiltrates. An EKG, an ECHO, cardiac enzymes × 3 every 6 to 8 hours, BNP, an ABG, and CT angiogram to rule out PE should be obtained to rule out cardiac and VTE etiologies.

2. Treatment is diuresis, O_2 supplementation, and correction of the underlying cause.

H. Hypertension is often not symptomatic.

1. Characteristics when symptomatic are a headache or change in vision.

2. Diagnosis is via BP assessment. If symptomatic, an EKG, cardiac enzymes × 3 every 6 to 8 hours, and CT head without contrast or MRI are indicated to rule out stroke.

3. Parameters

Category	Systolic	Diastolic	Follow-Up	Status
Mild	140–159	90–99	2 months	
Moderate	160–179	100–109	1 month	
Severe	180–209	110–119	1 week	Urgent
Crisis	210	120	Immediate	Crisis

4. Treatment for crisis range HTN can include: nitroprusside (Nipride) 1 to 10 mcg/kg/min IV; an angiotensin-converting

enzyme (ACE) inhibitor (enalapril) 12.5 mg PO or 1.25–2.5 mg IV every 6 hours; a beta blocker (labetalol) 20 mg IV, repeated at 40 to 80 mg q 10 minutes with a maximum dose 300 mg and a maintenance dose of 0.5 to 2 mg/min; an alpha blocker (Hydralazine): 5 to 20 mg IV.

5. Management of HTN, other than crisis range, is with single-agent or combination agents. First-line drugs are often diuretics (hydrochlorothiazide). Beta-blockers can be first- or second-line, as can be calcium channel blockers (a better response is seen with these drugs in African Americans). ACE inhibitors and angiotensin receptor blockers (ARBs) can be used if there are contraindications to other medications, or they can be used in combination with the above.

I. Arrhythmias are abnormal rhythms of the heart rate. It is important to always rule out a MI. If the patient is unstable, cardioversion should always be performed. Secondary investigation is directed at abnormal electrolytes, endocrine issues (TSH), and drug toxicity. Most arrhythmias are transient.

1. Atrial fibrillation is a tachyarrhythmia. Diagnosis is via EKG, which shows an irregularly irregular rhythm with no P wave. Treatment with IV diltiazem. A beta blocker can be helpful if there is a rapid ventricular response. Amiodarone has a lower incidence of recurrent atrial fibrillation. Digoxin can also be used. If there is persistent atrial fibrillation, ASA prophylaxis or consideration of anticoagulation. The $CHADS_2$ score is based on patient risk factors. These include: HTN greater than 140/90; age greater than 75; DM; history of CVA or TIA; or history of VTE. All risk factors are given a score of 1 except for the CVA and VTE components which are scored at 2 each. If the score is $\geq$ to 2, warfarin is recommended.

The risk of CVA annually based on CHADS2 score is:

Score	CVA risk
0	1.9
1	2.8
2	4
3	5.9
4	8.5
5	12.5
6	18.2

2. Atrial flutter is a tachyarrhythmia. Diagnosis is via EKG, which shows a saw tooth pattern. ASA prophylaxis is indicated.

3. Supraventricular tachycardia is a tachyarrhythmia. Diagnosis is via EKG, which shows tachycardia with no P waves. Treatment is initiated with vagal maneuvers. If this is unsuccessful, adenosine can be administered up to 3 times (given IV at 6 mg, again at 6 mg, then at 12 mg if no initial response).

4. Bradycardia is defined as a pulse less than 60 bpm. Diagnosis is via EKG. If the patient is symptomatic and not stable, the patient should be paced transcutaneously until a permanent pacemaker can be placed or the etiology diagnosed. If the patient is stable, treatment is with atropine dosed at 1 mg IV.

III. Shock and Sepsis

A. Shock is defined as a decrease in tissue perfusion. There are 5 types of shock: septic, cardiogenic, hemorrhagic, neurogenic, and iatrogenic. Diagnosis is via physical examination, vitals, EKG, and lab tests. Treatment generally consists of IVF and type directed support.

1. Cardiogenic shock can be due to ischemic heart disease (MI), HTN yielding a heavy afterload and severe cardiac strain, or pump failure from too much volume. Cardiogenic shock is managed by diuretics to reduce the preload, dopamine or dobutamine to increase cardiac function, norepinephrine if dopamine fails, and nitroprusside or a nitroglycerine drip for venous capacitance. Angiography with angioplasty, stent placement, LVAD, or CABG surgery can be employed for acute management.

2. Hemorrhagic shock is managed by IVF replacement (3:1 ratio of IVF to blood loss) and blood products, surgery for hemostasis, or embolization.

3. Neurogenic shock often occurs from embolic or hemorrhagic stroke, head trauma or metastatic disease. It is managed by IVF, pressor support, hyperventilation with intubation if necessary, radiation with steroids to reduce local inflammation, and potential surgery if a mass effect is present.

4. Iatrogenic shock is usually related to anaphylaxis. Treatment is to stop the offending medication/infusion, administration of steroids, antihistamines, O_2, and pressor support as indicated.

5. Septic shock, see section C below.

B. Generally, the systemic inflammatory response syndrome (SIRS) occurs when two or more of the following are documented in the setting of a known cause of inflammation: a body temperature greater than 38 degrees or less than 36 degrees Celsius; a pulse greater than 90 bpm; a respiratory rate greater than 20 bpm or a $PaCO_2$ less than 32; a WBC greater than $12 \times 10^3/\mu L$, or less than $4 \times 10^3/\mu L$, or greater than 10% band forms. In 2001, additional criteria were added for an inclusive approach to SIRS. These include: an altered mental status, oliguria, skin mottling, coagulopathy, hypoxemia, hyperglycemia without a diagnosis of diabetes, thrombocytopenia, and altered LFTs.

C. Sepsis is SIRS due to a known infection. Septic shock is sepsis with hypotension despite adequate fluid resuscitation. There are two stages: early hyperdynamic and late hypodynamic. The crude mortality is 28% to 50%.

  1. Intervention is needed with management in the ICU. An arterial line is needed to measure the MAP; consideration of a PA catheter for measurement of the CO, a Foley catheter to measure urine output; an ABG to measure the $PaCO_2$ and $O_{2;}$ laboratories to include: CBC, electrolytes, liver and renal panels, lactate and coagulation parameters, and cultures for bacteria, fungus, and virus. Goals are a CVP of 8 to 12; a MAP greater than 65, a urine output greater than 0.5 mL/kg/hr; and a mixed venous oxygen saturation greater than 70%. If oxygen saturation goals are not met in 6 hours, it may be beneficial to transfuse PRBC to a hemoglobin greater than 10 g/dL, and/or add dobutamine.

  2. Septic shock is managed with antibiotics, IVF, oxygen with intubation if indicated, and pressor support. All catheters should be changed and cultured. Any site of infection should be explored and drained if possible, with up to an 80% percutaneous success rate. Surgical exploration can access those sites not amenable to needle drainage. Fever and leukocytosis, respectively, are absent in 35% and 5% of peritoneal infections. Fungal infections should be treated with appropriate antibiotics. An eye examination should also be part of the workup. Viral infections should also be ruled out with appropriate culture when all other cultures are negative. Antibiotics should be continued for 14 days after negative blood culture.

  3. Multiple organ dysfunction syndrome (MODS) is development of the progressive physiologic dysfunction of 2 or more organ systems. This usually occurs after an acute threat to systemic homeostasis. Treatment is support of individual organ function and aggressive therapies aimed at correcting the underlying process.

IV. Renal: The definition of acute renal failure is not standardized.

A. A patient is usually diagnosed with a rising creatinine, or with a urine output of less than 400 mL/24 hr.

B. There are three types of acute renal failure: prerenal, renal (intrinsic), and postrenal. Lab tests should be ordered to include a CMP, urine analysis for microscopy, urine electroyltes to include Na and creatinine, specific gravity, and urine osmolality. The next step is to calculate the FeNa: The equation is UNa × SCr/SNa × UCr × 100%. The renal failure index is another calculation: (Urinary Na concentration × Plasma Cr concentration)/Urinary Cr concentration.

1. If the FeNa is less than 1% and the urine specific gravity is greater than 1.025, the diagnosis is prerenal failure and often due to hypoperfusion. If the FeNa is greater than 4% and the urine specific gravity (SG) is less than 1.01, the diagnosis is often due to renal ischemia. It is important to remember that a FeNa cannot be calculated if diuretics, mannitol, or IV contrast material have been given.

2. Prerenal failure: the etiology is often volume depletion from surgical blood loss, third spacing from removal of ascites, extensive bowel preparation and NPO status, congestive heart failure, severe liver disease, or other edematous states. Laboratory findings include: a urinary sodium concentration < 20 mEq/L, a urine:plasma creatinine ratio > 30, urine osmolality > 500 mOsm/kg. The renal failure index is < 1.

3. Intrinsic renal failure: the etiology can be aminoglycoside antibiotics, IV contrast material, cytolytic drug exposure, statin medication, rhabdomyolysis, hyperuricemia, multiple myeloma, and streptococcal infection. Findings include: a urinary sodium concentration > 40 mEq/L, a urine:plasma creatinine ratio < 20, and urine osmolality < 400 mOsm/kg. The urinary analysis can show eosinophils (acute interstitial nephritis), red blood cell casts (glomerulonephritis or vasculitis), or renal tubular epithelial cells and muddy brown casts (acute tubular necrosis). The cause is sloughing of renal

tubular cells into the lumen, demonstrating casts called Tamm-Horsfall bodies. Management is with support including volume repletion until euvolemia is reached, monitoring and restriction of potassium agents. A diuretic challenge can be offered if volume overload becomes evident. Dialysis should be considered if volume overload, acidosis, uremia, or EKG changes occur. Treatment is to stop the offending drug. A desired urinary output is 0.5 mL/kg/hr.

4. Postrenal failure is usually obstructive. This can occur with bilateral hydronephrosis from cervical cancer, nephrolithiasis, urethral obstruction, bladder compression from tumor, or ureteral obstruction from tumor/stone/surgery. Lab tests include: serum BUN:Cr > 20:1, a urine osmolality < 400 mOsm/kg and a urinary sodium concentration > 40 mEq/L. The Foley catheter should be checked and flushed. A renal ultrasound can be obtained to document hydronephrosis. A CT urogram can be obtained to evaluate for ureteral obstruction from surgical injury or tumor. Nephrolithiasis and retroperitoneal fibrosis can also cause this complication. Reduction of the obstruction with surgical correction or placement of a percutaneous nephrostomy tube is indicated. It is important to follow for *postobstructive diuresis*: postobstructive diuresis is defined as diuresis of more than 200 mL/hr for at least 2 hours. Electrolytes should be checked every 8 hours and the urine output replaced with intravenous fluids in the form of half normal saline at 80% of the hourly urine volume for the first 24 hours, then 50%. Postobstructive diuresis usually lasts 24–72 hours. Cardiac status should be observed for potential tachycardic failure.

C. Chronic kidney disease is defined as a GFR of less than 60 mL/min/1.73 m^2. End-stage renal disease (ESRD) is often caused by DM and HTN (68%). These patients are immunocompromised. The morbidity from surgery can be up to 54%, with a mortality of 4%. For renal patients, it is important to obtain a cardiac workup, manage fluids and electrolytes vigilantly, exercise caution for anemia and bleeding diatheses, and maintain both glycemic and blood pressure control.

D. Cardiac disease causes the most deaths in patients with end-stage renal disease, and 23% to 40% have no cardiac symptoms. Patients need to be euvolemic prior to surgery. They need dialysis without heparin 24 hours prior to surgery, and they need postoperative dialysis, the day of surgery if a large fluid load was given.

E. It is important to check electrolytes immediately after surgery and every 6 to 8 hours until they are normalized.

F. If the patient is uremic, platelets do not work well. Cryoprecipitate or dDAVP should be considered to prevent bleeding during surgery. IV estrogen can also be administered (0.6 mg/kg) 4 to 5 days prior to surgery.

G. Indications for dialysis include (AEIOU): acidemia, electrolyte abnormalities (hyperkalemia resistant to prior interventions), EKG changes, intoxication with dialyzable substances (aspirin, lithium), volume overload, uremia, and mental status changes. A large central venous catheter may need to be placed if there is an acute need for dialysis.

H. Daily management of renal complications include: strict I/Os, daily weight, and a low-sodium, and low-nitrogen diet.

V. Acid–Base Disorders

Disorder	Primary Change	pH	Compensatory Change
Metabolic acidosis	Decreased HCO_3	Decreased	Decreased pCO_2
Metabolic alkalosis	Increased HCO_3	Increased	Increased pCO_2
Respiratory acidosis	Increased PCO_2	Decreased	Increased HCO_3
Respiratory alkalosis	Decreased PCO_2	Increased	Decreased HCO_3

A. Metabolic acidosis: the anion gap is calculated by subtracting the serum concentrations of chloride and bicarbonate (anions) from the concentrations of sodium and potassium (cations): $= ([Na^+] + [K^+]) - ([Cl^-] + [HCO_3^-])$.

   1. Anion Gap: The etiology is based on the mnemonic "PLUMSEEDS." These stand for: Paraldehyde, Lactate, Uremia, Methanol, Salicylates, Ethylene glycol, Ethanol, Diabetic ketoacidosis, Starvation. Another mnemonic is "MUDPILES": Methanol, Uremia (chronic renal failure), Diabetic ketoacidosis, Propylene glycol, I (infection, iron, isoniazid, inborn errors in metabolism), Lactic acidosis, Ethylene glycol, Salicylates

   2. Nonanion Gap: The two main causes are diarrhea or renal tubular acidosis. Other causes include acetazolamide, saline administration, hyperalimentation, and ureteral conduit.

B. Metabolic alkalosis: Usually occurs from renal dysfunction due to the loss of hydrochloric acid from nausea/vomiting, volume contraction, exogenous bicarbonate administration, hypokalemia, or hyponatremia.

C. Respiratory acidosis: Occurs when there is a failure of ventilation usually due to mental status changes. These changes can occur because of a mass effect, medications, stroke, infection, or inappropriate mechanical ventilation settings.

D. Respiratory alkalosis: Occurs as a result of hyperventilation, including iatrogenic causes from excessive mechanical ventilation.

VI. Electrolyte Abnormalities

A. Sodium abnormalities

   1. Hyponatremia (serum sodium < 135 mEq/L):

   a. Pseudohyponatremia: an erroneously low measurement of sodium caused by elevations of plasma lipids, sugars, or proteins

   b. Hypotonic hyponatremia: increase in free water relative to sodium in extracellular fluids

   c. Hypovolemic hyopnatremia: characterized by loss of sodium and water, with a net loss of sodium relative to water. Caused by diuretics, adrenal insufficiency, diarrhea or vomiting

   d. Isovolemic hyponatremia: characterized by increase in water with the same sodium content. Caused by inappropriate ADH secretion or psychogenic polydipsia

   e. Hypervolemic hyponatremia: characterized by excess of sodium and water, with a net gain of water relative to sodium. Caused by heart, renal, or hepatic failure

   f. Signs/symptoms: hyponatremic encephalopathy associated with cerebral edema, increased intracranial pressure and seizures

   g. Treatment: based on low, normal, or high extracelluar volume. Avoid rapid correction to prevent central pontine myelinolysis

   2. Hypernatremia (serum sodium > 145 mEq/L):

   a. Hypovolemic hypernatremia: caused by inadequate intake of water, excessive loss from urinary tract, sweating or diarrhea. Treatment: volume replacement

b. Hypertonic syndromes: are characterized by impaired renal water conservation. This can be caused by: diabetes insipidus, either central or nephrogenic. Treatment: replace free water deficits

c. Hypervolemic hypernatremia: characterized by an increase in hypertonic fluid. This is caused by: excessive hypertonic saline resuscitation, sodium bicarbonate infusions, ingestion of seawater or excessive amounts of table salt. Treat with sodium restriction or diuretic with fluid replacement

d. It is important to avoid rapidly lowering the sodium concentration with free water to avoid cerebral edema.

B. Potassium abnormalities

   1. Hypokalemia (serum potassium < 3.5 mEq/L):

      a. Causes:

         i. Transcellular shift of potassium into cells from insulin, beta agonists, furosamide, or alkalosis

         ii. Diminished intake

         iii. Increased potassium losses from gastrointestinal or urinary tracts

      b. Signs: Fatigue, myalgia, muscular weakness, hypoventilation, paralysis, and arrhythmias

      c. Symptoms: EKG changes include: T wave inversion, U waves, ST depression, prolonged QT interval, prolonged PR interval, widening of QRS complex

      d. Treatment: Address the underlying cause

         i. Each 0.1 mEq/L of deficiency on laboratory value needs replacement with 10 mEq of potassium chloride (KCl).

         ii. The maximum rate of KCl in a peripheral IV is 10 mEq/hr; for a central line the rate is 20 mEq/hr.

         iii. Magnesium: Magnesium depletion can promote urinary loss of potassium, so it is recommended to also correct for magnesium deficit.

   2. Hyperkalemia (serum potassium > 5.5 mEq/L):

      a. Causes:

         i. Pseudohyperkalemia caused by hemolysis from traumatic blood draw

    ii. Transcellular shift from acidosis; rhabdomyolysis; cytotoxic cell death or drugs such as digitialis or beta receptor antagonists

    iii. Impaired renal excretion from adrenal insufficiency or drugs such as ACE inhibitors, angiotensin receptor blockers, NSAIDs, or potassium-sparing diuretics

    iv. Massive blood transfusions

  b. Symptoms: Cardiac toxicity, paralysis, and hypoventilation

  c. Signs: EKG changes including increased T waves, peaked T waves, prolonged PR and QRS intervals, loss of P waves

  d. Treatment is recommended if the serum K is greater than 6.5 mEq/L, the patient is acidotic, fluid overloaded, mental status changes are present, or EKG changes are present. Treatment:

- Kayexalate PO 15 g daily to QID or PR 30 to 50 g q 4 hours
- Sodium bicarbonate: 44 to 132 mEq IV
- Calcium chloride or calcium gluconate 10 to 30 mL of a 10% solution
- Glucose: 50 g IV
- Regular insulin: 10 units IV
- Dialysis if the patient does not respond to the above measures.

C. Magnesium abnormalities

  1. Hypomagnesemia:

    a. Causes: diuretic therapy, antibiotics, alcohol-related illness, diarrhea, diabetes mellitus, acute myocardial infarction, drugs such as digitalis or cisplatin

    b. Symptoms: generalized weakness and altered mentation. It is commonly associated with other electrolyte abnormalities, including hypokalemia, hypophosphatemia, hypocalcemia. It is also associated with hypokalemia that is refractory to treatment.

    c. EKG changes: torsades de pointes, increased PR and QT intervals, atrial and ventricular arrhythmias

    d. Treatment: magnesium sulfate IV or magnesium oxide PO

2. Hypermagnesemia

   a. Causes: impaired renal function or excessive administration

   b. Symptoms: hyporeflexia, EKG changes include first-degree AV block, complete heart block

   c. Treatment: calcium gluconate, intravenous fluids with Lasix, and hemodialysis if refractory

D. Calcium abnormalities

 1. Hypocalcemia:

   a. Causes: hypoalbuminemia, tumor lysis syndrome, renal failure, hypoparathyroidism, hypomagnesemia, hypermagnesemia, acute pancreatitis, rhabdomyolysis, or blood transfusion (due to citrate chelating calcium)

   b. Symptoms/signs: tetany, Trousseau's sign, Chvostek's sign

   c. Signs: EKG changes: increased QT interval, ventricular tachycardia

   d. Treatment: IV calcium gluconate or calcium chloride 10 mL of a 10% solution; PO calcium carbonate; or calcium gluconate 1 to 2 g orally 3 times a day with meals

 2. Hypercalcemia:

   a. Causes: bone metastasis, hyperparathyroidism, clear cell cancer of ovary or cervix, small cell cancers

   b. Symptoms: GI disturbances, hypotension, polyuria, confusion, depressed consciousness, coma

   c. Signs: EKG changes: shortened QT interval

   d. Treatment: rehydration with normal saline or one-half normal saline IV; diuresis with Lasix 40 mg IV q 2 hr after IV hydration; pamidronate (Aredia) 60 to 90 mg IV over 2 to 24 hr for 7 days; glucocorticoids such as hydrocortisone 250 to 500 mg IV q 8hr; calcitonin: lowers calcium by 1 to 3 mg/dL for 6 to 8 hr (perform skin test first to check for hypersensitivity, start at 4 IU/kg SQ or IM q 12 to 24 hr); Mithramycin dosed at 25 mcg/kg via slow IV push daily.

E. Phosphorus abnormalities

 1. Hypophosphatemia:

   a. Causes: impaired intestinal absorption, increased renal excretion, redistribution of phosphate into cells, diabetic ketoacidosis (DKA), glucose loading, oncogenic osteomalacia, hyperparathyroidism, and the diuretic phase of acute tubular necrosis

b. Symptoms/signs: muscular weakness, heart and respiratory failure, anemia

c. Treatment: sodium or potassium phosphate IV or PO

2. Hyperphosphatemia:

a. Causes: renal failure, tumor lysis syndrome, metabolic and respiratory acidosis, hypoparathyroidism

b. Symptoms/signs: deposition of calcium-phosphate complexes into soft tissue and tetany

c. Treatment: promote phosphorus binding with sucralfate or aluminum-containing antacids. Dialysis for patients with renal failure

VII. Fluids and Blood Products

TBW = 0.5 × kg body weight

Intracellular fluid = 0.4 × kg body weight

Extracellular fluid = 0.2 × kg body weight

Interstitial fluid = 0.15 × kg body weight

Plasma volume = 0.5 × kg body weight

Blood volume = 75 mL/kg

Electrolytes

Electrolyte	Plasma	Interstitial	Intracellular
Na	142	145	10 mEq/L
K	4	–	156 mEq/L
Cl	104	114	2 mEq/L
HCO_3	27	31	8 mEq/L
Ca^{2+}	5	0	3.3 mEq/L
Mg^{2+}	2	0	26 mEq/L
Phos	2	–	95 mEq/L

Body Fluid Composition

Fluid	Na	Cl	K	HCO₃	Daily Production
Gastric juices	60–100	100	10	0	1500–2000 mL
Duodenum	130	90	5	0–10	300–2000 mL
Bile	145	100	5	15–35	100–800 mL
Pancreatic	140	75	5	70–115	100–800 mL
Ileum	140	100	5	15–30	2000–3000 mL

A. Daily fluid management

1. Daily physiologic fluid intake is composed of the following: endogenous water production from oxidation (approximately 250 mL/day); healthy PO intake (approximately 2,000 to 2,500 mL/day).

2. Daily physiologic fluid losses: 2,000 to 2,500 mL. This is composed of water from the: urine 800 to 1,500 mL; stool 200 mL; insensible losses to include; respiratory 200 mL; and skin 800 mL.

3. Daily fluid requirement: 1,500 mL/m² body surface area (BSA)

4. Daily body weight loss if maintenance is with on IVF only: one-half kg/day

5. Increased fluid is needed when the patient is febrile. There should be a 15% increase in IVF for each degree above normal body temperature

B. IV Fluids:

1. D5W: 50g dextrose in 1,000 mL of fluid; provides 170 calories per liter.

2. LR: Multiple electrolyte concentration, similar to that of plasma. It is used to expand the plasma volume in hypovolemic states in the first 24 hours.

3. NS (0.9% NaCl): This is an isotonic solution. It is used to expand volume and correct mild hyponatremia.

4. ½ NS (0.45% NaCl): This is a hypotonic solution. It is used for postoperative IVF replacement after the first 24 hours. It is used when volume expansion is not required.

5. NaCl 3%: This is a hypertonic solution and is used to treat severe hyponatremia.

C. IV Fluid Composition

	Na	Cl	K	HCO₃	Ca	Glu	AA	Mg	PO₄	Ac	Osm
Plasma	140	102	4.0	28	5			2			290
NS	154	154									308
½ NS	77	77									154
¼ NS	34	34									78
LR	130	109	4.0	28	3						272
D5W						50 g					252
D10W						100 g					505
PPN	47	40	13			100 g	35 g	3	3.5	52	500
TMP	25	30	44			250 g	50 g	5	15	99	1900
D50						500 g					2520

D. Fluid Deficits

1. Presurgical deficit: From being NPO there is a 2 mL/kg/hr loss.

2. Intraoperative fluids: The rule of 1:3 blood loss to crystalloid fluid replacement should be followed. Blood transfusion should occur based on NIH transfusion guidelines, medical comorbidities, and anticipated adjuvant therapies. Third spacing fluid loss: Removal of significant ascites and water retained as tissue edema is difficult to quantify.

    It is usually assumed:

    a. 4 mL/kg/hr for minimal surgical procedures (e.g., wide local excision)

    b. 6 mL/kg/hr for moderate surgical procedures (e.g., appendectomy, hernia repair)

    c. 8 mL/kg/hr for major surgical procedures (e.g., radical hysterectomy, bowel resection)

    d. Insensible losses intraoperatively are 2 mL/kg/hr

3. Postoperative fluid replacement: Calculation should include output from surgical drains, urine, and insensible losses. Diuresis from extensive third spacing takes 1 to 3 days. Management can be with D5LR for the first 24 hours. No potassium is added to the IVF because of the possibility of tumor cell lyses and extracellular release from operative cell destruction. Then

D5½ NS is started POD 2 for continued volume replacement. Serum potassium should be checked daily. 10 mEq of potassium is added for each 1,000 mL of NGT drainage obtained.

E. Blood Component Therapy

1. Whole blood: has a volume of 517 mL. It is only indicated for acute blood loss that is severe enough to cause hypovolemic shock.

2. PRBC: has a volume of 300 mL. One unit can survive 21 days if refrigerated. The hematocrit increases 3% to 5% per unit. It contains: plasma (78 mL), citrate (22 mL), plasma protein (42 g), Na (15 mEq), potassium (5 mEq), and acid (25 nanoEq). It is important to check a Ca^{2+} level after significant transfusion due to the citrate chelation of divalent ions.

3. Platelets: one unit has a volume of 20 to 50 mL. One unit has 5.5×10^{10} platelets. They can be stored for only 72 hours. One unit increases the platelet count 7,000/mcL in 1 hour. The guideline for transfusion is 0.1 unit/kg; so a normal transfusion is 6 to 8 units.

4. Fresh frozen plasma (FFP): contains all clotting factors except platelets. FFP should be given after 10 to 12 units of blood. Components are: 250 mL of plasma; 200 units of factor VIII; and 200 units of factor IX.

5. Cryoprecipitate is obtained from the thawing of FFP at 4 degrees Celsius. Factors VIII, XIII, fibrinogen are the main factors in cryoprecipitate. Cryoprecipitate is mainly used for factor replacement in the treatment of hemophilia and von Willebrand's disease. It is transfused in a pack of 4–6 units. each having a volume of 15cc.

6. Albumin: used for volume resuscitation and hypoproteinemia. It is infused as a 5% or 25% solution and 25 g are commonly infused. The volume effects last for 12 hours. It increases the intravascular volume by 500 mL.

7. Artificial colloids include:

    a. Hetastarch: this is a 6% chemically modified starch polymer in isotonic saline. The volume effects last for 24 hours. Side effects can be significant and include: pruritis secondary to extravascular starch deposits (not allergy) and anaphylaxis (rare, 0.006% infusions).

b. Dextran: this is composed of glucose polymers produced by a bacterium. 10% Dextran-40 has a volume effect for 6 hours. Allergic reactions occur in 0.032% of infusions.

Blood Products

Blood Products	Contents	Volume	Indication
PRBC	Red cells	1 unit = 250 mL, raises Hct 3%	Acute or chronic blood loss
Platelets	Platelets	One unit = 50 mL. Raises platelets by 6×10^5.	Platelets < 20 nonbleeding patient, < 50 in bleeding patient
FFP	Fibrinogen, Factors II, VII, IX, X, XI, XII, XIII, and heat labile V and VII	1 unit = 150–250 mL, 11g albumin, 500 mg fibrinogen, 0.7–1.0 units clotting factors	DIC, Tx > 10 units of blood, liver disease, IgG deficiency, 1 unit raises fibrinogen by 10 mg/dL
Cryo precipitate	Factors VIII, XIII, von Willebrand's disease, fibrinogen	1 unit = 10 mL, 250 mg fibrinogen, 80 units factor VIII	Hemophilia A, von Willebrand's disease, fibrinogen deficiency

8. Risk of transfusion infection per unit of blood:

  a. Hepatitis C   1:2 million

  b. Hepatitis B   1:350,000

  c. HIV   1:2.3 million

  d. Bacterial   1:5,000 per unit of platelets

  1:1 million PRBC

VIII. Neurologic

  A. Neuromuscular blockage is often used to paralyze the patient. Pancurnium is chosen for its long-acting properties. It lasts for up to 90 minutes after an IV dose of 0.06 to 0.1 mg/kg. Continuous infusion is vagolytic and can cause a heart rate increase of 10 bpm or more. It is important to use vecuronium if the patient cannot tolerate an increased heart rate. An electronic twitch monitor is used to assess the degree of paralyzation. Acute quadriplegic myopathy is a potential adverse event causing postparalytic quadriparesis, which consists of the triad of acute paresis, myonecrosis with increased CPK, and abnormal electromyography.

B. Delirium is often seen in ICU patients. Haldol can be used to counteract delirium because of its minimal anticholinergic and hypotensive effects. It is given at a loading dose of 2 to 10 mg IV q 20 min, followed by scheduled dosing every 4 to 6 hr at 25% of the necessary loading dose.

C. Sedation is used to medically control the ICU patient for rest, recovery, and safety in the ICU environment. Daily interruption of sedation is necessary. This is associated with a shortened duration of ICU stay, less PTSD, and shorter mechanical ventilation. Propofol is used often as a sedative. It has no analgesic properties. It does count as lipid calories at 1.1 kcal/mL. Care should be taken in patients with hypertriglyceridemia, and so it is necessary to monitor triglycerides (TG) after 2 days of use.

D. Glascow Coma Scale

Response	Score
Eye opening	
Spontaneous	4
To verbal	3
To pain	2
None	1
Verbal response	
Oriented and talking	5
Disoriented and talking	4
Inappropriate talking	3
Incomprehensible	2
None	1
Motor response	
Obeys commands	6
Localizes pain	5
Normal flexion withdrawal	4
Decortical signs (flexion)	3
Decerebrate signs (extension)	2
None	1

Score
15 Normal
11 Normal if intubated
8 or less Coma

IX. Abdominal compartment syndrome: can occur due to ascites, bowel obstruction, ileus, peritonitis, or pancreatitis. It can also occur after massive fluid resuscitation in the setting of septic or hypovolemic shock. Diagnosis is by measurement of the intra-abdominal pressure via a Foley catheter with documentation of a pressure of greater than 12 mm Hg on 3 or more occasions 4 to 6 hours apart, or a single pressure of 20 mm Hg or greater. It can manifest as systemic hypotension, reduced urinary output, or decreased pulmonary compliance. On occasion, surgery to decompress the abdomen and temporary closure with a vacuum pack may be necessary

X. Risk stratification of morbidity and mortality in the ICU by different quantitative scales has been documented as reliable and reproducible in gynecologic oncology patients. Two scales are used the most often: the APACHE IV and the SOFA (sequential organ failure assessment). An increase of the SOFA score during the first 48 hours of ICU admission predicts a mortality of 50% or more.

REFERENCE

1. POISE Study Group. Effects of extended-release metoprolol succinate in patients undergoing non-cardiac surgery (POISE trial): a randomised controlled trial. *Lancet.* 2008;371(9627):1839–1847.

Chemotherapy

I. One Letter and Combination Chemotherapy Abbreviations

A: Dactinomycin

ABVD: Adriamycin/doxorubicin, bleomycin, vinblastine, dacarbazine

AcFucy: Dactinomycin, 5-FU, cyclophosphamide

AI: Aromatase inhibitor

B: Bleomycin

BEP: Bleomycin, etoposide, cisplatin

C: Cyclophosphamide

CDDP: cisplatin; cis-diamminedichloroplatinum

CHOPP-R: Cyclophosphamide, hydroxyurea, vincristine, procarbazine, prednisone, retuximab

CMFV: Cyclophosphamide, methotrexate, 5-FU, Vinblastine

D: Doxorubicin

E: Etoposide, VP-16

Epi: Epirubicin

F: 5-FU

H: Hydroxyurea

L: Chlorambucil

Lev: Levamisole

L-PAM: L-phenylalanine mustard

M: Methotrexate

MAC: Methotrexate, dactinomycin, cyclophosphamide or chlorambucil

MMC: Mitomycin

MOPP: Nitrogen mustard, vincristine, procarbazine, prednisone

O: Oncovin/vincristine

P: Cisplatin

Pr: Prednisolone

T: Tamoxifen

TVPP: Thiotepa, vinblastine, procarbazine, prednisone

V: Vinblastine

MVPP: Nitrogen mustard, vinblastine, procarbazine, prednisone

VAC: Vincristine, doxorubicin cyclophosphamide

VBM: Vinblastine, bleomycin, methotrexate

VBP: Vinblastine, bleomycin, cisplatin

VDC: Vincristine, doxorubicin, cyclophosphamide

II. Chemotherapy Definitions

A. Dose: Amount of chemotherapy administered

B. Intensity: The amount of drug administered over time

C. Schedule: Time interval for delivery of chemotherapy

D. Chemotherapy cycle: One treatment of single or combination agents in the full course of therapy

E. Chemotherapy course: Sequence of cycles for treatment

F. Planning of treatment: Must take into consideration tumor type, extent of disease, patient's comorbidities including renal function, age, social and emotional function, or if therapy is primary or salvage

III. Delivery

Routes are IV, IM, PO, intraperitoneal (IP), or regional. Most chemotherapy is administered systemically, by IV. It can be given regionally to primary tumors or their metastasis. Intraperitoneal chemotherapy is administration of chemotherapy directly into the abdominopelvic cavity. Regional chemotherapy can be used to treat solitary organ lesions, such as liver metastasis. This occurs by obstruction of the outflow tract for a limited amount of time so that the chemotherapy can penetrate the tumor mass directly. It can also be directly administered to a cavity such as for pleural or pericardial lesions.

IV. Metabolism

A. Pro-drugs can be bio-transformed into active metabolites. This includes cyclophosphamide. It is important to know those drugs that are activated by the liver because intraperitoneal administration may have no effect.

B. Excretion: Hepatobiliary or renal excretion are the main routes of excretion. Drugs can be metabolized to pro-drugs, to inactive states, remain unchanged, or accumulate in body tissues.

V. Principles of Chemotherapy Tumor Kill

The patient needs two cycles after resolution of tumor markers and/or no evidence of disease with complete clinical remission (CCR) to eliminate microscopic systemic disease.

VI. Chemotherapy Regimens

A. Primary: Chemotherapy is the initial treatment.

B. Adjuvant: Chemotherapy is used following primary treatment with surgery or radiation.

C. Neoadjuvant: Chemotherapy is used for initial treatment to be followed by surgery, radiation, or a combination of therapies.

D. Secondary: Any chemotherapy regimen given after primary chemotherapy.

E. Salvage: Chemotherapy is used in the treatment of recurrent or persistent disease after previous chemotherapy.

F. Consolidation: Chemotherapy that is used after primary or adjuvant chemotherapy to decrease the chance of cancer recurrence in patients with CCR. This is usually a short duration of treatment.

G. Maintenance: Chemotherapy that is used after primary or adjuvant chemotherapy to decrease the chance of cancer recurrence in patients with CCR. This is usually of a longer duration than consolidation therapy.

VII. Platinum Sensitivity/Resistance

Tumors are classified as platinum sensitive, resistant, or refractory.

A. Platinum Sensitive: if the tumor recurs 6 or more months after completion of primary platinum-based chemotherapy, it is said to be platinum sensitive.

B. Platinum Resistant: If the tumor recurs within 6 months of primary platinum-based chemotherapy, it is considered platinum resistant.

C. Platinum Refractory: If the tumor does not respond to initial platinum chemotherapy and growth continues during primary treatment, it is considered platinum refractory.

D. For germ cell tumors, the time interval is different and resistance is specified at 6 weeks. Germ cell tumors are designated as refractory if no response is seen at 4 weeks of ongoing chemotherapy.

VIII. Toxicity

A. Side effects from chemotherapy are graded according to severity. The most commonly affected organ systems are the gastrointestinal system, the hematopoietic system, and the integumentary system. Please refer to the common toxicity criteria (CTC) website for the full classification of toxicity grades. Management of toxicity due to chemotherapy is with a reduction in the total dose of drug per cycle, called a dose reduction. This is usually a 20–25% dose reduction, or a decrease in the AUC by 1 level.

B. Cardiac toxicity mainly occurs with doxorubicin. A history and exam can diagnose CHF. Confirmation is with an echocardiogram or with a multiple gated acquisition scan (MUGA) scan.

C. Pulmonary toxicity has been seen mainly with bleomycin. A pretreatment carbon monoxide spirometry diffusion capacity test (DLCO) is recommended. A 15% change in the FEV indicates toxicity. Pulmonary toxicity can also be determined clinically with an exam. Clinical symptoms such as rales, hypoinflation, or a lag in the inspiratory phase on exam, as well as dyspnea occur before a documented drop in FEV.

D. Secondary malignancies can occur after administration of chemotherapeutic agents. The rate is about 1% to 2%. Leukemias can occur from alkylating agents and include melphalan, the podophyllotoxins, etoposide, cyclophosphamide, and the platinum compounds. The development of leukemias is dose-dependent (2 g for etoposide). The median latency is 4 years after chemotherapy for epithelial ovarian cancer (EOC), with an overall incidence of 0.17% (1).

IX. The Cell Cycle

A. The cell cycle is broken into interphase and mitosis. Interphase consists of the G_1, S, and G_2 phases. G_1 is a variable period, where protein, RNA, and DNA, repair occur. The cell can terminally differentiate or continue in the cell cycle from this phase. S phase is when new DNA is synthesized. The G_2 phase occurs after the S phase and thus the cell contains 2 times the amount of DNA. This is a short phase. It is the variation in the length of the G_1 phase that affects the proliferative behavior of cell populations.

B. Mitosis consists of 5 phases. Prophase, the first phase, is when chromosomes condense. Metaphase is when chromosomal division occurs. This is the most radiosensitive phase. Anaphase is when sister chromosomes move to opposite cell poles. Telophase demonstrates polarization of chromosomes and disassembly of the cytoskeleton occurs. Cytokinesis follows with division of the cell into separate daughter cells. Cell cycle times vary from 10 to 31 hours.

C. Masses are usually palpated at 10^9 cells, or 1 cm in size. The 1-cm size usually occurs after 30 doublings of one tumor cell.

X. Growth Fraction
This consists of the fraction of cells in a tumor that are actively proliferating. This fraction ranges from 25% to 95%.

XI. Cell Death
Cell death has been seen with some tumors. This has been documented in some breast cancers associated with febrile episodes. (2)

XII. Log Kill
A constant amount of cells are killed with each dose of therapy—not a constant number of cells. To achieve substantial tumor reduction, a repetitive insult has to be delivered to the tumor. Single-agent chemotherapy can be curative in this fashion, but is not as effective as multiagent chemotherapy. Multiagent chemotherapy uses different drugs which target separate cellular pathways. The effect can be additive or synergic.

XIII. Cell Cycle Nonspecific Chemotherapeutic Agents
These agents kill cells in all phases of the cell cycle.

XIV. Cell Cycle Specific Agents
These agents depend on the proliferative fraction of the tumor and a specific cell cycle phase. These agents are usually more effective against tumors with a high proliferative rate and a high growth fraction.

XV. Cell Growth
Growth is usually demonstrated via a Gompertzian log tumor growth curve.

A. There are four phases to cell growth:

1. Lag growth phase

2. The log growth phase

3. Stable growth phase

4. Death phase

XVI. Mechanisms of Cytotoxicity

Chemotherapeutic agents can target cellular DNA, proteins (such as enzymes, receptors, or the metabolic respiratory chain), and RNA.

XVII. Mechanisms of Resistance

A. The Goldie-Coldman hypothesis is a mathematical model that predicts the probability of a tumor harboring drug resistant clones. The number of drug-resistant clones depends on the mutation rate and the size of the tumor.

B. Documented mechanisms of drug resistance include:

1. The MDR-1 and MDR-2 P-glycoproteins, which are components of the ABC (ATP Binding Cassette) transporters. These proteins transport drugs out of cells.

2. Cells can decrease the entry of the drug into the cell via down regulation of cellular receptors.

3. Metabolic inactivation of the drug can occur via up-regulation of the glutathione sulfate and DHFR enzymes.

4. Genomic change can occur:

a. via altered DNA repair mechanisms

b. gene point mutation

c. gene frameshift mutation

d. gene deletion

e. gene amplification

5. There can be altered binding affinity of the drug to albumin or intracellular targets.

XVIII. Prior to Chemotherapy Administration

The patient should have adequate laboratory values.

A. This is considered a white blood cell count (WBC) greater than $3 \times 10^3/\mu L$ with an ANC greater than $1.5 \times 10^3/\mu L$

B. Platelets greater than $100 \times 10^3/\mu L$

C. Normal LFTs

D. Creatinine less than 2 mg/dL or creatinine clearance greater than 50 mL/min

E. GOG status of either 0, 1, or 2 with an estimated survival of more than 2 months

CLASSES OF CHEMOTHERAPY AGENTS AND INDEPENDENT MECHANISMS OF ACTION

I. Alkylating Agents

Work by intercalating or cross-linking DNA—making DNA adducts. They are cell-cycle nonspecific.

A. Carboplatin (Paraplatin): A platinum compound. It is dosed with the following equation: Carboplatin total dose (mg) = AUC × (GFR + 25). It can be given at an AUC of 7 as single agent or at an AUC of 5 to 6 in combination therapy. Its mechanism of action is intercalation with DNA and is administered via the IV or IP route. It is eliminated via the renal system. Its toxicities are primarily thrombocytopenia, hypersensitivity reactions, leukopenia, nausea, and vomiting. The platelet nadir is usually around 21 days. Secondary toxicities can include nephrotoxicity 7%, peripheral neuropathy 6%, ototoxicity 1%. Vitamin B_6 can prevent some neurotoxicity. Hypersensivity can occur in 25% of patients if more than 6 cycles are received. There is an increased risk of leukemia with a relative risk of 6.5. Amifostine can reduce the amount of thrombocytopenia at a dose of 910 mg/m².

B. Cisplatin (Platinol): A platinum compound that works by intercalating with DNA and creating G-G adducts. It is administered either IV or IP. It can be given as a single agent to radiosensitize certain tumors at 40–50 mg/m² weekly. It can be given as single-agent therapy at 50 to 100 mg/m², or at 75 mg/m² in combination with other drugs every 3 weeks. 90% is eliminated by the renal system and 10% by the hepatic/biliary system. Primary toxicities are leukopenia and anemia. Nephrotoxicity occurs in 21%, ototoxicity in 10%, and some patients have peripheral or autonomic neuropathy. Secondary toxicities are allergic reactions, low sodium (Na), potassium (K), calcium (Ca), and magnesium (Mg). The pancytopenia nadir occurs between days 18 and 23. To reduce some nephrotoxicity, prehydrate with normal saline IVF and consider mannitol diuresis with an additional 3 g of $MgSO_4$.

C. Cyclophosphamide (Cytoxan): It is a pro-drug that is activated by liver metabolism and then the active drug intercalates with DNA. It is administered either IV or PO. It can be given as a single agent or in combination with other agents. The dosing is usually 10 to 50 mg/kg IV every 1 to 4 weeks, or 600 to 1,000 mg/m² every 4 weeks. 85% is eliminated by the liver and 15% by the renal system. Primary toxicities include pancytopenia (this is the most marrow-suppressive drug), nausea, vomiting, and alopecia. Secondary toxicities are hemorrhagic cystitis from the acrolein metabolite, SIADH if the dose is greater than 50 mg/kg, interstitial pneumonia, cardiomyopathy, and leukemia with a relative risk of 5.4% after 10 years. The nadir occurs at days 8 to 14. To diagnose hemorrhagic cystitis, obtain a urine analysis: confirmation is with gross hematuria or 20 RBC/HPF. Mesna should be coadministered to decrease the incidence of hemorrhagic cystitis. Methylene blue bladder irrigation can also decrease complications.

D. Dacarbazine (DTIC): Administered IV usually at a dose of 2 to 4.5 mg/kg/day for 5 to 10 days every 4 weeks. Elimination is via the renal system. Primary toxicities include pancytopenia, nausea, vomiting, and alopecia. Secondary toxicities include mucositis, stomatitis, myalgias, and hepatotoxicity. The nadir occurs 2 to 4 weeks after administration.

E. Ifosfamide (Ifex): Also a pro-drug; it is activated by hepatic metabolism and is administered IV at a dose of 1.2 to 1.6 g/m^2/day for 5 days every 3 to 4 weeks, 700 to 900 mg/m^2/day for 5 days every 3 weeks, or 1000 mg/m^2 on days 1 and 2 every 28 days as part of the ICE protocol. Elimination is via the renal system for 73% of the drug. Primary toxicities are hemorrhagic cystitis, pancytopenia, nausea, vomiting, and alopecia. Secondary toxicities are nephrotoxicity, SIADH, and CNS toxicity. CNS toxicity is increased with baseline dementia or a low serum albumin. The neurotoxin chloroacetaldehyde is a byproduct of this drug. The nadir is days 5 to 10 after administration and this drug also needs coadministration of mesna to decrease the incidence of hemorrhagic cystitis.

F. Melphalan (Alkeran): Cross links DNA and can be administered IV, PO, or IP. Dosing occurs at 16 mg/m^2 IV every 2 weeks for 4 doses then at 4-week intervals, or 1 mg/kg IV every 4 weeks. The PO dose is 6 mg/day for 2 to 3 weeks followed by a 4-week holiday. There is 63 times greater exposure via the IP route. Elimination is 99% renal. Primary toxicity is pancytopenia with secondary toxicities to include nausea, vomiting, and leukemia (11.2% cumulative 10-year risk). The nadir occurs at days 28 to 35 and there is increased drug bioavailability if taken after fasting for 8 hours. Drug resistance is via increased intracellular glutathione S-transferase, and buthionine sulfoximine (BSO) can reverse this resistance.

G. **Altretamine (Hexalen, Hexamethylmelamine):** This is a pro-drug that is metabolically activated by the liver. It is important to not take supplements with B_{12} because this inactivates the drug. It is administered PO at a dose of 260 mg/m^2/day in 4 daily divided doses for 14 to 21 days every 4 weeks. 85% is eliminated via the renal system. Primary toxicities are pancytopenia, neuropathy, nausea, vomiting, and nephrotoxicity. Secondary toxicities include rash, neurotoxicity, and seizures. The nadir occurs at days 21 to 28.

II. **Antitumor Antibiotics:** These agents intercalate with DNA, inhibit RNA synthesis, and interfere with DNA repair. They are cell-cycle nonspecific except for bleomycin.

A. **Bleomycin (Blenoxane):** Complexes with iron to form an oxidase and produces free radicals. These free radicals produce DNA strand breaks in the G2 and M phases. It can be administered either IV, IM, or intracavitary for effusions. Dosing is calculated at 1 unit = 1 mg. The IV dose is bolused at 30 mg/week for 12 weeks, or 10 mg/m^2/day for 4 days every 4 weeks. Do not exceed 400 mg total. For pleural effusions, 60–120 mg can be instilled into the cavity. 70% is eliminated by the kidneys. Primary toxicities are interstitial pneumonitis (10%), pulmonary fibrosis (1%), alopecia, mucositis, and non-neutropenic fever. Secondary toxicities are nausea, vomiting, pancytopenia, hyperpigmentation, and allergic reactions. The nadir occurs at day 12. Pulmonary toxicity occurs due to the iron free radicals targeting first the type I alveoli followed by the type II alveoli. DLCO (carbon monoxide diffusion capacity spirometry) is the test to determine pulmonary toxicity. A 15% change from pretreatment value signifies toxicity and thus the need to discontinue treatment. A chest x-ray should be obtained prior to each course along with a DLCO, but it is important to rely on physical examination and patient symptoms. Risk factors for pulmonary toxicity are prior mediastinal irradiation, age greater than 70, and hyperoxia during surgical anesthesia. Steroid therapy may help with acute pneumonitis.

B. **Doxorubicin (Adriamycin):** Inhibits the strand passing activity of topoisomerase-II, and also intercalates with DNA. It is administered via IV and chelates with iron and copper. These heavy metal chelations contribute to the cardiomyopathy toxicity of the drug. It is dosed at 60 to 75 mg/m^2 as a single agent or 40 to

60 mg/m^2 in combination every 3 to 4 weeks. Elimination is hepatobiliary for 40% of the drug. It is a vesicant. Primary toxicity is pancytopenia and secondary toxicities are radiation recall, cardiomyopathy, and palmar plantar erythema (PPE). To avoid PPE, consider treatment with vitamin B$_6$, avoid hot tubs and high friction activities. The nadir is at days 10 to 14. With a total dose greater than 500 mg/m^2, the patient has an 11% risk of cardiomyopathy. If the total dose is greater than 600 mg/m^2, there is a 30% risk. Dexrazoxane (Zinecard) is a cardioprotective agent. It is administered at a 10:1 ratio, but if there is renal compromise, it should be dose reduced (to a 5:1 ratio). Risk factors for development of cardiomyopathy are age greater than 70 years, prior cardiac disease, and prior mediastinal radiation. Pretreatment tests include a baseline multigated acquisition (MUGA) scan or echocardiogram, EKG, and a chest x-ray. If symptoms present during treatment, obtain a MUGA scan or an echocardiogram.

C. **Liposomal Doxorubicin (Doxil):** The mechanism of action is similar to the nonliposomal form. It is given IV every 4 weeks at 40 to 50 mg/m^2. It is not a vesicant. Drug is found highly concentrated in tumor tissue (4 times the serum amount). Toxicity is primarily pancytopenia. Secondary toxicity is palmar plantar erythema (PPE).

D. **Dactinomycin (Actinomycin D):** The mechanism of action is DNA intercalation and it is administered IV. Dosing can be 9 to 13 mg/kg IV per day for 5 days every 2 weeks or 1.25 mg/m^2 every 2 weeks for nonmetastatic GTD, 90% is eliminated via the hepatobiliary system. Primary toxicities are pancytopenia, nausea, vomiting, and mucositis. Secondary toxicity is alopecia. The nadir is days 7 to 10. The mode of resistance is via MDR P-glycoprotein.

E. **Mitomycin C (Mutamycin):** A pro-drug that crosslinks DNA. It is selectively activated by hypoxic cells. It is administered IV and dosed as a single agent at 10 to 20 mg/m^2 or in combination at 10 mg/m^2 every 6 to 8 weeks. Elimination is by the hepatobiliary system for 90% of the drug. Primary toxicity is pancytopenia and secondary toxicities are nausea, vomiting, nephrotoxicity, microangiopathic hemolytic anemia, hemolytic uremic syndrome (HUS), and multiorgan failure. The nadir is 4 to 6 weeks. There is cumulative myelosuppression so the total lifetime dose should be less than 60 mg/m^2.

F. **Mitoxantrone (Novantrone):** Inhibits topoisomerase-II and is administered IV or IP at a dose of: 12 to 14 mg/m^2 IV; or 10 mg/m^2 in 2 liters of NS IP every 3 weeks. Elimination is hepatobiliary and primary toxicities are nausea, vomiting, diarrhea, and myelosuppression. The nadir is day 10. This drug may cause the "Smurf" syndrome and can turn the bowel and sclera blue.

G. **Levamisole (Ergamisol):** A synthetic imidazothiazole derivative initially used for helminthic infections. It is administered PO at a dose of 50 mg PO TID × 3 days per week, weekly for 1 year in combination with chemotherapy (5-FU). It is eliminated via the renal system. Primary toxicities are stomatitis, diarrhea, nausea, vomiting, and a metallic taste. Secondary toxicities are fever, chills, fatigue, myalgias, agranulocytosis, telangiectasia, seizures, edema, and chorea. The nadir is days 7 to 10. The tablets contain lactose: Lactaid may be necessary in those with lactose intolerance.

III. **Antimetabolites**
These drugs antagonize folate, purines, pyrimidines, or ribonucleotide reductase. They therefore interfere with DNA synthesis. These agents are cell cycle specific for the S phase.

A. **5-Fluorouracil (5-FU, Efudex):** A pro-drug that is metabolized to FUDR. FUDR is a pyrimidine antimetabolite that inhibits thymidylate synthase and is incorporated into DNA and RNA. Administration is IV or topical. Dosing as a single agent is with a loading dose of 12 mg/kg (maximum of 800 mg) daily for 4 to 5 days, then after 28 days, a weekly maintenance dose of 200 to 250 mg/m^2 every other day for 4 days every 4 weeks. It can also be dosed at 800 to 1,000 mg/m^2 IV daily for 4 days, repeated every 3–4 weeks. Oral dosing of 15 to 20 mg/kg/day for 5 to 8 days can be used. Topical/vaginal application is given as a 5% cream; apply 1/2 vaginal applicator of 5% 5-FU (2.5 g) deep in the vagina at bedtime every 2 to 3 weeks. Elimination is 80% by the liver and 15% by the kidneys. Primary toxicities are granulocytopenia, thrombocytopenia, mucositis, nausea, vomiting, alopecia, and hyperpigmentation. Secondary toxicities are photosensitivity, cerebellar syndrome from the metabolite fluorocitrate, palmar plantar erythrodysesthesia (occurs in 42% to 82% and can be reversed with B$_6$ dosed at 50 to 150 mg), and cardiotoxicity. The nadir is days 9 to 14. Patients with a genetic deficiency of DHFR should not receive this drug.

B. **Capecitabine (Xeloda):** A pro-drug that is metabolized to 5-FU. It is administered PO with a starting dose of 1250 mg/m² administered as a divided BID dose. A reduced starting dose (950 mg/m² bid) is required for patients with a creatinine clearance equal to 30 to 50 mL/min). It is given for 14 days of a 21-day cycle. Elimination is renal and primary toxicities are diarrhea, nausea, and vomiting. Secondary toxicities are hand-and-foot syndrome, rash, dry skin, and fatigue. If the patient is taking warfarin concomitantly, frequent monitoring of the INR is recommended.

C. **Methotrexate (Trexall):** Blocks DHFR and can be administered IV, PO, IM, or intrathecally. The dose can be weekly at 30 to 50 mg/m² IM or IV; 0.4 mg/kg IV or IM daily × 5 days every 14 days; 1 mg/kg IM or IV, days 1, 3, 5, and 7 with leucovorin given 15 mg orally on days 2, 4, 6, and 8 every 14 days; or 100 mg/m² IV bolus followed by 200 mg/m² 12-hour continuous IV infusion with leucovorin given 15 mg orally every 12 hours × 4 doses (beginning 24 hours after start of MTX infusion) every 14 days; or 12 to 15 mg/m²/week intrathecally. Elimination is mainly renal. Primary toxicities are nausea, vomiting, pancytopenia, mucositis, and hepatotoxicity. Secondary toxicities are nephrotoxicity, alopecia, and interstitial pneumonitis. The nadir is days 4 to 7. Resistance is via elevated DHFR or mutated transport mechanisms into the tumor cells. Methotrexate accumulates in pleural effusions, so it is necessary to drain effusions before administration. It is also helpful to alkalinize the urine with 3 g of sodium bicarbonate 12 hours before therapy.

D. **Hydroxyurea (Hydrea):** S-phase specific and inhibits ribonucleotide reductase. It is administered IV or PO. Dosing is 1 to 3 mg/m²/day every 2 to 6 weeks; 80 mg/kg twice weekly; or 2–3 g/m² twice weekly. Elimination is mainly renal and toxicity is myelosuppression. The nadir occurs at 10 days.

E. **Gemcitabine (Gemzar):** A synthetic nucleoside analog. It is a pro-drug and is metabolized to its active diphosphate and triphosphate states by the liver. These metabolites are then incorporated into DNA and cause masked chain termination. In addition it is a radiosensitizing agent. It can cause radiation recall. Dosing is IV. It can be given as a single agent at 800 to 1000 mg/m² IV weekly for 7 weeks of an 8-week cycle; 1000 mg/m² weekly for 3 weeks of a 4-week cycle, or at 1000 to 1250 mg/m² days 1 and 8 with cisplatin at 75 to 100 mg/m² on day 1 given prior to gemcitabine by 24 hours of a

3-week cycle. Elimination is 90% renal. Primary toxicities are neutropenia, elevated LFTs, alopecia, and mucositis. Secondary toxicities are subcutaneous edema, hemolytic uremic syndrome, and acute respiratory distress syndrome (ARDS).

IV. **Plant Alkaloids:** These agents inhibit microtubule function and arrest cells in M phase. They are cell-cycle specific.

    A. Etoposide (VP-16, VePesid): The mechanism of action is inhibition and stabilization of topoisomerase-II. It arrests cells in the G_2 phase. There are multiple regimens but it can be given at a dose of 100 mg/m² days 1–5 the first week of a 3 week cycle, or 50 mg/m²/day × 21 days PO. Elimination is primarily renal with 98% being cleared by the kidneys. Primary toxicities are pancytopenia, nausea, and vomiting. Secondary toxicities are alopecia, neurotoxicity, and hypotension; therefore, give over 30 minutes. It can also cause secondary leukemia above a total dose of 2 g. The nadir is day 16.

    B. Paclitaxel (Taxol): Stabilizes microtubules and promotes their formation. It can be given IV or IP and should be administered before platinum agents. Single-agent dosing is usually 175 to 250 mg/m² but in combination it is usually dosed at 175 mg/m² every 3 weeks or 80 mg/m² weekly every 3 weeks. Dose reduction is usually to 135 mg/m². Elimination is 90% hepatic/biliary and 10% renal. Primary toxicities are neurotoxicity (distal extremities), pancytopenia, hypersensitivity reactions to the vehicle cremophor, arrhythmias, and alopecia. Secondary toxicities are nausea, vomiting, mucositis, arthralgias, and an abnormal EKG. The nadir is days 8 to 11. Always premedicate before chemotherapy with dexamethasone 20 mg PO 12 and 6 hours prior to administration, Benadryl 50 mg IV/PO, and cimetidine 300 mg IV both 30 minutes before initiation.

    C. Albumin-Bound Paclitaxel (Abraxane, ABI-007): Stabilizes microtubules and promotes their formation. The albumin-bound drug has a superior toxicity profile because it lacks the castor oil-base that paclitaxel is mixed with. Dosing is 260 mg/m² IV every 3 weeks without needed premedications. Cardiotoxicity occurs in 3% of patients, neutropenia occurs in 9% of patients, and neuropathy is dose dependent.

    D. Topotecan (Hycamtin): Inhibits topoisomerase-I and is usually given IV. Dosing as a single agent is 1.25 to 1.5 mg/m²/day for 3 to 5 days/week every 3 weeks. Elimination is both renal and hepatic. Primary toxicities are myelosuppression and alopecia with secondary toxicity being asthenia. The nadir is days 9 to 15.

E. **Irinotecan (Camptosar):** A pro-drug and inhibits topoisomerase-I. It is given IV at doses of: 125 mg/m² every week, 240 mg/m² every 3 weeks, or 350 mg/m² every 3 weeks. Elimination is hepatobiliary. Primary toxicities are anemia, nausea, vomiting, elevated liver enzymes, and alopecia. Secondary toxicity is diarrhea. Use antimotility agents (e.g., loperamide at 16 mg/day) as soon as diarrhea appears. The nadir is days 15 to 27.

F. **Docetaxel (Taxotere):** Inhibits the depolymerization of tubulin and stabilizes microtubules. It is given IV as: a single agent at 60 to 100 mg/m² every 3 weeks; or in combination at 85 to 100 mg/m² every 3 weeks. Its elimination is primarily hepatobiliary at 99.4%. Primary toxicities are neutropenia, edema, and hypersensitivity reactions. Secondary toxicity is a maculopapular rash. The nadir occurs at 5 to 9 days. To decrease the rate of hypersensitivity reactions and third spacing edema, premedicate with corticosteroids 8 mg bid starting 1 day prior to and continuing up to 4 days after administration.

G. **Vinblastine (Velban):** Inhibits microtubule assembly by binding to tubulin and is given IV at a dose of: 0.1 to 0.5 mg/kg/week (4 to 20 mg/m²); 6 mg/m² days 1 and 15 every 3 weeks; or 0.15 mg/kg days 1 and 2 every 3 weeks. It is eliminated via both the renal (30%) and the hepatobiliary (20%) systems. Primary toxicities are pancytopenia, constipation, abdominal pain, and adynamic ileus. Secondary toxicities are nausea, vomiting, mucositis, alopecia, neurotoxicity, Raynaud's syndrome, and transient hepatitis. The nadir is days 4 to 10.

H. **Vincristine (Oncovin):** Inhibits microtubule assembly. It is administered IV at a dose of: 1 mg/m², or 0.01 to 0.03 mg/m² given every 1 to 2 weeks. Elimination is primarily renal (90%), with hepatobiliary elimination at 10%. Primary toxicities are neurotoxicity, and alopecia. Secondary toxicities are pancytopenia, constipation, and SIADH. The nadir is day 7.

I. **Vinorelbine (Navelbine):** Inhibits microtubule assembly and is given IV: as a single agent at a dose of 30 mg/m² every week; or in combination at 25 mg/m² weekly. Elimination is hepatobiliary. Primary toxicities are granulocytopenia, neurotoxicity, nausea, vomiting, alopecia, and chest pain. Secondary toxicities are arthralgias, SOB, and constipation. The nadir is days 7 to 14. It is incompatible with 5-FU, mitomycin C, thiotepa, antibiotics, and antivirals and can exacerbate pulmonary toxicity.

V. Hormonal Agents

These agents bind hormone receptors and either stimulate or inhibit DNA transcription depending on the agonist/antagonist properties of the drug. They are cell-cycle nonspecific.

A. Leuprolide Acetate (Lupron): A GnRH superagonist administered as a depot IM injection. Dosing can be 3.5 to 7.5 mg monthly, or 11.25 to 22.5 mg every 3 months. Elimination is renal. Primary toxicity is hot flashes with secondary toxicities of headache, edema, and bone pain.

B. Megestrol (Megace): A progestin given PO at doses of 160 to 320 mg daily. Elimination is renal. Primary toxicity is edema and weight gain. Secondary toxicities are DVT/VTE, and a Cushing-like syndrome.

C. Tamoxifen (Nolvadex): An estrogen receptor agonist/antagonist administered PO at a dose of 20 mg daily. Elimination is hepatobiliary and primary toxicity is hot flashes. Secondary toxicities are vaginal bleeding, DVT/VTE, rash, and endometrial cancer.

D. Anastrozole (Arimidex): A nonsteroidal aromatase inhibitor given PO. The dose is 1 mg daily. Elimination is renal. Primary toxicities are anorexia, vaginal dryness, and hot flashes. Secondary toxicities are DVT/VTE, osteopenia, and osteoporosis.

E. Letrozole (Femara): A nonsteroidal aromatase inhibitor. It is given PO at a dose of 2.5 mg a day. Primary toxicities are bone pain and hot flashes, arthralgias, and dyspnea in 20% of patients. It does not increase serum FSH and does not impact adrenal steroid synthesis.

F. Exemestane (Aromasin): A steroidal aromatose inhibitor. It is an irreversible inhibitor. It is dosed at 25 mg/day. Primary toxicity is hot flashes, fatigue, and arthralgias.

VI. Receptor and Signaling Targeted Therapies

A. Bevacizumab (Avastin): A monoclonal antibody against vascular endothelial growth factor (VEGF) that interferes with tumor angiogenesis. It is administered IV at a dose of 5, 7.5, or 15 mg/kg every 1 to 3 weeks. Elimination is renal. Primary toxicities are HTN (28%), nephrotic syndrome, gastrointestinal perforation (1% to 11%), wound dehiscence, and CHF.

B. **Imatinib Mesylate (Gleevec):** Inhibits the protein tyrosine kinase Bcr-Abl and is administered PO daily. It is eliminated via the hepatobiliary system and is dosed at 400 mg/day for chronic myeloid leukemia (CML), and at 600 mg/day for blast crisis CML or gastrointestinal stromal tumor (GIST). Primary toxicities are nausea, vomiting, muscle cramps, skin rash, diarrhea, and heartburn with a secondary toxicity of fluid retention.

C. **Trastuzumab (Herceptin):** A monoclonal antibody to the *HER-2/neu-erb2* receptor. It is administered IV as a loading dose of 4 mg/kg over 90 minutes. It is given in combination with chemotherapy every 3 weeks. Maintenance monotherapy continues after completion of cytotoxic chemotherapy at 2 mg/kg every 3 weeks. Elimination is renal and toxicities are a rash or CHF (1% to 29%).

VII. **Protective Agents:** These agents protect against the cytotoxic effects of chemotherapeutic drugs.

A. **Leucovorin:** Has two mechanisms of action. It is protective against MTX and it modulates and prolongs the effects of 5-FU. Dosing is: 370 mg/m^2/day for 5 days during 5-FU infusion plus an additional infusion of 500 mg/m^2/day beginning 24 hours before the first dose of 5-FU and continuing 12 hours after completion of 5-FU therapy; or 5 to 15 mg PO or 10 to 20 mg/m^2 given IV 10 minutes before 5-FU infusion. It is eliminated by the renal system. Primary toxicities are pancytopenia, nausea and vomiting. The nadir is days 7 to 14.

B. **Dexrazoxane (Zinecard):** Chemoprotective against doxorubicin induced cardiomyopathy. It chelates divalent heavy metals and is administered IV, 30 minutes prior to chemotherapy at a dose of 10:1 (500 mg/m^2 dexrazoxane to 50 mg/m^2 of doxorubicin). Consider administration when the cumulative dose of doxorubicin rises to 300 mg/m^2. Elimination is primarily renal with primary toxicities of granulocytopenia, nausea, vomiting, and alopecia.

C. **Amifostine:** A radioprotective and cytoprotective compound. It has a highly selective transport mechanism into normal cells and there it scavenges free radicals. It can reduce the renal toxicity of cisplatin as well as the neurotoxicity of other agents. It is administered IV 30 minutes prior to chemotherapy at a dose of 740 to 910 mg/m². Toxicity is mucositis, nausea, vomiting, arterial hypotension, and hypocalcemia. The dosing interval is with chemotherapy and elimination is renal.

D. Sodium Thiosulfate: Protects against cisplatin-induced nephrotoxicity. It is administered IV at a dose of 16 to 20 mg/m² given 2 hours after cisplatin. The dose interval is with chemotherapy and elimination is renal.

E. Mesna: Chemoprotective against hemorrhagic cystitis and inactivates the metabolite acrolein. It can be administered IV or SC at a dose that is 20% of the total cytotoxic alkalator dose. Dosing is prior to chemotherapy with two additional doses 4 and 8 hours after chemotherapy treatment. Elimination is renal.

F. Buthionine Sulfoximine (BSO): Enhances the cytotoxicity of alkylator agents by modifying GSH and GST, thus depleting intracellular levels of glutathione. It is administered IV. Dosing is with a loading dose of 3 g/m² over 30 minutes, followed by 3 consecutive 24-hour infusions at 18 mg/m². Chemotherapy should be given after 48 hours of buthionine sulfoximine. Elimination is via the renal system.

VIII. Treatment of Extravasation Injury

A. Cisplatin: Thiosulfate should be injected into the skin site at 1/3 to 1/6 molar solution. 2 mL should be injected for every 100 mg extravasated.

B. Doxorubicin: Cold compresses should be applied immediately to the site for 60 minutes with consideration of an injection of 150 U hyaluronidase into the site. Cold topical DMSO can also be applied. This agent can cause extensive ulceration and treatment is debridement of the primary and recurrent ulcers.

C. Etoposide: Consider an injection of 150 U of hyaluronidase into the site.

D. Mitomycin C: Topical DMSO should be applied every 6 hours × 14 days.

E. Vinblastine: Warm compresses should be applied immediately to the site for 60 minutes with consideration of an injection of 150 U of hyaluronidase into the site. Corticosteroids can also help if injected into the site.

    F. Vincristine: Warm compresses should be applied immediately to the site for 60 minutes with consideration of an injection of 150 U of hyaluronidase into the site.

REFERENCES

1. Vay A, Kumar S, Seward S. Therapy-related myeloid leukemia after treatment for epithelial ovarian carcinoma: an epidemiological analysis. *Gynecol Oncol.* 2011;123(3):456–460.
2. Hobohm U. *Cancer Immunol Immunother.* 2001 Oct; 50(8):391–396.

Radiation Therapy

I. Radiation Types

There are different types of radiation currently used in medicine.

A. X-rays are extranuclear radiation. They occur from bombardment of an atom/target by another source—usually high-speed electrons.

B. The alpha particle demonstrates cluster decay where a parent atom ejects a defined daughter collection of nucleons. These have a typical kinetic energy of 5 MeV. Because of their relatively large mass, their $+2$ electric charge, and relatively low velocity, alpha particles are very likely to interact with other atoms and lose their energy. Their forward motion is effectively stopped within a few centimeters of air or paper. This particle is the same as a Helium^4 particle (2 protons and 2 neutrons).

C. Beta particles are high-energy, high-speed electrons emitted by certain types of radioactive nuclei. Beta particles are ionizing radiation. They are stopped by millimeters of tissue. The production of beta particles is termed beta decay.

D. Gamma particles are a form of ionizing radiation that originates from the decay of the nucleus of a radioactive isotope. Energies range from ten thousand (10^4) to ten million (10^7) electron volts.

E. An isotope is one of two or more atoms having the same number of protons but a different number of neutrons. This makes the nucleus unstable. The atom then spontaneously decomposes/decays and excess energy is given off by emission of a nuclear electron or helium nucleus and radiation, to achieve a stable nuclear composition. Some of these isotopes include radium-226, cesium-137, iridium-192, cobolt-60, and gold-198.

F. Electron energy comes from outside the nucleus. Electrons are used to treat tumors en face—close to the skin.

II. Definitions

A. Roentgen: is the amount of photon radiation that causes 0.001293 g of air to produce 1 electrostatic unit of positive or negative charge. This number is the mass of 1 mL of air at 769 mm Hg and 0 degrees C.

B. Kinetic Energy Related to Mass (KERMA): is the transfer of energy from photons to particles. Particles transfer this energy to tissue and this is defined as absorbed dose.

C. Relative biologic effectiveness (RBE): is the ratio of the dose required for a given radiation to produce the same biologic effect induced by 250 kV of x-rays.

D. Isodose: is the line that connects structures which receive equal radiation dose.

E. Source to skin distance (SSD): is usually defined at 80 to 100 cm from the machine to the patient. Radiation is dosed at a fixed point from the patient and thus there needs to be standardization of distance for treatment.

F. Isocenter: is a fixed point in the patient around which treatment is rotated.

G. Dmax: is the point where the maximum amount of dose from one beam is deposited. The dose at Dmax is defined at 100%. The depths of Dmax for some common energies are: 4 MV, 1.2 cm; 6 MV, 1.5 cm; 10 MV, 2.5 cm; 18 MV, 3.2 cm.

H. Percent depth dose: is the change in dose with depth within the patient.

I. Gross tumor volume (GTV): direct tumor volume by measurement. The GTV requires a high dose of radiation to treat the primary or bulky tumor. This dose is usually 80 to 90 Gy.

J. Clinical target volume (CTV): this includes any region that has a high likelihood of harboring malignancy but appears clinically normal. The CTV requires a lower dose than GTV. This dose is usually around 45 to 54 Gy and is adequate to treat occult or microscopic disease.

K. Planning target volume (PTV): is a margin added to account for organ motion and daily setup error.

III. Radiation Effects

There are two basic types of energy transfer that may occur when X-rays interact with matter:

- Ionization, in which the incoming radiation causes the removal of an electron from an atom or molecule leaving the material with a net positive charge.

- Excitation, in which some of the X-ray's energy is transferred to the target material leaving it in an excited (or more energetic) state.

There are 3 important processes that can occur when X-rays interact with matter. These processes are: the Photoelectric effect; the Compton effect; and Pair Production

A. The Photoelectric effect produces energy in the eV–keV range. This type of radiation occurs when atoms absorb energy from light and emit electrons. This form of radiation is used for diagnostic x-rays and to simulate radiation treatment beams. The photoelectric effect occurs when photons interact with matter with resulting ejection of electrons from the matter. Photoelectric (PE) absorption of x-rays occurs when the x-ray photon is absorbed resulting in the ejection of electrons from the atom. This leaves the atom in an ionized state. The ionized atom then returns to the neutral state with the emission of an x-ray characteristic of the atom. Photoelectron absorption is the dominant process for x-ray absorption up to energies of about 500 KeV.

B. Pair Production occurs when the x-ray photon energy is greater than 1.02 MeV. An electron and positron are created with the annihilation of the x-ray photon. Positrons are very short lived and disappear (positron annihilation) with the formation of two photons of 0.51 MeV energy. Pair production is of particular importance when high-energy photons pass through materials with high atomic numbers. This type of energy is not used clinically.

C. The Compton effect is when an incident photon interacts with an outer electron. The energy that results is shared between the ejected electron and the scattered photon. Compton Scattering is important for low atomic number specimens. At energies of 100 keV–10 MeV the absorption of radiation is mainly due to the Compton effect. This type of energy is used for the radiation treatment of cancers. Photons are harvested from the decay of a source. First, the source has intrinsic decay. The electrons from this decay are used to bombard tungsten causing the Compton effect. The resultant photon is the radiation we use in linear accelerator machine.

IV. Energy Equivalences

1 Gray (Gy) is equal to 1 Joule per kg of tissue.

1 Gray (Gy) is equal to 100 cGy.

100 radiation absorbed doses (Rads) are equal to 1 Gy.

1 Rad is equal to 1 cGy.

V. Radiation Delivery

A. External beam radiation is delivered using a linear accelerator machine. These machines deliver 4 to 24 mega electron volts (MeV). Total radiation dose is administered via a daily divided dose called a fraction. Common daily doses/fractions are 1.8-2 Gy. A total dose of 90 Gy is needed to sterilize most tumors. Non cancerous tissues cannot tolerate this total dose from external beam radiation, so brachytherapy is needed to locally deliver radiation directly to the tumor.

B. Brachytherapy is the local, and often internalized, delivery of radiation. For gynecologic cancers, radiation is often delivered using tandem and ovoids, vaginal cylinders, or interstitial needles. Brachytherapy is delivered at a low-dose rate or a high-dose rate.

   1. LDR is defined as 0.4 to 2 Gy/hr. HDR is defined as a dose greater than 12 Gy/hr or greater than 20 to 250 cGy/min (12 to 15 Gy/hr). The dose conversion from LDR to HDR is 0.6.

   2. HDR is more common now because of a number of patient based reasons: treatment time is shorter; treatment is delivered on an outpatient basis; there is no need for bed rest, there is better ability to retract the rectum for shorter periods of time, and therefore better patient acceptance and comfort. Clinically, there is better implant reproducibility and a greater degree of certainty that the sources will remain stable during treatment. The HDR applicators are less bulky so patients with narrow vaginas don't necessarily have to be treated with interstitial implants. The smaller source size also allows for finer increments in source location and weighting and a better ability to shape the dose distribution.

   3. Isotopes: Iridium-192 is the most commonly used isotope. The half-life of iridium is 74 days. Cesium-137 is no longer available but its half-life is 30 years. Cobalt-60 is also no longer used but its half-life is 5.26 years. Radium-226 has a half life of 1626 years and has little use in modern radiation oncology.

VI. Tumoricidal Basics

A. Radiation dose is proportional to the time the patient is exposed to the dose. The dose is also proportional to the distance from the source (the inverse square law): $1/r^2$. Dosing used to be mg/hr based. It is now dosimetry based.

B. In the log cell kill model each dose—called a fraction—kills a fixed amount of cells. Radiation works by causing breaks in the

DNA backbone via one of two types of energy, a photon or a charged particle (an electron). This damage is either direct or indirect with ionization of the atoms which make up the DNA chain. Indirect ionization is the result of the ionization of water, forming free radicals, notably hydroxyl radicals, which then damage the DNA. Direct ionization is the result of electrons causing single stranded DNA breaks. These single stranded breaks need to be on opposing strands of DNA in close proximity to each other in order to create a double stranded break. Oxygen free radicals modify radiation damage making irreparable. Oxygen is transported to tumors via the blood system, so adequate Hg levels are needed. Without oxygen, the cell survival curve shifts to the right.

C. There are two cell survival/dose response curves, the linear and the linear-quadratic. The linear "curve" is a straight line and this is represented by LDR. LDR is delivered over a protracted period of time and cell kill is by a single electron. The linear quadratic curve demonstrates cell kill initially principally by 2 breaks in the DNA caused either by the same electron or by 2 different electrons. This cell survival curve is straight initially and then curves representing HDR type delivery.

D. The linear quadratic equation: $-\ln S = alphaD + betaD^2$. The alpha component is the nonreparable damage, whereas the beta component represents reparable damage. S is the surviving fraction of cells. The dose at which the cell kill is due to equal linear and quadratic components is called the alpha beta ratio.

E. The BED is the biologically equivalent dose and is used as a guide to determine optimal dosing. The BED = D[1 + d/(alpha/beta)] where D is the total dose, and d is the dose per fraction. Early side effects demonstrate an alpha/beta ratio of 10 whereas late side effects and tumor control assume an alpha/beta of 3.

F. The cell can respond to radiation differently depending on its phase in the cell cycle. Late S phase is the most radioresistant phase and M phase is most radiosensitive. There are two possible outcomes after exposure to radiation: survival, or death. If the cell survives there is cell cycle arrest and DNA repair.

G. There are 3 types of cell death. The first is apoptotic which is ordered programmed cell death. A lot of tumors have mutations in apoptotic pathways and thus do not respond to apoptotic signals easily. The second type of cell death is mitotic. Mitotic death may take days. The third is senescence: Senescence is when cell proliferation is irreversibly arrested and death eventually ensues.

VII. The 4 R's of Radiation

A. Repair: radiation in fractionated doses is not as lethal as if it were delivered in one high dose. Sublethal repair occurs when a certain percentage of cells are killed, and those that survive can repair their damage and continue to divide.

B. Re-assortment: radiation kills cells best when they are in the late G_2 and M phases, which are the most radiosensitive cycles. Other cycles are relatively radioresistant. After a dose of fractional radiation, the cells which were in the more radioresistent phases (and survived) reassort themselves into their next cell cycle. They then become more radiosensitive and when the next dose of radiation is delivered they have a higher likelihood of death.

C. Repopulation: is when the surviving population of cells which are not lethally damaged divide and replace those that were killed.

D. Re-oxygenation: is when the tumor generates new blood vessels to bring in a higher oxygen tension via hemoglobin. Oxygen must be present during radiation to generate the free radical that yields DNA damage. Low oxygen tension makes cells more radioresistant.

DISEASE SITE RADIATION TREATMENT

I. **Cervical Cancer:** All stages of cervical cancer can be treated with definitive radiotherapy. Anatomical dosing is based on the paracervical triangle—the lateral vaginal fornices and the apex of the anteverted uterus. Dosing is directed at 2 common points. Point A is 2 cm superior and 2 cm lateral to the external cervical os. This correlates anatomically to where the ureter and the uterine artery cross. Point B is 2 cm superior and 5 cm lateral to the external cervical os. This point corresponds to the obturator lymph node basins. Point T is inside point A. It is 1 cm superior to the external cervical os and 1 cm lateral to the tandem; it receives a dose 2 to 3× the dose to point A. Point P is located along the bony pelvic sidewall at its most lateral point and represents the minimal dose to the external iliac lymph nodes. Point C is 1 cm lateral to point B and is approximate to the pelvic sidewall. Point H is an HDR point: it originates from a line that connects the middwell position of the ovoids and intersects with the tandem. Then move superiorly the radius of the ovoids (to top of ovoids) + 2 cm, and then 2 cm perpendicularly. The vaginal surface is where the lateral radius of the ovoid and ring applicator fall. This receives a dose 1.4 to 2.0 times the point A dose.

A. Current dosing for cervical cancer prescribes a total dose to point A of 85 to 90 Gy with 60 Gy dosed to point B.

  1. External beam radiation can provide 50.4 Gy to the point A via whole pelvic radiation with a 15 Gy boost when appropriate. The dose to point A is brought up from 50.4 Gy using external beam radiation to the total desired dose of 85 to 90 Gy with brachytherapy.

  2. If LDR is used, the brachytherapy dose is 50 to 60 cGy/hr with 40 Gy total given. If HDR is used, the dose is 30 Gy. The brachytherapy dose per HDR fraction to point A is 3 to 10.5 Gy. The total number of fractions is 2 to 13. The number of fractions per week is 1 to 3. The morbidity is lower for fractions less than 7 Gy. GOG protocols use 6 Gy × 5 fractions to point A. RTOG protocols allow more variation depending on the external beam radiation dose with brachytherapy fraction sizes of 5.3 to 7.4 Gy using 4 to 7 fractions. Platinum-based chemotherapy should be used in the definitive management of cervical cancer.

B. Sequencing of brachytherapy with external beam radiation is based on tumor size, patient anatomy, and practitioner discretion. For non-bulky disease, HDR is often integrated after 20 Gy of external beam therapy, around the second week of treatment. Alternatively, some deliver whole pelvic radiation to 50.4 Gy followed by 5 HDR insertions.

C. Brachytherapy most commonly uses the tandem and ovoid system. There are 48 dwell positions in the tandem. The radiation sources are usually spaced 2.5 to 5 mm apart. The dwell position is where the source is driven to stop. The longest tandem possible should be used. The tandem should be loaded so the sources reach the uterine fundus. This enables adequate distribution to the lower uterine segment, the paracervical tissues, and obturator lymph nodes. The tandems have 3 curvatures (15, 30, and 45 degrees), the greatest curvature is used in cavities measuring >6 cm. A flange is added to the tandem after insertion into the uterine cavity and approximates the exocervix. The keel is then added and prevents rotation of the tandem after packing.

D. Vaginal ovoids come in four different sizes. The largest sized ovoid that the patient can tolerate is placed as far laterally and cephalad as possible. This gives the highest tumor dose possible. The mini sized ovoid is 1.6 cm in diameter, the small is 2 cm in diameter, the medium is 2.5 cm in diameter, and the large is 3 cm in diameter. The mini does not have any shielding to protect the bladder. A wide separation of the ovoids is desired as this increases the dose to the pelvic sidewall. A 10-mg protruding source is recommended if the vaginal ovoids are separated by more than 5 cm. Optimal positioning is: on the AP view the tandem is midline and unrotated, the tandem is midway between the colpostats, the keel is in close proximity to the gold seed markers, and the colpostats are placed high in the vaginal fornices; on the lateral view the tandem bisects the colpostat, there is sufficient anterior and posterior packing, and the tandem is equidistant from the sacral promontory and the pubis.

E. The anterior bladder point is determined by placement of a Foley catheter with 7 mL of radiopaque material placed into the balloon. The balloon is then pulled down against the urethra creating this point.

F. The posterior rectal point is determined by packing the vagina with radiopaque packing and moving 5 mm posterior to that line. The vaginal surface dose should be kept below 140 Gy.

G. In the postoperative setting, patients can be broken into 2 risk categories: (1) those with intermediate risk factors (LVSI, stromal DOI, and tumor size per GOG 92 (2) those with high risk factors (2+ positive lymph nodes, lesion size greater than 2 cm, positive margins, or parametrial involvement proven histologically) per GOG 109. Whole pelvic EBRT should be considered for those with intermediate risk factors, and concurrent platinum-based chemotherapy in addition to whole pelvic EBRT for those with high risk factors. Some centers treat both groups with combination therapy. The adjuvant dose is 45 to 50.4 Gy external beam radiotherapy.

H. Types of applicators:

1. Fletcher-Suit and Henschke tandem and ovoids are commonly used. The Delclos applicator uses the mini ovoids. The Henschke applicator uses hemispheroidal ovoids and the tandem and ovoids fixed together. This creates an easier applicator for shallow vaginal fornices.

2. The Fletcher-Suit and Delclos cylinders are used for narrow vaginas, when ovoids are contraindicated. They are also used to treat varying lengths of the vagina mandated by vaginal spread of disease. Cylinders vary in size from 2 to 4 cm in diameter.

3. Ring applicators are an adaption of the Stockholm technique. There are 3 sizes: the small is 36 mm, the medium is 40 mm, and the large is 44 mm diameter. It is important to not activate all positions in the ring, as this will increase the dosing to the bladder and rectum. Often 4 dwell positions are activated on each side of the smallest ring, 5 dwell positions on each side of the medium ring, and 6 dwell positions on each side of the largest ring. Tandems are available in lenths of 2–8 cm and the tandem angels are available with 30, 45, 60, and 90 degrees.

4. Interstitial applicators are used if there is a narrow or obliterated vagina, obliterated vaginal fornices, bulky or barrel shaped cervical tumors, parametrial disease, vaginal disease, or if there is recurrent unresectable disease. This method of radiation delivery uses iridium loaded stainless steel or plastic needles. There are a few different applicators. One is the Martinez universal perineal interstitial template (MUPIT). Another is the Syed-Neblett template which has 3 different templates consisting of 36, 44, or 53 needles. If LDR is used, the dosing is 60 to 80 cGy/hr with a total dose of 23 to 40 Gy over 2 to 4 days. If HDR is used, the dosing is 60% of the total LDR dose given in 1 to 2 fractions per day over 2 to 5 days. External beam radiation usually precedes implantation.

II. Uterine Cancer

A. Brachytherapy for uterine cancer is commonly used in the adjuvant setting. Fletcher colpostats or a variety of vaginal cylinders are used. The upper one-half to one-third of the vagina is treated after a hysterectomy.

B. When using Delclos or Burnett vaginal cylinders, treatment is to the upper 4 to 5 cm of the vagina. The dose distribution conforms to shape of the cylinder. The dose is specified either at the mucosal surface or to 0.5 cm deep. Studies have shown that 95% of the vaginal lymphatics are located within 3 mm of the vaginal surface. The LDR dose is 80 to 100 cGy/hr to the surface and 50 to 70 cGy/hr if treated to 0.5 cm deep. For recurrent disease, the tumor may need more than 80 Gy in total dose. More than 80 Gy to vagina in the adjuvant setting is not needed and treatment is usually limited to a total HDR dose of 21 Gy in 3 doses of 7 Gy to the surface, or 5 Gy in 6 doses to 0.5 cm deep.

C. Bulky Stage 2 or 3B uterine cancer should be preoperatively treated with radiotherapy. Radiation is dosed at 85–90 Gy with 45–50.4 delivered by EBRT and 21–30 Gy by brachytherapy.

D. Medically inoperable uterine cancer is a rare occurrence. Radiation treatment is with the placement of double or triple intrauterine tandems, or Heyman-Simons capsules in combination with external beam radiation. Total dosing follows that for the primary treatment of cervical cancer.

E. Residual postoperative vaginal disease less than 0.5 cm, may be treated with brachytherapy cylinders or ovoids to 45–50.4 Gy. If there is thicker residual vaginal disease, external beam or interstitial radiation therapy is needed.

F. Recurrent vaginal disease should be treated with external beam radiation followed by brachytherapy. Doses over 80 Gy are usually needed. Recurrent pelvic disease can be treated with external beam radiation.

G. Indications for treatment in the adjuvant setting are based on stage and patient risk factors.

   1. For high-intermediate risk disease, patients are stratified by age and pathological risk factors to include: G2/3, LVSI, or outer one-third myometrial involvement.

   2. If there is cervical stromal involvement, a combination of external beam and brachytherapy are used.

   3. For Stage 3A with adnexal metastasis, external beam radiation alone can give an 85% 5-year survival (YS). For Stage 3B parametrial or pelvic peritoneal disease, external beam radiation with brachytherapy can be considered. For Stage 3C, a combination of external beam radiation and chemotherapy can be considered.

   4. For early-stage patients with aggressive histology (serous or clear cell), radiotherapy in combination with platinum-based chemotherapy has been used. For those with Stage 1 disease and any residual tumor, brachytherapy and chemotherapy have been used. For those staged 2 or higher, external beam radiation has been used with chemotherapy (1).

III. Vulvar Cancer

A. Indications for treatment of the pelvic and groin lymph node (LN) basins are:

   1. FIGO Stage 3B and greater lesions

   2. In the neoadjuvant setting in combination with platinum based chemotherapy for advanced T3/T4 lesions. If the patient has clinically negative or resectable groin LNs, recommendation is to undergo pretreatment groin LN dissection. If all groin LNs are negative, patients can receive radiation therapy to only the primary tumor.

3. Adjuvant primary tumor bed radiation can be considered if positive margin(s) are present after resection, although this has not been shown to increase OS.

B. Treatment: Radiation is prescribed to a total dose of 45–57.6 Gy. A narrow posterior field is used with 15 to 18 MV and a wide anterior field is used with 6 MV and an additional 12 Mev dose is prescribed to each groin. A photon thunderbird with a deep match, or a photon through and through field, can also be designed. If the patient is thin and the depth of the inguinal vessels is less than 3 cm, an electron patch may be used. There is an 11% rate of femoral neck fracture or necrosis with these doses.

IV. Vaginal Cancer

A. Treatment is indicated for all FIGO stages, and definitively for Stage 2 and higher. Treatment is usually a combination of EBRT dosed at 45–50.4 Gy in 180 cGy fractions daily for 4 to 5 weeks, followed by brachytherapy or interstitial implants with an additional 21 to 30 Gy. Concurrent platinum based chemotherapy should be considered.

V. Ovarian Cancer

A. There are minimal uses for radiation therapy for epithelial ovarian tumors. Isolated local recurrence or residual tumor after completion of chemotherapy are debatable indications.

B. For germ cell tumors, radiation has a slightly higher indication. Dysgerminomas are highly radiosensitive and treatment can be considered for primary or recurrent disease.

C. Sex cord stromal tumors can also benefit from radiation therapy. This has been studied in recurrent granulosa cell tumors. There is data to support a 43% response rate (2).

DESIGN OF EXTERNAL BEAM RADIATION FIELDS

The external beam fields are designed in a 4 field box as anterior-posterior/posterior-anterior (AP/PA) fields plus lateral fields. These are customarily outlined as 15 × 15 cm squares for the APPA fields and 8 to 9 cm wide for the lateral fields. The intent of the four fields is to use narrow lateral beams to avoid some small bowel and a portion of the rectum posteriorly. CT or MRI based planning can accurately outline the radiation targets and simultaneously spare vital organs using mobile blocks called collimators. A collimators is a device that narrows a beam of particles and multiple collimators are used to vary the radiation fields. Radiation is dosed with a 0.7–1 cm expansion around the involved LN, bone, and muscle (CTV) except for the groin LN where there should be a 2 cm margin. The PTV should have an additional 1 cm margin. In general, the principle of extending node treatment volume one nodal echelon proximal to the level of clinical involvement is a prudent guideline. IMRT is now being used in a significant number of centers to decrease side effects to vital structures. IMRT uses computer-controlled x-ray accelerators to distribute precise radiation doses to malignant tumors or specific areas within the tumor. The pattern of radiation delivery is determined using highly tailored computing applications.

I. Cervical Cancer

    A. For cervical cancer, the superior border for non-bulky Stage 1B/2A disease is S1/L5. For bulky or more advanced disease the border is L4/5. There is data to suggest that in 87% of patients the bifurcation of the common iliac vessels was above the L5 prominence (3). Thus, it may be necessary to extend the upper field border to L2/3. Other studies have shown with CT-based planning that 79% of patients treated with conventional fields had inadequate coverage. CT-based planning was then able to cover 95% of patients appropriately. The inferior border is the mid or lower border of the obturator foramen or 3 to 4 cm below the most distal vaginal component of disease. It is important to cover the inguinal LN if the distal vagina is involved. The lateral borders are 2 to 2.5 cm lateral to the pelvic brim. The anterior border is the pubic symphysis. It may be necessary to extend this coverage to 2 cm anterior to the pubis in order to cover the external iliac arteries. The posterior border is conventionally set posterior to S2/S3. A study found that in Stages 1B and 2, the most common inadequate margin was the posterior border at the S2/3 interface and there was no increase in rectal complications when the entire sacrum was included in the radiation field (4). Treatment is 85–90 Gy using combined external beam radiation and brachytherapy. External beam radiation is dose at 45–50.4 Gy and brachytherapy is dosed at 30 Gy for HDR and 40 Gy for LDR.

    B. Midline blocks are used to increase the dose to the parametria or pelvic sidewalls while shielding the bladder, distal ureters, and rectosigmoid. Some customize the midline block at the 50% isodose line that passes through point A. Some feather the block at specific isodose intervals. Most use rectangular blocks 4 to 5 cm in width, as this is the distance between the distal ureters. A margin of 0.5 cm lateral to the lateral ovoid surface is recommended in designing the width of the midline block.

C. A parametrial boost of an additional 15 Gy is recommended if there is bulky parametrial disease or pelvic sidewall disease. This is done after completion of whole pelvic radiation. Doses needed to eradicate parametrial disease are about 60 Gy.

D. A lymph node boost is dosed at 15 Gy to enlarged or known positive LN. Data has shown that 16% of patients with biopsy proven positive LN, treated with chemotherapy and radiation, had residual disease after 45 Gy even with a 15 Gy boost (5).

E. Extended field radiation defines coverage of the para-aortic LN basins. The superior margin of this field is T12/L1 and the inferior margin is L4/5, laterally the spinous vertebral processes, and 2 cm anterior to the vertebrae. The dose is 45 Gy plus an extra 15 Gy boost for positive LN.

II. Uterine Cancer

A. Uterine cancer fields are: superiorly the L4/5 interface, inferiorly the mid or lower obturator foramen, laterally 2 to 2.5 cm lateral to the pelvic brim, anteriorly the pubic symphysis, and posteriorly S2/3 of the sacrum. External beam radiotherapy covers the upper one-half to two-thirds of the vagina, the parametria, and the pelvic LNs. Treatment is to 50.4 Gy, with a 15 Gy boost to involved parametria or positive LN.

B. To decrease vital organ complications, the patient can be treated in the prone position with a full bladder or use of a belly board.

C. Brachytherapy to the vaginal cuff alone can be given up to 50 Gy. If used in the adjuvant setting, HDR brachytherapy is usually dosed at 21 Gy: consisting of 7 Gy for 3 fractions or 5 Gy for 6 fractions to a vaginal depth of 0.5 cm.

III. Vulvar Cancer Vulvar cancer fields are: superiorly the L4–5 interface unless positive LN were documented above the inguinal ligament and if so the superior border is the L3/4 interface; inferiorly 2.5 cm below the ischial tuberosity or 2 cm below the most inferior portion of the primary vulvar tumor medially 3 cm from the body's midline and laterally extending in a line connecting the femoral head and the ASIS to include the inguinal nodes with an additional 2 cm lateral margin. The total dose is 45 to 57.6 Gy, with a 20 Gy boost to each groin. Gross tumor probably requires a dose of at least 70 Gy. Patients should be simulated supine in the frog-leg position with a full bladder.

IV. Vaginal Cancer: The fields are similar to that of cervical cancer: superiorly the L5–S1 interface; inferiorly to 2 cm below the lesion, and then 2 cm lateral to the pelvic brim. For lesions that include the lower one-third of the vagina the groins should be included and those fields, lateral margins extend in a line connecting the femoral heads and the ASIS to include the inguinal nodes.

V. **Ovarian Cancer:** The fields are that of site directed radiation or whole abdominal radiotherapy.

VI. **Whole Abdominal Radiotherapy (WAR):** WAR is not commonly given as adjuvant therapy. It can be given for salvage treatment. The total dose is 30 Gy in fraction sizes of 150 to 170 cGy/day. The field margins are 1 to 2 cm above the diaphragm superiorly (with heart shielding), 1 to 2 cm lateral to the peritoneal reflection, and inferiorly 2 cm below the inguinal ligament. Usually, whole pelvic radiation follows with a dose of 45 to 50 Gy. The kidneys should be blocked at 15 Gy and the liver blocked at 25 Gy.

RADIATION EFFECTS

I. The definition of an **early complication** is occurrence less than 3 months after completion of radiotherapy. A **late complication** is defined as onset after 3 months. Late effects are usually due to capillary damage (endarteritis obliterans).

II. **Skin toxicity** is usually delayed for 2 to 3 weeks. Most patients get moist desquamation about 2 weeks into treatment. There can also be erythema. Dry desquamation can occur after the 4th week. Toxicity is enhanced by actinomycin D and doxorubicin. Treatment is sitz baths, diarrhea control, and sulfa-based barrier creams. The epidermis returns in 14 days. Late effects can be depigmentation and telangiectasias.

III. **Vaginal toxicity** can be manifested with a yellow-white discharge due to mucositis. This can continue for 6 months. Treatment is with hydrogen peroxide douches, antibiotics, or hyperbaric therapy. Remember to rule out radiation necrosis and possible fistula— these complications may require a flap or even exenteration. The distal vagina is less tolerant with a maximum dose of 80 to 90 Gy vs. a maximum dose of 120 to 150 Gy for the proximal vagina. Narrowing and shortening of the vagina is a late effect and can occur in 80% of patients. Symptoms are pain. Diagnosis is with examination. Treatment is with frequent intercourse, vaginal dilators, and estrogen cream. Neovaginal reconstruction is complicated with high rates of failure and potential fistula.

IV. **Urinary tract toxicity** can present with frequency, urgency, and dysuria from decreased bladder capacity. Pyridium may help.

A. Spasms can be relieved by smooth muscle relaxants such as B&O suppositories or urospas. Always rule out infection. The UA can show radiation cystitis with WBC and RBC present but without bacteria. Focal ulcerations, hyperemia, and edema occur at greater than 30 Gy. Above 60 Gy hematuria occurs due to telangiectasias.

B. Hemorrhagic cystitis occurs in 1 to 5%. Treatment is with continuous irrigation with normal saline, cautery ablation via cystoscopy, methylene blue instillation, formalin instillation, Alum 2% instillation, hyperbaric oxygen, or Elmiron. Surgical diversion with a conduit is a last resort.

C. Ureteral stricture occurs at a rate of 2.5% at 20 years. A unilateral stricture is more common. Symptoms include pain, or an increasing BUN/creatinine. Diagnosis is via laboratories, IVP, or CT imaging. Treatment is with stenting, dilation, or surgical resection and reanastomosis.

V. Fistula formation can occur from the GI or urinary systems. Symptoms are spontaneous stool or urinary loss from an improper orifice. Diagnosis is with a full clinical examination, EUA with biopsies if necessary. A fistulogram, CT, MRI, or PET scan may be helpful.

A. Conservative management of bowel fistula is with: NPO status, TPN, somatostatin 50 to 200 mcg SC TID, H_2 blockers, Questran, and tincture of opium BID. Surgical intervention is with colostomy, repair, and excision of the fistulous tract. TPN and bowel rest is often tried but rarely efficacious.

B. Treatment of urinary fistula require diagnosis of the location of the fistula, diversion with a Foley catheter or nephrostomy tube, and resection of the fistula and tract. A neobladder can be constructed as last resort.

VI. Bowel toxicity is primarily diarrhea which is due to shortened villi and loss of their absorptive function. The dose tolerance of the small bowel is 45 Gy, the large bowel 70–75 Gy, and the anus 60–65 Gy.

A. Acute radiation enteritis is demonstrated by watery diarrhea which starts during the 2nd or 3rd week of treatment at about 20 Gy. There is increased flatulence and noisy bowel sounds. Treatment is with a low-residue diet, hydration, and antimotility agents. Somatostatin and bowel rest may be indicated. Chronic diarrhea is managed with dietary changes.

B. Small bowel injury can occur as stricture or stenosis. It can present as a partial SBO or a complete SBO. These occur in 5% of patients, with the terminal ileum and cecum being the most common site because they are anatomically fixed. Symptoms of a partial obstruction are delayed postprandial cramping, nausea, vomiting, and diarrhea. Diagnosis is with clinical examination, UGI, and SBFT. Treatment is with bowel resection and re-anastomosis.

C. Malabsorption can occur from excess bile salts reaching the colon. These are cathartics so treatment with cholestyramine may help.

D. Rectosigmoid toxicity can be symptomatic with a stricture causing a partial or complete large bowel obstruction. Diverting colostomy may be a treatment of last resort.

E. Rectal toxicity can present with tenesmus, mucus production, pain, worsening of hemorrhoids, and proctitis. It occurs in 2% to 3% of patients. Treatment is with antispasmodics or steroid suppositories or enemas. Telangiectasia's can cause bleeding and ulceration. Treatment of these is with cortisone rectal suppositories, sulfasalazine enemas, mesalamine (Rowasa) suppositories bid for 6 weeks, and hyperbaric oxygen.

F. Gastric outlet obstruction can occur from progressive fibrosis and can even lead to perforation.

VII. **Ovarian failure occurs** between 2.5 to 6 Gy for the germ cell components, presenting as permanent sterility. The stromal support cells fail at 24 Gy. Attempts to prevent ovarian failure are occasionally successful. Options include midline oophoropexy (surgical placement behind the uterus), surgical transposition to the upper pelvis (with a 40%–71% rate of success), cortical stripping and cryopreservation, oocyte retrieval with cryopreservation, or in vitro fertilization and embryo cryopreservation.

VIII. **Bone marrow toxicity** can present as:

A. Pancytopenia. This is because 40% of the marrow is in the pelvis. Symptoms can include fatigue (anemia), increased susceptability to infections (leukopenia), and bruising or bleeding (thrombocytopenia). Patients need weekly monitoring of the complete blood count (CBC).

B. Insufficiency fractures can also occur. The tolerance for the femoral head is 45 Gy. Fractures most commonly occur in the sacrum, ileum, pubic bones, and acetabulum. Asymptomatic fractures occur at a rate of 34% to 39% and symptomatic fractures at a rate of 13%. Symptoms are the sudden onset of pain which worsens with weight bearing. MRI is the best means for diagnosis. Treatment is surgical stabilization.

C. The femoral neck can develop avascular necrosis. Treatment for this is hip replacement.

IX. Liver toxicity can present as:

   A. Veno occlusive disease. This is due to platelet coagulation causing congestion and thrombocytopenia.

   B. Radiation hepatitis may occur and present with an elevated alkaline phosphatase 3 to 10× normal. Small portions of the liver can receive up to 70 Gy. The whole liver should not receive more than 30 Gy.

X. Renal toxicity usually manifests as a nephrotic syndrome. Toxicities present as HTN, leg edema, proteinuria, or a normocytic normochromic anemia. The kidney should not receive more than 18 to 20 Gy. To avoid toxicity, preferentially load 70/30 AP PA and block the kidneys completely after 18 to 20 Gy.

XI. Fetal toxicity: In utero exposure of the fetus invariably occurs during the diagnosis and treatment of gynecologic malignancies in pregnancy. If treatment occurs at 1 to 2 weeks of pregnancy, the effect is all or nothing with spontaneous abortion or continuation of pregnancy without effect. At 2 to 6 weeks, congenital anomalies and death can occur, with a 2 Gy dose yielding 70% mortality. At 6 to 16 weeks growth retardation and mental retardation occur with a risk of 40% per Gy. After 30 weeks, no gross malformations tend to occur. The risk of leukemia is increased if exposure is in the 3rd trimester. The risk is about 6% per Gy. A dose less than 1 mGy is negligible. For the entire gestational period, no more than 0.5 cGy exposure should occur.

Radiation Tolerance of Different Organs	
Organ	TD50 (Gy)
Bone marrow	5
Ovary	10
Kidney	25
Lung	30
Liver	50
Heart	60
Intestine	62
Spinal cord	60
Brain	65
Bladder	65

Cervical Cancer and Radiotherapy Delivery Time

The prolongation of overall treatment time and timing of brachytherapy can impact the outcome of radiation therapy.

The pelvic recurrence rate when treatment time is:

Stage	< 7 weeks	7–9 weeks	> 9 weeks	P values
IB	7%	22%	6%	$P < .01$
IIA	14%	27%	36%	$P = .08$
IIB	20%	28%	34%	$P = .09$
III	38%	44%	49%	$P = .18$
III when point A dose > 80 Gy	32%	40%	51%	$P = .08$

10-Year Cause-Specific Survival by Treatment Time

Stage	< 7 Weeks	7–9 Weeks	> 9 Weeks	P Value
IB	86%	78%	55%	$P = .01$
IIA	73%	41%	48%	$P = .01$
IIB	72%	60%	70%	$P = .01$
III	42%	42%	39%	$P = .43$
III (pt A dose > 80 Gy)	46%	44%	37%	$P = .016$

REFERENCES

1. Kelly MG et al. *Gynecol Oncol* 2005; 98(3):353–9.
2. Wolf JK et al. Radiation treatment of advanced or recurrent granulosa cell tumor of the ovary. *Gynecol Oncol* 1999; 73(1):35–41.
3. Greer BE, Koh WJ, Figge DC. Gynecologic radiotherapy fields defined by intraoperative measurements. *Gynecol Oncol*. 1990;38(3):421–424.
4. Greer BE. Expanded pelvic radiotherapy fields for treatment of local-regionally advanced carcinoma of the cervix: outcomes and treatment complications. *Am J Obstet Gynecol*. 1996; 174(4):1141–1149.
5. Houvenaeghel G, Lelievre L, Rigouard AL. Residual pelvic lymph node involvement after concomitant chemoradiation for locally advanced cervical cancer. *Gynecol Oncol*. 2006;102(3):523–529.

Sexual Function and Cancer

I. Sexual dysfunction is common in patients undergoing diagnosis of and treatment for gynecologic malignancies. This is due to pain, discomfort, bleeding, and/or psychological stress that may make intimacy difficult. Sexual disorders are typically not screened for effectively, thus masking the problem. Even for patients in whom sexual dysfunction is identified, there is little support to manage the problem.

II. Comprehensive screening questionnaires have been validated as effective screening tools for different sexual disorders (1). Sexual disorders can be classified as disorders of desire, arousal, orgasm, or sexual pain disorders.

   A. Chronic medical condition such as hypertension, diabetes, anxiety, and depression can have a negative impact on desire and should be addressed.

   B. Surgical disfigurement may also be a factor in desire. For women with ostomies the 4 Ps approach has been applied: prepare (adjust diet in preparation for intimacy to reduce gastrointestinal problems), pouch (pouch covers are available in multiple different fabrics, including lace or silk), position (avoid positions that cause pressure on ostomy to prevent compression or spillage), and pleasure (communicate with the partner that the goal is pleasurable intimacy) (2).

III. Treatment-induced menopause and altered gonadal function from radiation or chemotherapy are among the factors that may contribute to disorders of arousal and orgasm. In most hormonally sensitive cancers, systemic estrogen therapy has generally been contraindicated. However, for lower-risk patients, topical estrogens have been found to be effective and relatively safe for the treatment of vaginal symptoms after menopause. Other nonhormonal therapies include vaginal moisturizers and lubricants. With regard to arousal, the prescription device EROS-CVD is used to create gentle suction over the clitoris and has been proven beneficial in women with female arousal disorders, including those who have undergone treatment for cancer.

IV. Patients experiencing pain during intercourse from vaginal shortening either due to surgery or radiation may benefit from the use of vaginal dilators along with the use of lubricants and possibly estrogen products, in order to lengthen and widen the vagina. Other methods that minimize dysparenuia are positional changes.

REFERENCES

1. Quirk F, Haughie S, Symonds T. The use of the sexual function questionnaire as a screening tool for women with sexual dysfunction. *J Sex Med.* 2005;2(4):469-477.
2. Perez K, Gadgil M, Dizon DS. Sexual ramifications of medical illness. *Clin Obstet Gynecol.* 2009;52(4):691–701.

Fertility and Cancer Treatment

I. Chemotherapeutic Drugs and Risk of infertility

Definite	Chlorambucil Cyclophosphamide L-Phenylalanine mustard Nitrogen mustard Busulfan Procarbazine
Probable	Doxorubicin Vinblastine Cytosine arabinoside Cisplatin Nitrosoureas m-AMSA Etoposide
Unlikely	Methotrexate Fluorouracil Mercaptopurine Vincristine
Unknown	Bleomycin

II. Radiation and Fertility

A. The ovaries are the most radiosensitive organs, with only 5 Gy to 15 Gy of radiation causing sterility.

B. Age does play a role in the risk of infertility with radiation. The older a woman is when receiving radiation to the ovaries, the higher her risk of ovarian failure.

C. Operative procedures performed to protect the ovaries from radiation include midline oophoropexy (moving the ovaries behind the uterus) or transposition above the pelvic brim.

D. Other efforts utilized to protect the ovaries from radiation damage are pelvic shielding.

E. Cortical stripping with cryopreservation, oocyte retrieval with cryopreservation, in vitro fertilization with embryo cryopreservation, or oophorectomy with cryopreservation and subsequent reimplantation of ovarian tissue are all other strategies used for fertility preservation.

Cancer in Pregnancy

I. Cancer occurs in 1 mother per every 1,000 live births, with approximately 4,000 cases of concurrent pregnancy and maternal malignancy each year. The most common cancer in pregnancy is breast cancer. The most common cancer of the female reproductive system in pregnancy is cervical cancer.

    A. If cancer is diagnosed prior to 24 weeks gestation the patient can decide to terminate the pregnancy.

    B. If a malignancy is diagnosed after fetal viability, treatment can be delayed until the late second trimester, third trimester, or after delivery, depending on the specific clinical situation.

II. **Radiation in Pregnancy**. Radiation has different effects on a fetus depending on the stage of fetal development at the time of radiation exposure.

    A. At preimplantation, the effects are "all or nothing" meaning that radiation will either kill the embryo or not affect it at all, although there are recent reports of increased rates of fetal malformations with radiation prior to implantation.

    B. Organogenesis occurs 8 weeks after fertilization. The main fetal effect of radiation during organogenesis is intrauterine growth restriction but a wide array of congenital structural deformities can occur. With doses of greater than 1 Gy, morphologic anomalies, and mental retardation, may develop.

    C. The main effect of radiation in the fetal stage, is resultant cognitive impairment. The CNS is the most sensitive until about 25 weeks. Intrauterine growth restriction can also occur with doses greater than 0.5 Gy.

D. The recommended maximum dose of radiation during pregnancy is 0.5 Gy.

Type of Examination	Fetal Dose Range in cGy
CXR	0.00006
KUB	0.15–0.26
Lumbar spine	0.65
Pelvis	0.2–0.35
Hip	0.13–0.2
IVP	0.47–0.82
Upper GI series	0.17–0.48
Barium enema	0.18–1.14
Mammography	0.00001
CT head	0.007
CT upper abdomen	0.04
CT pelvis	2.5
99Tc bone scan	0.15

E. There are three principal sources of radiation exposure to the fetus during maternal radiation: photon leakage through the treatment head of the machine, scatter radiation emanating from the imaging equipment, and internal scatter within the mother from the treatment beams. Fetal radiation exposure can be reduced by external shielding, but internal scatter cannot be modified.

III. Chemotherapy in Pregnancy

A. The background rate of fetal anomalies for all pregnancies is 2% to 3%. The risk of anomalies with chemotherapy in the first trimester is 6% using a single-agent drug regimen and 17% with combination therapy. If folate antagonists are excluded, the risk is reduced to 6%.

B. Chemotherapeutic agents commonly used during pregnancy are vinca alkaloids, doxorubicin and cisplatin. Alkylators such as cisplatin and doxorubicin can carry a 14% risk of fetal anomalies in the first trimester and 4% in the second trimester. Vinca alkaloids are particularly useful during the first trimester and do not cross the placenta. Doxorubicin can be used in the first trimester of pregnancy. The multidrug resistance (MDR1) P-glycoprotein is found in higher amounts of the endometrium and placenta. MDR1 may provide protection for the fetus. Cisplatin can cause a 50% risk of intrauterine growth restriction, bilateral neonatal hearing loss, or leucopenia. Antimetabolites can cause cranial nasal dystocia, auditory malformations, micrognathia, and limb deformities.

C. Chemotherapy administration should be avoided within 3 weeks of the expected date of delivery because of: maternal myelosuppression; nadirs of blood components; increased risk of infection; and decreased wound healing for procedures such as episiotomy and cesarean section. Breastfeeding is contraindicated for women who are on active chemotherapy regimens to avoid transmission to the baby through breast milk.

IV. Cervical Cancer in Pregnancy

A. Cervical cancer occurs in approximately 1.2 to 10.6 cases per 10,000 deliveries. Pregnant patients are 3.1 times more likely to be diagnosed with Stage I disease vs. nonpregnant patients. There is no difference in survival in pregnant vs. nonpregnant patients. Treatment of preinvasive lesions can be delayed until after delivery as the progression of dysplasia to a higher grade postpartum is 7%.

B. Cervical cancer in pregnancy is diagnosed via cervical biopsy of gross lesions or colposcopic directed biopsy of lesions concerning for invasion. Endocervical curettage is not performed during pregnancy.

C. Conization is indicated if: there is persistent severe cervical dysplasia suggestive of an invasive lesion; minimal stromal invasion found on cervical biopsy; or if invasive disease cannot be ruled out by colposcopy and biopsy alone. In the first trimester, 24% of patients undergoing cervical conization experienced fetal loss (3). In the third trimester, conization was complicated by high blood loss but no loss of pregnancy, a 10% pregnancy loss in the second trimester, and 0% pregnancy loss in the first trimester (4). Another report (5) detailed a 9% risk of hemorrhage and a 4% risk of delayed bleeding. There may be an increased rate of preterm deliveries. Cold knife cervical conization (CKC) is possibly better than LEEP in pregnancy because it is easier to control the size of the specimen with a CKC. Furthermore, a loop is difficult to pass through the more edematous cervix that occurs with pregnancy. A coin-shaped biopsy is preferred in pregnant patients rather than a cone-shaped biopsy. The timing of the biopsy should be between 14 and 20 weeks gestation. Placement of a McDonald cerclage at the time of a cervical excision procedure may be considered.

D. Progression of cancer during pregnancy is probably rare. Treatment delay can be considered for early-stage cancers diagnosed after 20 weeks. Longer delay to let an earlier pregnancy proceed to term is controversial. Spontaneous abortion occurs at doses of 40 Gy. 27% of patients do not pass the conceptus spontaneously and require evacuation. In patients with advanced stage cancers, near term, a short delay is permissible, followed by radiotherapy within 2 to 3 weeks of delivery. The mode of delivery of pregnant patients with cervical cancer is controversial. Vaginal delivery may be possible with small volume tumors. Cesarean delivery can decrease the risk of hemorrhage and obstructed labor, especially in cases where there is a large friable tumor. However, incisional recurrence has been reported. There have been 10 cases of episiotomy site recurrence in women who have had vaginal deliveries. 14% of patients who had a cesarean section had local metastasis following delivery compared to 59% of patients who delivered vaginally. Some studies showed decreased survival with vaginal delivery (75%, vs. 55% for cesarean delivery) (6).

E. If a cesarean section is performed, a classical cesarean hysterotomy should be made. This can be followed by radical hysterectomy and/or ovarian transposition. A cesarean that is planned and timed is better than an unplanned delivery because of the possibility of hemorrhage and need for emergent hysterectomy, likely eliminating the opportunity for staging.

V. Ovarian Neoplasms in Pregnancy. Ovarian neoplasms are detected in approximately 2% of all pregnancies and 1 in 8000 to 20,000 deliveries. Most ovarian neoplasms found in pregnancy are simple ovarian cysts with approximately 70% resolving by the second trimester. Surgical evaluation is indicated in the second trimester if the mass persists and is greater than 6 to 8 cm, rapidly increasing in size, or complex. Torsion can occur in 5% to 15% of pregnant patients and can often occur during the time when the uterus is rapidly growing during the first 16 weeks of pregnancy or during the time of uterine involution postpartum. 17% of these masses can cause obstruction of labor, necessitating cesarean delivery. Surgical treatment, if indicated, is usually unilateral cystectomy. If malignant, at minimum, unilateral oophorectomy with staging procedures and cytoreduction is indicated.

A. Malignancy is found in 2% to 6% of adnexal masses. Most ovarian cancers in pregnancy are found at Stage I, likely due to incidental early detection during fetal ultrasound.

B. A tumor marker that remains unchanged during pregnancy is LDH. CA-125 has limited usefulness in pregnancy because it is non specific and levels can fluctuate throughout pregnancy.

C. Teratomas are the most common histologic type of ovarian neoplasm found during pregnancy. The second most common ovarian neoplasm in pregnancy is serous cystadenoma. Most ovarian tumors are benign.

D. Germ cell tumors are the most common ovarian neoplasms found during pregnancy and mature teratomas are the most common histologic type. The most common malignant germ cell tumor is a dysgerminoma. Dysgerminomas comprise about 30% of all ovarian malignancies found during pregnancy. They have a significant rate of bilaterality (10%–15%). Because these neoplasms can rapidly increase in size, they have a tendency to cause pain, become incarcerated in the pouch of Douglas, and can acutely torse. In a study of pregnant patients with dysgerminoma, obstructed labor occurred in 33% of patients and fetal death occurred in 24% (7). Treatment of dysgerminomas is primarily surgical. At minimum, a unilateral salpingo oophorectomy is performed along with ipsilateral pelvic and para-aortic lymph node dissection and staging biopsies. The rate of recurrence is approximately 10% for disease confined to one ovary. Other germ cell tumors that can occur during pregnancy are immature teratomas and endodermal sinus tumors. Treatment is primarily surgical and fertility preserving surgery is usually feasible.

In patients with advanced dysgerminoma, adjuvant chemotherapy is indicated. All patients with nondysgerminoma tumors except for stage 1A grade 1 immature teratoma should receive adjuvant chemotherapy. Regimens include bleomycin, etoposide, cisplatin and vinblastine, cisplatin, bleomycin, which have had favorable outcomes during pregnancy for the mother and infant.

E. Sex cord stromal tumors such as granulosa cell tumors and Sertoli-Leydig tumors are uncommon during pregnancy, but when they do occur, they are associated with rupture, hemoperitoneum, and labor dystocia. Treatment is surgical, with staging and fertility preserving surgery.

F. Epithelial ovarian cancers diagnosed during pregnancy have the same prognosis as in nonpregnant patients. Surgical staging should be performed. The administration of chemotherapy during the second and third trimesters is feasible if indicated for advanced disease. Ovarian tumors of low malignant potential are usually found at Stage I and clinical outcomes are favorable.

VI. Other Gynecologic Cancers in Pregnancy. Other gynecologic malignancies quite rare during pregnancy.

A. Vaginal cancer, if diagnosed during pregnancy, may be of clear cell histology, especially if the patient had a history of diethylstilbestrol (DES) exposure. Symptoms/signs include a vaginal mass and abnormal vaginal discharge or bleeding. Treatment is with chemotherapy and radiotherapy starting postpartum for most stages.

B. Vulvar cancer may present with symptoms of vulvar irritation and puritis, or with a visible mass. Surgical treatment should be delayed until the second trimester, with the groin node dissection occurring after delivery in order to minimize the surgical morbidity during pregnancy. Vaginal delivery is feasible after surgical excision as long as the vulvar wound is healed and there is no potential for dystocia from introital scarring.

C. Endometrial cancer associated with pregnancy is usually diagnosed postpartum. The prognosis is usually favorable as most tumors are focal and well differentiated.

REFERENCES

1. Averette HE, Nasser N, Yankow SL. Cervical conization in pregnancy. Analysis of 180 operations. *Am J Obstet Gynecol.* 1970;106(4): 543–549.
2. Hannigan EV. Cervical cancer in pregnancy. *Clin Obstet Gynecol.* 1990;33(4):837–845.

3. Robinson WR, Webb S, Tirpack J. Management of cervical intraepithelial neoplasia during pregnancy with LOOP excision. *Gynecol Oncol.* 1997;64(1):153–155.

4. Jones WB, Shingleton HM, Russell A. Cervical carcinoma and pregnancy. A national patterns of care study of the American College of Surgeons. *Cancer.* 1996;77(8):1479–1488.

5. Karlen JR, Akbari A, Cook WA. Dysgerminoma associated with pregnancy. *Obstet Gynecol.* 1979;53(3):330–335.

Surveillance Recommendations

Endometrial Cancer Surveillance Recommendations

Variable		Months			Years	
		0–12	12–24	24–36	3–5	> 5
Review of symptoms and physical examination						
	Low risk (Stage IA Grade 1 or 2)	Every 6 mo	Yearly	Yearly	Yearly	Yearly
	Intermediate risk (Stage IB–II)	Every 3 mo	Every 6 mo	Every 6 mo	Every 6 mo	Yearly
	High risk (Stage III/IV, serous or clear cell)	Every 3 mo	Every 3 mo	Every 6 mo	Every 6 mo	Yearly
Papanicolaou test/cytologic evidence		Not indicated	Not indicated	Not indicated	Not indicated	Not indicated
CA-125		Insufficient data to support routine use	Insufficient data to support routine use	Insufficient data to support routine use	Insufficient data to support routine use	Insufficient data to support routine use
Radiographic imaging (CXR, PET/CT, MRI)		Insufficient data to support routine use	Insufficient data to support routine use	Insufficient data to support routine use	Insufficient data to support routine use	Insufficient data to support routine use
Recurrence suspected		CT and/or PET scan; CA-125	CT and/or PET scan; CA-125	CT and/or PET scan; CA-125	CT and/or PET scan; CA-125	CT and/or PET scan; CA-125

298

Epithelial Ovarian Cancer Surveillance Recommendations

Variable	Months				Years	
	0–12	12–24	24–36	3–5	> 5
Review of symptoms and physical examination	Every 3 mo	Every 3 mo	Every 4-6 mo	Every 6 mo	Yearly
Papanicolaou test/cytologic evidence	Not indicated	Not indicated	Not indicated	Not indicated	Not indicated
CA-125	Optional	Optional	Optional	Optional	Optional
Radiographic imaging (CXR, PET/CT, MRI)	Insufficient data to support routine use	Insufficient data to support routine use	Insufficient data to support routine use	Insufficient data to support routine use	Insufficient data to support routine use
Recurrence suspected	CT and/or PET scan; CA-125	CT and/or PET scan; CA-125	CT and/or PET scan; CA-125	CT and/or PET scan; CA-125	CT and/or PET scan; CA-125

Nonepithelial Ovarian Cancer (Germ Cell and Sex-Cord Stromal Tumors) Surveillance Recommendations

Variable		Months			Years	
		0–12	12–24	24–36	3–5	> 5
Review of symptoms and physical examination						
	Germ cell tumors	Every 2–4 mo	Every 2–4 mo	Yearly	Yearly	Yearly
	Sex-cord stromal tumors	Every 2–4 mo	Every 2–4 mo	Every 6 mo	Every 6 mo	Every 6 mo
Serum tumor markers						
	Germ cell tumors	Every 2–4 mo	Every 2–4 mo	Not indicated	Not indicated	Not indicated
	Sex-cord stromal tumors	Every 2–4 mo	Every 2–4 mo	Every 6 mo	Every 6 mo	Every 6 mo
Radiographic imaging (CXR, CT, MRI)						
	Germ cell tumors	Not indicated unless tumor marker normal at initial presentation	Not indicated unless tumor marker normal at initial presentation	Not indicated	Not indicated	Not indicated
	Sex-cord stromal tumors	Insufficient data to support routine use	Insufficient data to support routine use	Insufficient data to support routine use	Insufficient data to support routine use	Insufficient data to support routine use
Recurrence suspected		CT scan, tumor markers	CT scan, tumor markers	CT scan, tumor markers	CT scan, tumor markers	CT scan, tumor markers

Cervical, Vulvar, and Vaginal Cancer Surveillance Recommendations

Variable		Months				Years	
		0-12	12-24	24-36	3-5	> 5
Review of symptoms and physical examination						
	Low risk (early stage, treated with surgery alone, no adjuvant therapy)	Every 6 mo	Every 6 mo	Yearly	Yearly	Yearly
	High risk (advanced stage, treated with primary chemotherapy/ radiation therapy or surgery plus adjuvant therapy)	Every 3 mo	Every 3 mo	Every 6 mo	Every 6 mo	Yearly
Papanicolaou test/ cytologic evidence		Yearly	Yearly	Yearly	Yearly	Yearly
Recurrence suspected		CT and/ or PET scan	CT and/ or PET scan	CT and/ or PET scan	CT and/ or PET scan	CT and/ or PET scan

Surveillance Visit Checklist

Checklist for Surveillance of Gynecologic Malignancies

Patient name _____

Visit date _____

Disease site and stage _____

Date of diagnosis/surgery _____

Date treatment completed _____

Symptoms review and treatment side-effects

- Pain (abdominal or pelvic, hip or back)
- Abdominal bloating
- Vaginal bleeding (also rectum, bladder)
- Weight loss
- Nausea and/or vomiting
- Cough or shortness of breath
- Lethargy/fatigue
- Swelling of abdomen or leg(s)
- Sexual dysfunction
- Neuropathy
- Fatigue

Physical examination

- General physical examination
- Lymph node assessment (axillary, supraclavicular, and inguinal)
- Pelvic examination (vulvar, vaginal speculum, bimanual, and rectovaginal exam)

Tumor markers _____

Disease status

- No evidence of disease
- Suspect recurrence
  - Radiographic imaging _____
- Biopsy _____
- Refer to gynecologic oncologist

Routine health maintenance

Breast cancer screening

- Yearly clinical breast examination _____
- Mammogram _____
  Every 1 to 2 years starting with ages 40 to 49 years, then yearly

Colon cancer screening

- Colonoscopy or flexible sigmoidoscopy _____
  Every 5 to 10 years beginning at age 50 years

Genetic screening

- Not indicated
- Recommended/completed _____

Menopausal assessment

Osteoporosis prevention

Calcium (1,200 mg–1,500 mg) and vitamin D (800 IU)

Bone mineral density testing: begin at age 65 years or sooner if on glucocorticoid therapy

Smoking cessation

Weight maintenance (exercise, diet)

REFERENCE

1. Salani R, Backes FJ, Fung MF. Posttreatment surveillance and diagnosis of recurrence in women with gynecologic malignancies: Society of Gynecologic Oncologists recommendations. *Am J Obstet Gynecol.* 2011;204(6):466–478.

Palliative Care

I. **Palliative care** is an area of health care that specifically focuses on relieving and preventing the suffering of patients.

   A. The ultimate goal is to provide the best possible quality of life for people facing the pain, symptoms, and stresses of serious illness. It is appropriate throughout all stages of an illness. It can be provided along with treatments that are meant to cure.

   B. Palliative therapies not only improve a patient's quality of life, but also have been shown to extend life. In a study of patients with metastatic non-small cell lung cancer, patients were randomized to receive either early palliative care integrated with standard oncologic care or standard oncologic care alone. Despite the fact that fewer patients in the early palliative care group than in the standard care group received aggressive end-of-life care (33% vs. 54%, $P = .05$), median survival was longer among patients receiving early palliative care (11.6 months vs. 8.9 months, $P = .02$) (1).

   C. Palliative surgical or medical intervention can relieve symptoms and lead to less pain for the patient. In these instances, correction of the terminal disease is not anticipated or achieved. Approximately 10% of procedures are performed for palliative intent, not cure.

II. **Hospice** care is palliative care that typically occurs when a patient is considered to be terminal, or within 6 months of death.

III. It can be quite difficult discussing the implications of a life-threatening illness with a patient and the family. There are a few things to keep in mind when discussing terminal disease and end-of-life care:

   A. Hope is important.

B. Emotions run high: Negative emotions such as fear, anxiety, frustration, and depression are common and are manifested in a variety of ways by patients and their caregivers.

C. Respect is important. Health care providers should listen to and honor the perspectives and choices of patients and their families.

IV. A multidisciplinary approach is important.

A. Effective palliative care involves a team approach. This involves the patient and her physician and may also include: palliative care physicians; specialists, general practitioners; nurses; nursing assistants or home health aides; social workers; chaplains; and physical, occupational, and speech therapists.

V. Communication is the most important factor in terminal care.

A. Timing of discussion: soon after the diagnosis of advanced or recurrent cancer. Options for palliative care should be discussed.

B. Ensure that legal documents are drawn up: these include a living will, power of attorney, advanced directive.

C. Specific issues to address with the patient: the need for ventilatory support; TPN; the need for emergent surgery; interventional procedures for relief of acute symptoms; invasive procedure endpoints and indications; DNR consent; timing for discontinuation of supportive measures; location for death (hospital vs. home).

ACTIVE DYING (I.E., TRANSITIONING)

I. Patients will have: increased somnolence; increased oral secretions from the inability to swallow; a decreased appetite; potential delusions and/or hallucinations; body temperature fluctuation; decreased urinary output, apnea, agonal breathing, and skin mottling.

ETHICAL ISSUES

I. When the wishes of a patient contradict the physician's management desires and compromise cannot be attained, transfer of care to another physician may be appropriate.

II. The involvement of a hospital ethical committee may be appropriate at times.

III. Ethical guidelines:

    A. Nonmaleficence

    B. Beneficence

    C. Autonomy

    D. Justice

IV. Medical futility: After having an open discussion with the patient about their terminal disease and realistic expectations, the physician needs to determine when it is advisable to move from an aggressive therapeutic approach to supportive care. The pathway for withdrawal of care, once a decision has been made, is as follows:

    A. Obtain informed consent

    B. Plan for the procedure and potential side effects

    C. Address the patient's distress

    D. Move the patient to an appropriate setting

    E. Use adequate sedation

    F. Document the procedure

    G. Review the outcomes

REFERENCE

1. Temel JS, Greer JA, Muzikansky A. Early palliative care for patients with metastatic non-small cell lung cancer. *N Engl J Med.* 2010;363(8): 733–742.

Statistics

I. Definitions

A. General definitions:

Variable—anything manipulated in an experiment

Independent variable—one varied by and under the control of the experimenter

Dependent variable—one that responds to manipulation

Nominal variable—a named category, e.g., sex, diagnosis

Ordinal variable—a set of ordered categories, e.g., stage of cancer, are ordered but the the significance between each step is not known

Interval variable—measurement in which the step between is meaningful (temperature, age)

Ratio—ratio of the numbers has some meaning

Parametric—data that follow a normal distribution

Nonparametric—data do not follow a normal distribution (nominal and ordinal)

Incidence—current number of new events/population at risk in same time interval

Prevalence—total number of events/population at risk. Prevalence should be more than the incidence

B. Measures of central tendency:

Mode—value most often reported

Median—value with half the responses below and half above (nonparametric)

Mean—average of all values

C. Measures of dispersion

Standard deviation (SD) of the mean is the square root of the variance. The smaller the SD, the less each score varies from the mean: 1 SD = 68%, 2 SD = 95.5%, 3 SD = 99%

Variance—(value of point − mean)^2/total number of data points

Range—is the difference between the highest value and the lowest value.

Percentile—where the result lands out of 100.

II. There are 2 methods to analyze data. Descriptive statistics communicate results, but does not generalize beyond the sample. Inferential statistics communicate the likelihood of these differences occurring by a chance combination of unforeseen variables.

A. Null hypothesis: By statistical convention it is assumed that the speculated hypothesis is always wrong, and that the observed phenomena simply occur by chance. It is this hypothesis that is to be either nullified or not nullified by the test. When the null hypothesis is nullified, it is possible to conclude that data support the alternative hypothesis.

B. The extent to which the test in question shows that the **"speculated hypothesis"** has or has not been nullified is called its significance level; the higher the significance level, the less likely it is that the phenomena in question could have been produced by chance alone.

C. Statistics for Inference (hypothesis) testing:

1. **Confidence intervals (CI)**—used to indicate the reliability of an estimate. The CI is calculated by 1-alpha.

2. **Standard error (SE)**—this is used to help determine if the result is true or occurs more by chance. SE = SD/square root of sample size. The SE can either be: systemic, where the wrong measure is taken each time or random, where the answer is different each time the experiment is run.

3. The margin of error—the amount the results are expected to change from one experiment to another.

4. **Central limit theory (CLT)**—if the sample size is sufficiently large (n > 10), the mean will normally distribute regardless of the original distribution. This theory allows the parametric assessment of nonparametric data.

5. **Z-test**—compares the sample mean with the known population mean.

D. Sensitivity: Sensitivity relates to the test's ability to identify positive results. The sensitivity of a test is the proportion of people who have the disease who test positive for it. For example, a sensitivity of 100% means that the test recognizes all actual positives—i.e., all sick people are recognized as being ill. Thus, in contrast to a high specificity test, a negative result in a high sensitivity test is used to rule out the disease.

This can be written as:

Sensitivity = Number of true positives/Number of true positives + Number of false negatives

True positives/All positive with disease

If a test has high sensitivity then a negative result would suggest the absence of disease.

E. Specificity: Specificity relates to the ability of the test to identify negative results. The specificity of a test is defined as the proportion of patients who do not have the disease who will test negative for it. This can also be written as:

Specificity = Number of true negatives/Number of true negatives + Number of false positives

True negatives/All negative with disease.

The specificity states the ability of a test to determine if the patient tests negative that the patient does not have the disease.

F. Positive Predictive Value: This test reflects the probability that a positive test reflects the underlying condition being tested for.

G. Negative Predictive Value (NPV): This test reflects the proportion of subjects with a negative test result who are correctly diagnosed. A high NPV means that when the test yields a negative result, it is most likely correct in its assessment.

	Disease Positive	**Disease Negative**
Positive exp/screen	A	B
Negative exp/screen	C	D

Sensitivity—True positives/All with disease	A/(A+C)
Specificity—True negatives/All without disease	D/(B+D)
Positive predictive value	A/(A+B)
Negative predictive value	D/(C+D)

H. **Type I error:** This occurs when one rejects the null hypothesis (H0) when it is true. A type I error may be compared to a false positive. The rate of the type I error is called the size of the test and denoted by the Greek letter α (alpha). It usually equals the significance level of a test. In the case of a simple null hypothesis, α is the probability of a type I error. If the null hypothesis is composite, α is the maximum of the possible probabilities of a type I error. The rate of a type I error is related to the confidence interval ($1 - \alpha = CI$).

I. **Type II error:** This occurs when one fails to reject a false null hypothesis. A type II error may be compared to a false negative. The rate of the type II error is denoted by the Greek letter β (beta) and is related to the power of a test ($1 - \beta$ = power).

Tabularized Relations Between Truth/Falseness of the Null Hypothesis and Outcomes of the Test:

	Null Hypothesis (H_0) Is True	Null Hypothesis (H_0) Is False
Reject null hypothesis	Type I error false positive (FP)	Correct outcome True positive (TP)
Fail to reject null hypothesis	Correct outcome True negative (TN)	Type II error false negative (FN)

False positive rate (α) = Type I error = 1 − Specificity = FP/(FP + TN)

False negative rate (β) = Type II error = 1 − Sensitivity = FN/(TP + FN)

Power = Chance of detecting a difference that is really there = $1 - \beta$

Confidence interval = The chance that a true value lies within the specified interval (1-alpha)

Confidence level = The chance that, with repeated sampling, the range of values actually contains the actual parameter

Likelihood ratio positive = Sensitivity/(1 − Specificity)

Likelihood ratio negative = (1 − Sensitivity)/Specificity

J. **Alpha** is the cutoff for the *P* value.

K. ***P* value:** a measure of the strength of the evidence against the null hypothesis.

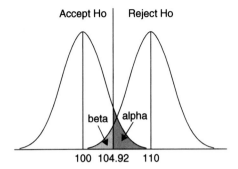

Accept Ho | Reject Ho

beta | alpha

100 104.92 110

L. One- and two-tailed tests: If the distribution from which the samples are derived is considered to be normal, Gaussian, or bell shaped, then the test is referred to as a one- or two-tailed T test.

1. **A one-tailed test** evaluates samples that fall within the curve and are excluded if they fall into one of the tails of the curve. For a standard deviation of 95%, the full 5% falls into the single tail of the curve.

2. **A two-tailed test** evaluates samples that fall within the curve and are only excluded if they fall into either one of the tails of the curve. For a standard deviation of 95%, 2.5% falls into each tail. It is recommended that most statistical analysis should be two-tailed.

3. A test is called two-tailed if the null hypothesis is rejected for values of the test statistic that fall into either tail of its sampling distribution, and it is called one-sided if the null hypothesis is rejected only for values of the test statistic falling into one specified tail of its sampling distribution.

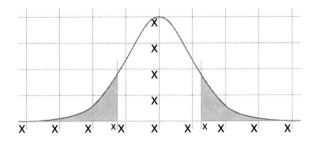

    4. If the test is performed using the actual population mean and variance, rather than an estimate from a sample, it would be called a one- or two-tailed **Z test**.

  M. **Power** is affected by: the significance criterion, the magnitude of effect, and the sample size. The beta level is usually set at 0.2. Thus, the power by convention is usually 0.8. There are two ways to perform a power analysis: a priori and post hoc. A priori (before) is the means to estimate for a sufficient sample size. Post hoc analysis is usually not recommended.

    1. To decrease the amount of type I error, the alpha level can be reduced (e.g., from 0.05 to 0.01).

    2. To decrease the amount of type II error, the sample size can be increased, the effect size can be changed, or the significance criterion can be changed.

  N. **Attributable risk**—risk of disease or death in a population exposed to some factor of interest minus the risk of those not exposed.

III. **The Receiver Operating Characteristic (ROC)**: is the graphical plot of the sensitivity (on the *x*-axis), or the true positive rate, versus 1 − specificity (on the *y*-axis), or the false positive, for a binary classifier system as its discrimination threshold is varied. The ROC can also be represented equivalently by plotting the fraction of true positives out of all positives (TPR = true positive rate) versus the fraction of false positives out of the negatives (FPR = false positive rate). It reflects the accuracy of the test. The area under the ROC curve is closely related to the Mann-Whitney U test, which tests whether the positives are ranked higher than the negatives. For an optimal test, all points should fall into the upper left quadrant.

IV. **Endpoints of a study** are important for evaluation of: PFS, OS, and clinical response. It is necessary to choose good primary endpoints to reflect the effectiveness of the experimental therapy. Surrogate endpoints are often chosen instead because of proposed study length, study cost, and known etiologic associations with the primary endpoint.

V. There are **4 phases of trials.**

    1. A **phase I trial** is a dose limiting trial. Doses of drugs are tested until a maximum tolerated dose. When 50% to 75% of patients have an adverse event (dose limiting toxicity, DLT), the dose one level prior to the DLT dose is chosen as the maximum tolerated dose (MTD). The MTD is chosen as the dose to proceed with to the next phase trial.

2. **A phase II trial** assesses the activity and toxicities of the drug chosen at the MTD in relation to the disease of interest.

3. **A phase III trial** assesses efficacy. There are two types of phase III trials; the noninferiority trial and the equivalency trial.

   a. The noninferiority trial evaluates two drugs to ensure their outcomes are similar (cisplatin vs. carboplatin with taxol in ovarian cancer).

   b. The equivalency trial evaluates an augmentation in care (adding platinum to radiation for cervical cancer vs. radiation alone).

   c. The randomized controlled trial is the most expensive type of study. It takes a large amount of time to complete, needs a large number of subjects (150 in each arm to reduce the type II error), is prospective, provides the best level of evidence, and is the only type of trial to prove causality. Two factors can be chosen for study design: either hypothesis based (efficacy/noninferiority/equal) or outcome of interest based (efficacy or application in everyday practice).

4. **A phase IV trial** is the postmarketing surveillance trial that ensures the drug is working appropriately with stated benefits.

VI. There are a number of **randomization techniques** that can be applied: simple/coin toss; sequential digits; permuted blocks; stratified blocks; dynamic randomization; systemic n-th; cluster; census; matching; restriction; quota; volunteer; cross over; split body; factorial.

VII. **Eligibility criteria** are the criteria to determine which patients to enroll in a study. These criteria serve 4 functions: scientific benefit; safety; logistic considerations; and regulatory considerations.

VIII. **To avoid bias or confounding**, patients and/or investigators can be: blinded; masked; adjusted for specific factors; randomized; the sample size can be increased; a placebo can be used; factors can be restricted, or matched.

IX. Trial Safety, Review, and Ethics

A. The **Data Safety Monitoring Board (DSMB)** is present for: quality control; administrative capacities; and endpoint monitoring. The knowledge of any benefit or harm tends to accumulate over time and the DSMB can monitor the safety and efficacy of the trial impartially. It can also perform an interim analysis for safety and outcomes.

B. The **Institutional Review Board (IRB)** was mandated in 1974 to be established locally for all government funded research.

C. Human subject rights have been established in two main doctrines. The **Belmont Report** (1979) outlines respect for persons; justice; and beneficence. The **Nuremberg Code** (1949) outlines human subject rights to include participation in the study be voluntary; the study be worthwhile; the study be unavailable by other means; the current state of knowledge is obtained from animals and cannot be obtained further from animal studies; there will be avoidance of unnecessary suffering; no deaths are to be expected; the risk is consistent with study benefits; appropriate precautions are taken for the study; the study is planned and reported by qualified persons; consent is ongoing; assessment of risks and benefits are ongoing; and the study is to be terminated if the risk of injury is imminent.

X.

Trials can be broken up into **prospective and retrospective** types. The prospective trials include the randomized controlled trials and the cohort trials. The retrospective trials include the case control and cross sectional trials. Another way to look at trials are the randomized trials versus the observational trials. The observational trials are the cohort trials, the case control trials, the ecologic trials, case series, and the case report.

XI. Trial Evaluation

A. **Validity** is described in two fashions. External validity means the study results apply to the entire population. Internal validity means the study results apply specifically to those individuals studied.

B. Symmetry means that all things between groups are similar.

C. Confounding is the distortion of the effect of one risk factor by the presence of another

D. **Bias is any process or effect that produces results that differ systematically from the truth.**

1. Nondifferential bias means that the biases are the same in all study groups.

2. Differential bais means that the biases are different between groups.

3. There are a number of types of bias. Confounding bias is the systematic error where there is failure to account for the effect of one variable on others. Ecological bias is the systematic error where the group average is applied to individuals. Measurement bias is when the measurement methods consistently differ between groups. Screening bias is when the disease is picked up earlier in the latent period by screening, but this screening does not affect the course of the disease. Reader bias is error of interpretation by reader inference. Sampling bias occurs when study design or execution produces errors in sampling. Zero time bias is when unintended differences exist from the beginning of the study, at enrollment.

XII. **Survival Analysis**: There are two main types of survival analysis.

A. The **time series analysis** is the parametric analysis.

B. The **Kaplan-Meier** (KM) analysis is nonparametric and allows right censoring. KM analysis is used because all patients cannot start the study at the same time, there is withdrawal or loss to follow-up, patients die, and the study must end.

C. The **Log Rank test** compares the survival curves of 2 or more groups. It is a nonparametric test.

D. The **Cox Regression** proportional hazards test allows analysis of several risk factors affecting survival. It is a nonparametric test as well.

E. The **Wilcoxon rank sum test** can be used when no censoring occurs.

XIII. **Causality**: There are a number of criteria for judging causality. There must be validity of the study; strength in the study; plausibility (there is current biological support); consistency (the study can be replicated); a temporal relationship; a dose response; and alternative explanations have been ruled out.

XIV. **WHO screening guidelines** are in place to provide support for optimization of screening tests. These include: the disease history is understood; the disease is an important health problem; there is a latent stage to the disease; there is a test for the disease; there are facilities available for diagnosis and treatment; the cost to diagnosis is low and acceptable to the patient; and the screening is a continuous process.

XV. **Parametric Versus Nonparametric Testing**

A. **Parametric** test means that there was random sampling, there is a normal distribution, the two populations are independent, there are quantitative variables (interval or ratio), and the variances of the normal distributions are equal. Parametric tests include: the Z test (which tests the means of the populations), the one sided t-test, the t-test, the paired t-test, and the unpaired t-test. Also included are the ANOVA (which measures differences between 2 or more groups), the ANCOVA (which measures the difference between 2 or more groups and combines regression), the FANCOVA (which is the factorial ANOVA and allows comparison between 2 or more groups with each variable having at least 2 levels).

B. **Nonparametric** tests are qualitative and measure associations. These tests include the binomial test, the sign test, the Wilcoxon test, the Mann-Whitney U test, the Fishers test, the Chi-square test, the Kruskal-Wallis test, and the Friedman test.

XVI. **To quantify associations**, three types of tests are commonly used. The Pearson's test is for parametric data. The Spearman's rank correlation is for nonparametric data. Kendall's correlation is often used to document concordance.

XVII. **Means of Magnitude** tests refers to three ratios.

A. The **Odds Ratio** (OR) is used in case control and logistic regression. It can be calculated as: ad/bc. It is the risk of an event happening. It can be reversed and 1/OR is the event free survival.

B. The **Relative Risk** (RR) is used in cohort and randomized controlled trials. It can be calculated as: exposed/unexposed, or a/a+b/c/c+d. The RR is cumulative over the entire study period or the patient or samples life span.

C. The **Hazard Ratio** (HR) is the instantaneous risk. It is the time to an event.

XVIII. Univariate Versus Multivariate Testing

  A. The univariate test evaluates data on a single variable. It facilitates more advanced analysis and is the first step in looking at data analysis.

  B. The multivariate test looks at greater than 1 variable at a time. This test can reduce a large number of variables to a smaller number of factors for data modeling. It can select a subset of variables based on which original variables have the highest correlation with the principle of interest. It validates a scale by demonstrating that items load on the same factor.

XIX. The following graph compares parametric tests to nonparametric tests for specific indications.

Type of Data

Goal	Measurement (From Gaussian Population)	Rank, Score, or Measurement (From Non-Gaussian Population)	Binomial (Two Possible Outcomes)	Survival Time
Describe one group	Mean, SD	Median, interquartile range	Proportion	Kaplan-Meier survival curve
Compare one group to a hypothetical value	One-sample *t* test	Wilcoxon test	Chi-square or binomial test	
Compare two unpaired groups	Unpaired *t* test	Mann-Whitney test	Fisher's test (Chi-square for large samples)	Log-rank test or Mantel-Haenszel
Compare two paired groups	Paired *t* test	Wilcoxon test	McNemar's test	Conditional proportional hazards regression
Compare three or more unmatched groups	One-way ANOVA	Kruskal-Wallis test	Chi-square test	Cox proportional hazard regression

(*Continued*)

Type of Data

Goal	Measurement (From Gaussian Population)	Rank, Score, or Measurement (From Non-Gaussian Population)	Binomial (Two Possible Outcomes)	Survival Time
Compare three or more matched groups	Repeated-measures ANOVA	Friedman test	Cochrane Q	Conditional proportional hazards regression
Quantify association between two variables	Pearson correlation	Spearman correlation	Contingency coefficients	
Predict value from another measured variable	Simple linear regression or nonlinear regression	Nonparametric regression	Simple logistic regression	Cox proportional hazard regression
Predict value from several measured or binomial variables	Multiple linear regression or multiple nonlinear regression		Multiple logistic regression	Cox proportional hazard regression

Reference Material

I. PERFORMANCE STATUS SCALES

A. GOG/ECOG/WHO/Zubrod (1)

0 – Asymptomatic (fully active, able to carry on all predisease activities without restriction)

1 – Symptomatic but completely ambulatory (restricted in physically strenuous activity but ambulatory and able to carry out light or sedentary work)

2 – Symptomatic, < 50% in bed during the day (ambulatory, capable of all self-care; unable to carry out any work activities. Up and about more than 50% of waking hours)

3 – Symptomatic, > 50% in bed, but not bedbound (capable of limited self-care, confined to bed or chair 50% or more of waking hours)

4 – Bedbound (completely disabled. Cannot carry on any self-care. Totally confined to bed or chair)

5 – Dead

B. Karnofsky Performancy Status Scale Rating Criteria (%)

100 Normal no complaints; no evidence of disease.

90 Able to carry on normal activity; minor signs or symptoms of disease.

80 Normal activity with effort; some signs or symptoms of disease.

70 Cares for self; unable to carry on normal activity or do active work.

60 Requires occasional assistance, but is able to care for most personal needs.

50 Requires considerable assistance and frequent medical care. Unable to care for self; requires equivalent of institutional or hospital care; disease may be progressing rapidly.

40 Disabled; requires special care and assistance.

30 Severely disabled; hospital admission is indicated although death not imminent.

20 Very sick; hospital admission necessary; active supportive treatment necessary.

10 Moribund; fatal processes progressing rapidly.

 0 Dead

II. ADVERSE EVENT GRADING

Common Terminology Criteria for Adverse Events (CTCAE): ctep .cancer.gov/reporting/ctc.html

III. RECIST (RESPONSE EVALUATION CRITERIA IN SOLID TUMORS)

A. Tumor response is measured via RECIST guidelines version 1.1 (2). These are easily applicable criteria for measuring tumor response using x-ray, CT, and MRI.

B. RECIST criteria are based on the presence of at least one measurable lesion, presuming that linear measures are an adequate substitute for 2-D methods. There are 4 response categories:

CR (complete response) = disappearance of all target lesions

PR (partial response) = 30% decrease in the sum of the longest diameter of target lesions

PD (progressive disease) = 20% increase in the sum of the longest diameter of target lesions

SD (stable disease) = small changes that do not meet above criteria

REFERENCES

1. Oken MM, Creech RH, Tormey DC. Toxicity and response criteria of the Eastern Cooperative Oncology Group. *Am J Clin Oncol.* 1982;5(6): 649–655.
2. Eisenhauer EA, Therasse P, Bogaerts J. New response evaluation criteria in solid tumours: revised RECIST guideline (version 1.1). *Eur J Cancer.* 2009;45(2):228–247.

IV. USEFUL FORMULAS

I. The Crockcroft-Gault equation: This equation provides an estimate of creatinine clearance based on: age, weight, sex, and serum creatinine without the need for a 24-hour urine collection.

$$\text{Cr Clearance} = \frac{[(140 - \text{Age}) \times \text{Weight (kg)}] \times 0.85}{[0.72 \times \text{Serum Cr (mg/dL)}]}$$

II. The Calvert formula calculates the carboplatin dosing using the GFR from the Crockcroft-Gault equation: Dose (mg) = Target AUC × (GFR + 25). The AUC is usually set from 5 to 7 for untreated patients, and 4 to 6 for previously treated patients

III. The Jelliffe formula is good for adult patients with normal muscle mass not on hemodialysis. This calculation is not applicable to patients less than 18 years old, serum creatinine less than 0.6 mg/dl, weight less than 35 or more than 120 kg, unstable creatinine, muscle mass less than 70% or more than 130% of normal.

CrCl (female) = $0.9 \{[98 - 0.8 \times (\text{A-20})]/\text{SCr (mg/dL)}\}$

Where: A = age in years; CLcr = creatinine clearance in mL/min/1.73 m^2.

The patient's BSA must be determined. The CrCl value obtained by the above equation must be multiplied by (BSA/1.73) to obtain the patient's creatinine clearance in absolute terms (i.e., mL/min). Weight is in kg and height is in cm.

IV. BSA: The most widely used formula is the Du Bois formula:
BSA = $0.007184 \times W^{0.425} \times H^{0.725}$
A commonly used and simple calculation is the Mosteller formula:
BSA = Square root of $(W \times H/3600) = 0.016667 \times W^{0.5} \times H^{0.5}$

V. The fractional excretion of sodium can help determine prerenal, intrinsic, or postrenal disease:

$FE_{Na} = (U_{Na} \times S_{Cr})/(S_{Na} \times U_{Cr}) \times 100$

Below 1% indicates prerenal disease.

A value above 2% or 3% indicates acute tubular necrosis or other kidney damage.

VI. Serum Osmolality = $2[Na] + [K] + BUN/2.8 + Glu/18$

Normal is 280–295 mOsm/kg.

VII. Fe deficit = $1000 + (15\text{-Hgb}) \times (\text{kg weight})$

Normal is: 2 grams

VIII. A-a Gradient = $PAO_2 - PaO_2$. The $PAO_2 = (FiO_2 \times (760 - 47)) - (PaCO_2/0.8)$. Normal is: 80–100 mm Hg.

IX. Corrected Serum Na: measured sodium $+ 0.016 \times$ (serum glucose in mg/dL $- 100$)

V. ABBREVIATIONS

5-FU: 5-fluorouracil

ABG: arterial blood gas

ACOG: American Congress of Obstetricians and Gynecologists

ACTION: Adjuvant Chemotherapy in Ovarian Neoplasms

ADH: antidiuretic hormone

AFP: alpha fetoprotein

AGC: atypical glandular cells

AGUS: abnormal glandular cells of unknown significance

AIS: adenocarcinoma in situ

AJCC: American Joint Committee on Cancer

ANC: absolute neutrophil count

ARDS: acute respiratory distress syndrome

ASA: acetylsalicylic acid

ASC-H: atypical squamous cells, cannot exclude high grade

ASC-US: atypical squamous cells of undetermined significance

ASD: atrial septal defect

ASIS: anterior superior iliac spine

AST: aspartate transaminase

ATHENA: Addressing The Need for Advanced HPV Diagnostics

ATP: adenosine triphosphate

AUC: area under the curve

AV: atrioventricular block

BEE: basal energy expenditure

BEP: bleomycin, etoposide, cisplatin

bid: twice a day

BiPAP: bilevel positive airway pressure

BMI: body mass index

BMP: basic metabolic panel

BNP: brain natriuretic peptide

BP: blood pressure

BSE: bovine spongiform encephalopathy

BSO: bilateral salpingo-oophorectomy

BUN: blood urea nitrogen

CABG: coronary artery bypass graft

CAP: cisplatin, doxorubicin, cyclophosphamide

CBC: complete blood count

CCC: clear cell carcinoma

CCR: complete clinical response

CD: cisplatin, doxorubicin

CDP: cisplatin, doxorubicin, paclitaxel

CEA: carcinoembryonic antigen

CHAMOCA: cyclophosphamide, hydroxyurea, actinomycin D,
    methotrexate, vincristine, leucovorin, doxorubicin

CHF: congestive heart failure

CI: confidence interval

CIN: cervical intraepithelial neoplasia

CIS: carcinoma in situ

CIWA: Clinical Institute Withdrawal Assessment

CK: creatine kinase

CKMB: creatine kinase-MB

CMP: comprehensive metabolic panel

CNS: central nervous system

COPD: chronic obstructive pulmonary disease

CPAP: continuous positive airway pressure

CPK: creatine phosphokinase

CPR: complete pathological response

CR: complete response

CT: X-ray computed tomography

CV: cardiovascular

CVA: costovertebral angle

CVP: central venous pressure

CXR: chest x-ray

D&C: dilation and curettage

DBP: diastolic blood pressure

dDAVP: desmopressin

DES: diethylstilbestrol

DFR: disease-free survival

DFS: disease-free survival

DHEA: dehydroepiandrosterone

DHEAS: dehydroepiandrosterone sulfate

DKA: diabetic ketoacidosis

DM: diabetes mellitus

DMSO: dimethyl sulfoxide

DNR: do not resuscitate

DOI: depth of invasion

DS: double-stranded

DSS: disease-specific survival

DTIC: dacarbazine

DVT: deep vein thrombosis

EBL: estimated blood loss

EBRT: external beam radiation therapy

ECC: endocervical curettage

ECHO: echocardiogram

EGD: esophagogastroduodenoscopy

EGFR: epidermal growth factor receptor

EIA: enzyme immunoassay

EKG: electrocardiogram

ELISA: enzyme-linked immunosorbent assay

EMA-CO: etoposide, methotrexate, actinomycin D–cyclophosphamide, and vincristine

EMA-EP: etoposide, methotrexate, actinomycin D–etoposide, cisplatin

EMACO: etoposide, methotrexate, actinomycin D, cyclophosphamide, and vincristine

EMB: endometrial biopsy

EOC: epithelial ovarian cancer

EORTC: European Organisation for Research and Treatment of Cancer

ER: estrogen receptor

ERT: estrogen replacement therapy

EUA: exam under anesthesia

FDG: fludeoxyglucose

FEV: forced expiratory volume

FFP: fresh frozen plasma

FIGO: Federation of Gynecology and Obstetrics

FNA: fine needle aspiration

FSH: follicle-stimulating hormone

GCSF: granulocyte colony stimulating factor

GFR: glomerular filtration rate

GI: gastrointestinal

GIS: gastrointestinal anastomosis

GnRH: gonadotropin-releasing hormone

GOG: Gynecologic Oncology Group

GSH: glutathione

GST: glutathione S-transferase

GTD: gestational trophoblastic disease

GU: genitourinary

HAART: highly active antiretroviral therapy

hCG: human chorionic gonadotropin

Hct: hematocrit

HDR: high-dose-rate intracavitary brachytherapy

HPF: high-powered field

HPV: human papilloma virus

HR: hazard ratio

HRT: hormone replacement therapy

HSIL: high-grade squamous intraepithelial lesion

HSV: herpes simplex virus

HTN: hypertension

HUS: hemolytic uremic syndrome

IBD: inflammatory bowel disease

ICE: ifosfamide, cisplatin, etoposide

ICON: International Collaborative Ovarian Neoplasm Trial

ICU: intensive care unit

IDS: interval debulking surgery

IM: intramuscular

IMA: inferior mesenteric artery

IMRT: intensity modulated radiation therapy

INH: isoniazid

INR: international normalized ratio

IP: intraperitoneal

IVC: inferior vena cava

IVF: intravenous fluid

IVP: intravenous pyelography

JGOG: Japanese Gynecologic Oncology Group

JP: Jackson-Pratt

JVD: jugular venous distension

JVP: jugular venous pressure

KUB: kidneys, ureters, bladder

LDH: lactate dehydrogenase

LDR: low-dose-rate intracavitary brachytherapy

LEEP: loop electrosurgical excision procedure

LFT: liver function test

LMP: low malignant potential

LMW: low molecular weight

LN: lymph node

LND: lymph node dissection

LSIL: low-grade squamous intraepithelial lesion

LV: left ventricular

LVSI: lymphovascular space invasion

MAC: methotrexate, actinomycin D, cyclophosphamide

METS: metabolic equivalents

MI: myocardial infarction

MMMT: malignant mixed Müllerian tumor

MPA: medroxyprogesterone acetate

MRI: magnetic resonance imaging

MTHFR: methylenetetrahydrofolate reductase

MTX: methotrexate

MVP: mitral valve prolapse

NCCN: National Comprehensive Cancer Network

NCI: National Cancer Institute

NCIC: National Cancer Institute of Canada

NFT: no further treatment

NGT: nasogastric tube

NPO: nothing by mouth

NPV: negative predictive value

NS: not statistically significant

NSAID: nonsteroidal anti-inflammatory drug

OCP: oral contraceptive pills

OR: overall response

ORR: overall response rate

OS: overall survival

PA LND: para-aortic lymph node dissection

PA: para-aortic

PAC: premature atrial contraction

PALN: para-aortic lymph node

PAOP: pulmonary artery occlusion pressure

PCR: polymerase chain reaction

PCWP: pulmonary capillary wedge pressure

PDA: patent ductus arteriosus

PDS: primary debulking surgery

PE: pulmonary embolus

PEEP: positive end-expiratory pressure

PEG: polyethylene glycol

PET: positron emission tomography

PFI: progression free interval

PFS: progression-free survival

PFT: pulmonary function test

PFTC: primary fallopian tube cancer

PICC: peripheral centrally inserted catheter

PLAP: placental alkaline phosphatase

PLND: pelvic lymph node dissection

PO: orally

POD: postoperative day

POISE: Perioperative Ischemic Evaluation Study

POMB-ACE: cisplatin, vincristine, methotrexate, bleomycin, actinomycin D, cyclophosphamide, etoposide

PPLND: pelvic and para-aortic lymphadenectomy

PPV: positive predictive value

PR: partial response

PRBC: packed red blood cells

PSTT: placental-site trophoblastic tumor

PT: prothrombin time

PTCA: percutaneous transluminal coronary angioplasty

PTSD: posttraumatic stress disorder

PTT: partial thromboplastin time

PTU: propylthiouracil

PVB: cisplatin, vinblastine, bleomycin

PVC: premature ventricular contractions

PVR: post void residual

qid: four times a day

QOL: quality of life

RBBB: right bundle branch block

RBC: red blood cells

RFS: recurrence-free survival

RR: response rate

RT: radiation therapy

RTOG: Radiation Therapy Oncology Group

SBP: systolic blood pressure

SC: subcutaneous

SCD: sequential compression device

SEER: Surveillance Epidemiology and End Results

SIADH: syndrome of inappropriate antidiuretic hormone secretion

SIMV: synchronized intermittent mandatory ventilation

SIRS: systemic inflammatory response syndrome

SL: sublingual

SLL: second-look laparotomy

SMA: superior mesenteric artery

SOB: shortness of breath

STD: sexually transmitted disease

TA: thoracoabdominal

TACO: transfusion-associated circulatory overload

TAH: total abdominal hysterectomy

TAP: paclitaxel, doxorubicin, cisplatin

TB: tuberculosis

TCA: trichloroacetic acid

TG: triglycerides

TID: three times a day

TNM: tumor, node, metastasis

TPN: total parenteral nutrition

TRALI: transfusion-related acute lung injury

TSH: thyroid-stimulating hormone

TVUS: transvaginal ultrasound

UA: urinalysis

USO: unilateral salpingo-oophorectomy

V/Q: ventilation/perfusion

VAC: vincristine, doxorubicin, cyclophosphamide

VAIN: vaginal intraepithelial neoplasia

VIN: vulvar intraepithelial neoplasia

VIP: etoposide, ifosfamide, cisplatin

VPB: vinblastine, cisplatin, bleomycin

VSD: ventricular septal defect

VTE: venous thromboembolism

WAR: whole abdominal radiation

WBC: white blood cells

WHO: World Health Organization

WP: whole pelvic

Y: Year

YS: year survival

Index